THE
SATURATED
SENSORIUM

THE
SATURATED SENSORIUM

**Principles of Perception and Mediation
in the Middle Ages**

*Edited by Hans Henrik Lohfert Jørgensen,
Henning Laugerud & Laura Katrine Skinnebach*

Aarhus University Press | 🏃

THE SATURATED SENSORIUM

Principles of Perception and Mediation in the Middle Ages

© The authors & Aarhus University Press 2015

Layout and cover design: Jørgen Sparre

The book is typeset in Adobe Garamond and Franklin Gothic

Production: Narayana Press, Gylling, Denmark

Printed in Denmark 2015

ISBN 978 87 7124 313 0

Aarhus University Press

www.unipress.dk

CONTENTS

Acknowledgements

The Saturated Sensorium was realised
through the generous financial support of:

The Novo Nordisk Foundation

Aarhus University Research Foundation

Faculty for Arts and Humanities,
Linnæus University

Department of Linguistic, Literary and Aesthetic Studies,
University of Bergen

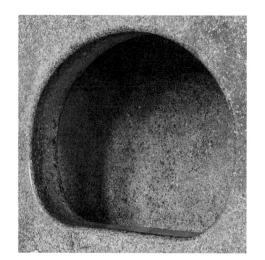

8

INTO THE SATURATED SENSORIUM

Introducing the Principles of Perception and Mediation in the Middle Ages

[Hans Henrik Lohfert Jørgensen]

Going Multimedieval

An interdisciplinary group of Scandinavian medievalists met in Aarhus, Denmark in the spring of 2009, to debate the concept of a seminar with a rather outlandish and experimental title: *Multimiddelalder*. This translates into something like 'Multiple Middle Ages', while also implying 'Multi Media Ages'. It would thus involve the recognition of a multiplicity of media and sense relations beyond established modern categories and across the accustomed thresholds of modern communication. In this sense, the *Medium Aevum* – originally a modern term for what is in principle not modern[1] – can be redefined and offered a new place in media history. Instead of just preceding or contrasting mediatised modernity, the 'age in the middle' may be appreciated as pivotal in the on-going development of epochal principles of perception and mediation: an 'age of the medium', both historically and in a broader perspective – suggesting diachronic and synchronic implications alike. A 'multimedieval', mixed-media culture, that is, of renewed inspiration to late- (or post-)modern fascinations with the transmedial hybridity, intersensorial entanglements, and multimodal cross-overs now challenging modern ontologies of autonomous, self-contained media.

For those no longer adhering to the ever more contested and untenable notions of 'pure' art forms, medieval media practices offer a plentiful reservoir of strategies for combining, blending, and fusing media modalities into rich and abundant wholes not forced into a priori categorisations. Here, we do not look for pure optical painting or listen to purely auditory music excluding other modes of sensation or signification. In place of such select ideals, we may hear of ceremonial soundscapes in compound spaces of sensation and mediation; we may reconstruct complex sensescapes of multisensory impressions generated by ritual practices, performers, and percipients; or we may encounter the miscellaneous materiality of touchable and kissable imagery featuring iconic appearances, precious objects, inserted relics, dramatised narratives, and written words to be hymned or read aloud. Here, various classes of media inform and include each other while various types of sense experience permeate and saturate each other. Media of perception and expression coincide and co-operate instead of policing their own inherent boundaries, isolating their own experiential dominions, or seeking to define their own particular properties. Here, we can study theories of, say, musical harmony, which integrate – with an admirable ease – what we are normally used to think of as entirely different arts. Indeed, this could include wholly different domains of existence, ranging from perceptual to mathematical proportion, from physical to spiritual harmony, from psychic to cosmic structures.

Therefore, the manifold multiplicity of medieval notions of music may serve to illustrate the integration and coalescence of areas of life and mediation otherwise seemingly apart or separate. Presently, this sonorous example will allow us to explain the basic idea and aim of the present book, itself intended to be a coherent and amiable amalgamation of several overlapping fields of investigation and facets of social and cultural history – secular as well as sacred, material as well as communicational, embodied as well as mental. It is a book about the senses and their media in the *Medium Aevum;* about perceptual principles, practices, and paradoxes; about what it implied to perceive and mediate something in given situations and concrete contexts. A series of individual but coordinated and correlated chapters each covers a principal branch of the cultural history of perception and mediation in order to highlight the integrated and unified nature of medieval media and senses. Taking their point of departure in either representative notions and problems signalled by the chapter headings, or in select exemplary cases of these general principles, they explore what sensing was, what it meant, what it did: how sensation operated within each area, how it was conceived, how it was performed, how it was mediated.[2] They discuss the multi- and intermediality of cultural or cultic artefacts as well as the sensorial and intersensorial dimensions of a wide array of distinctive concepts and practices within medieval religion, art, material culture, public life, social conventions, monastic living, miraculous events, texts, tales, images, literature, architecture, music, food, ritual, devotion, cognition, corporeality, memory, and thinking. *The saturated sensorium* nurtured the worldly and unworldly practices of presentation, representation, and mediation; the corporeal and spiritual concepts of sensation, sanctity, and incarnation; the physical and ceremonial spaces of environment, cult, and commemoration; the emotional and intellectual body of love, meditation, and recollection; the material and visual culture of sacraments, celebration, and consumption. Across a number of academic disciplines, these intertwined domains of sensory and media history are addressed from the interdisciplinary, intermedial, and intersensorial perspective informing the book as a whole, thus contributing to a new vision – and a new version – of the Middle Ages, emerging in some of the most recent scholarship: an *age of intermedia*.

Age of Intermedia

Returning now to the broad and mixed medium of music – or, as it was perhaps rather perceived and practiced – the *intermedium* of music, it will allow us to suggest what is at stake in this revision. The medieval perception and understanding of music exceeds and challenges the boundaries that define the realm of aesthetics in the modern sense. For Boëthius (c. 475-524), author of the widely influential *De institutione musica*, for instance, the three primary kinds of music comprised sensory, extra-sensory, and infra-sensory modes of mediation and sensation. In an extended field of music, a comprehensive continuity of harmonies was linked by the same elemental modulations and proportions, from the microcosm of man to the macrocosm of the universe: 1) the physical, corporeal, and vocal sounds of actually performed music, which would issue from its appropriate instruments (also counting the voice) to be absorbed as "a unified multiplicity" by the external senses, seeking beauty in numerical and emotional relationships alike; 2) the supersonic music of all the world and natural creation, theoretically inherited from antiquity as *musica mundana*, generated by the spherical motions of celestial bodies and the universal concord of elements; 3) the self-reflective music of man, *musica humana*, residing in our bodily and mental constitution as an extension of our inner and outer nature, only perceived by the one descending into the depths of himself.[3] In this generally accepted trichotomy, comparing and melding music in nature, music in man, and music in art (i.e. music made by man), the audible *musica instrumentalis* was sounded to accord with – *ad imitationem* – the higher inaudible kinds of music from which it all originated.[4] It was a doctrine of unity in diversity, an axiom, not of purity but of plurality, not of a single sonic modality but of sensory multimodality, not of media autonomy, but of interconnection, interdependence, and intermediality.

Thus, the ample system was reproduced by, among others, Aurelian of Réomé in the ninth century, who observed "that a wondrous harmony [*mira harmonia*] joins together and unites all creatures. [...] music radiates from the whole of creation".[5] Since everything that exists is arranged in an overall conformity, a composite yet concordant composition, "there is music [*consonantia*] in all things".[6] Sound was sensed to mediate an ultrasonic principle, namely an admirable synthesis of all perceptible things and creatures. Within this totalising synthesis, auditory beauty itself was nothing less than a universal concept including music as well as poetry and literature. These were joined together because they were all intended for instrumental and/or vocal performance, and were hence received by the ear in unison with other senses. "[O]ne kind of music uses instruments", according to Boëthius, "and another composes poetical works" – seamlessly merging media today belonging to different realms.[7] Among the liberal arts, music was considered to be a general property of things and could be found everywhere in the world, not only in chanted *carmina*, melodious verses, aural poems, oral recitations, and dramatised plays, but also in motion, dance, gesture, bodily posture, architecture, and other visual pleasures. The musical *modulatio* of contrasting components created a sensible order in structured vocalisations, verbalisations, and visualisations: in arranged words, coordinated movements, pictorial compositions, materialised edifices, and even social bodies, all of which manifested the underlying conception of a manifold whole, a multiple unity. In a deeper institutional sense, everything was saturated with music, harmonising superficial differences into an ineffable *concordia*. It was a 'multimedium' on a very extensive and far-reaching scale, exceeding the modern limitations and classificatory restrictions of the worlds of sound, senses, and media. In a way, the whole sensory sphere was experienced as a medium – or indeed, an intermedium – for God's comprehensive self-revelation, glimpsed in the divine order, which lended some measure of proportion to all things created, whatever sensorial instrument they played in the grand polyphony of perception. As a result, the world of sensation provided the model for human intermedia of all kinds, exploring their own creative potential within the order of creation.

In order for us to grasp this syncretistic sensibility, we may just lend an ear to the *Speculum musicae*, that is, a voluminous treatise of music theory from the early fourteenth century: "Music in the general, objective sense applies in a way to everything [*quasi ad omnia se extendit*] – to God and His creations, incorporeal and corporeal, heavenly and human, and to the theoretical and practical sciences".[8] Or we may listen to Grosseteste (c. 1168-1253) on the liberal arts: "It is not only the harmony of the human voice and movements which is subject to musical examination, but also the harmony of instruments and everything which, by sound or movement [*in motu sive in sono*] affords pleasure".[9] Or we may take a dance to the visible music of Roger Bacon, presented in his monumental *Opus Maius* around 1267: "Apart from those branches of music which concern sounds, there are others dealing with visible things, that is, human movements [*gestus*] which include movements in the dance and all bending of the body".[10] In such an audio-visual and kinaesthetic conformity of categories, the consonance of movable man, visual world, and somatic sound was manifested to the senses – at least ideally – in a synaesthetic *symphonia* of sensory values. Emblematic of this concomitance of perceptual values, Johannes Cotton in his early twelfth-century *De musica* expressed the emotional and sensorial effect of one sense modality spilling over into the other: "The organic tonus and its accompanying feeling are intensified by certain tastes and odors, weakened by others. This is true of colors as well as of sounds".[11] In other words, sensory impulses were actually felt to permeate and inundate one another across their assumed areas of perception, olfactory and gustative stimuli able to effect visual and auditive responses, and vice versa. Within this sensual synaesthesia – which may be perceived as one subordinate variant of a greater pattern of multimodality – perception, so it seems, was experienced as polymorphous and peripatetic. Likewise, Guido of Arezzo observed that music crossed modalities and had certain qualities in common with colour, odour, and savour. In his *Micrologus*, "Short treatise on music", written around 1025, he sings out loud the copious concordance of this entire paradigm of intermingled and interchangeable sensation:

> It is no wonder that the ear [*auditus*] should take delight in the variety of sounds, just as the eye [*visus*] takes pleasure in the variety of colours, the nose [*olfactus*] is excited by the variety of smells, and the tongue [*lingua*] rejoices at different tastes. The sweetness of delightful things penetrates wondrously, as through the window of the body, into the depth of the heart.[12]

Sight, hearing, olfaction, and gustation come together in touching body and heart with the "sweetness" so often hailed as a unifying feature of both physical and spiritual experience. A suggestive vocabulary of sweet sounds and perfumed sensations ("suavitas", "dulcis", "dulcissimum", "florata" etc.) bears witness to the polyphonic communion of sensory values so deeply felt by past percipients. In the *saturated sensorium*, the sweet senses blended into each other and saturated one another, just like the perception of music was saturated with feelings and savoury suggestions, with sensuous motions and emotions, with odoriferous smells and tastes, with flowery tones, colours, and chromatic shades coupling nuances of vision and audition. Offering a continuous window onto the perceptible world, the bodily senses inundated the overwhelmed recipient with interrelated impressions, hearing saturated with feeling and flavour, seeing and moving saturated with phonics and rhythm. In the end, there was far more to perceptual experience than indicated by the reductive Aristotelian systematisation of the five 'classical' senses.[13] However neat and tidy, the sensory order of *visus* (sight), *auditus* (hearing), *tactus* (touch), *olfactus* (smell), and *gustus* (taste) did not – and does not – describe the compound and braided operation of human sense perception.

Euphony of Sense and Media Modalities

From the perspective of media interaction it is not just what Edgar de Bruyne, when speaking about the Carolingian intermediality of rhythm and proportion, has termed "the perfect unity of dance, song, and poetry" – hence anticipating one of the chapters in this book (on the intermediality of the medieval popular ballad).[14] It is also that these media and forms of expression were conceived of as more or less the same thing, or at least that they conformed to the same rules and the same domain, bridging variable modes of signification and sensory stimulation: music usually consisted of both melody and meaningful words, lyric was habitually intoned or sung, and texts typically recited as oral–aural compositions in a social space of embodied sensory presence. When responding to the plural impact of what Werner Faulstich has called "Menschmedien", percipients could readily see, hear, feel, and smell the performers' present bodies, regardless of whether these communicated through vocal, verbal, gestural, rhythmical, theatrical, or other corporeal means.[15] In a media history, not of mutual segregation and compartmentalisation, but of reciprocal interchange and fusion, "[…] there was no poetry unaccompanied by music, nor music without words".[16] In the resonant proclamations of Guido, this medial and modal interrelationship explains the sensual charm of congruous plural forms – the mixed melody of multimodality, so to speak:

> Consider, then, that just as everything that is spoken can be written [*omne quod dicitur scribitur*] so everything that is written can be made into song again. Thus, everything that is spoken can be sung [*canitur omne quod dicitur*] for writing is depicted by letters [*scriptura litteris figuratur*]. [...] So a sweet blending [*suavis concordia*] is found in the different parts. In verse we often see such concordant and mutually congruous lines that you wonder, as it were, at a certain harmony of language [*symphoniam grammaticae*]. And if music be added to this, with a similar interrelationship, you will be doubly charmed by a twofold melody.[17]

This is a remarkable "euphony" – as Guido terms it – of basic media modalities: song, speech, writ, language, and their figuration or depiction, one leading to or containing the other, as when depicted letters (exemplified by the vowels) were pronounced and made into notes, transmitted back and forth between the sensory domains of the eye, the ear, and the mouth. In an almost cyclical intercommunication, these modes were all functionally interdependent and operationally interlaced, sometimes absorbing and assimilating each other, sometimes sustaining and underpinning each other. Written letters figured images of script harbouring both the euphonic intonations of spoken language and the diaphonic movements between sounding syllables and exclaimed neumes.

Accordingly, there was also an iconic, figurative, or even pictorial component of this entangled media matrix – a visual or 'intervisual' element in the amalgam of communicative configurations. In the first instance, there was neither music without acoustic images nor images without acoustic resonance. Likewise, there were no pictures without words, either those painted in them (e.g. speaking scrolls or inscriptions), those narrated by them (e.g. biblical accounts or stories), or those preached before them (e.g. sermons, prayers, or readings). In a performative culture of *oral intermediality*, music was always also a tale, a tale was always also music. Moreover, an image was always also a tale; a tale was always also an image, performed by a living body. In addition, there was another dimension as well to this prolific and untroubled amalgamation of basic media. In a corporeal culture of *material intermediality*, an image was always also a text, and a text was always also an image, due to the physically inscribed materiality of both handwritten texts and handmade imagery. In principle, both manual script and crafted pictures were concrete objects or vehicles of representation transmitting their semantic information or content by graphic marks – that is, visible and readable signs – materialised in a solid palpable form. The perceptual tangibility of spoken words was crystallised into the physical image of writ in stone, metal, ivory, mosaics, manuscripts, or dyed parchment, in order to be treated as ornate pictures of words. "Writing is depicted by letters", so Guido says: visualised, shaped, carved, incised, engraved, illuminated, coloured, gilt, and adorned with calligraphy to achieve the visual and tactile materiality of writing that Rosario Assunto has labelled "objektive Anschaubarkeit des Geschriebenen" and "Schrift als Schaubild".[18] As a 'Schau image', a display object, a sensory manifestation, the tangible text was meant both to be seen *as* a body (i.e. displayed like an image) and to be vocalised *by* a body (i.e. read aloud and voiced like music). In the age of intermedia, writing, picturing, speaking, singing, and performing joined each other and formed part of a continuous communicative repertoire aimed at inundating all the bodily senses "to the point of saturation".[19]

Thus the verbal and the visual, paramount in modern media hierarchies based on representation and referentiality, were employed as *contact media* as well. Both words and images provided perceptible and palpable presence alongside their encoded semantic utterance, hence challenging any notion of a monochord *homo spectator*, allegedly sustained by a Western civilisation of spectacles and printing. Both integrated and interwove two complementary principles of transmission to the recipient: intelligible reference and signification, operating mostly in the 'higher' representational senses, as opposed to transference of corporeal or incorporeal contact, operating mostly – but not exclusively – in the bodily proximity senses. When the ill sought cure by absorbing the sensory power and presence of holy books, either through the touch of their skin, through the kiss of their mouth, or through the oral consumption of liquids in which the powerful books had been washed, they deliberately confused sense and media domains that we today tend to consider distinct and separate.[20] Pictures for their part were expected to address their beholders not just visually, as shimmering scenes of sight and optical perception, but also in a highly corporeal, tactile, textural, aural, and even olfactory manner. It was not unusual for images to manifest the perceptual presence of the figured prototype across the threshold of representation – sometimes embracing, caressing, or sounding a voice to the onlooker, sometimes exuding, bleeding, or emitting a sweet-smelling odour of sanctity.[21] Such sensory mediations and materialisations transgress logical thresholds and eclipse fundamental conceptual and ontological distinctions: between representation and presentation/presence, between signifying and being, between the sign and the thing, between the medium and the mediated, between mediality and reality, between mediate distance senses and immediate contact senses, between reading/viewing and consuming/absorbing. A book of Christ or an image of Christ also *was* Christ and should be perceived and taken in as such. This interweaving of seeming opposites let the real be present in mediation, the senses in the medium, the haptic in the optic, the somatic and sensual in the visual and textual.

Conversely, these integrated media manifestations substantialised and texturised the senses, bringing them "to the point of saturation" – that is, "the point of integration." In a communal production of perception, integrated senses and intermedia invoked an *integrated sensorium*. (The anthropological designation 'sensorium' is here taken to mean the perceptual system as a whole, in its social situation, cultural construction, and historical formation).[22] Discussing a medieval mixed-media context amalgamating all of the available perceptual channels into a mesmerising multisensory enactment, Bissera Pentcheva has recently pointed out that the time has now come for investigations of the full spectrum of sensation and for assessing sense experiences in their mutual interaction: "[T]he Eastern Orthodox liturgy maintained its late antique tradition of *saturation of the senses*. This synaesthetic experience is characteristic of Byzantium, yet it is rarely discussed in medieval studies".[23] In order to meet this scholarly shortage, she herself takes on the Byzantine icon – that exemplary archetype of medieval cult medium – showing how its shifting material and sensory appearance was affected by the solemn and reverent words said to it, by the reverberation of liturgical music and prayer in front of it, by the radiance of oil lamps reflected from its gilded surfaces, by the changing highlights and shadows of flickering candles stirred by the approaching percipient's breath and *proskynesis*, by the bodily movements and kisses of prostrate devotees, and by wafting scents of holy fragrance, ceremonial smoke, or burning incense enveloping the animated apparition. Its inspiriting effect resided in "the simultaneity of senses":

> The icon is in fact a surface that resonates with sound, air, light, touch, and smell. [...] In saturating the material and sensorial to excess, the experience of the icon [...] offers us a glimpse into what vision meant: [...] a synesthetic vision [...] in which the whole body is engaged. [...] This performance inundates and saturates the human corporeal apprehension. The effect of sight and touch is coupled with hearing and smell [culminating in] taste. Through it emerges the climax: partaking in the sacred.[24]

Confronted with the dense materiality and mediality of such an appealing object, generating such intersensorial excesses in such a condensed ambience, icon perception inevitably became mixed and multimodal. Sight was experienced also as touch, hearing, smell, and taste – all integral to and part of "seeing" an *eikon*.[25] Even if the title and concept of the present volume are not expressly inspired by Pentcheva, and even if its focus is not Byzantine, it still shares the same ambition of exposing medieval cultural production in all its riveting richness of multimedial, intersensorial, and synaesthetic saturation. *The saturated sensorium* was permeated by a proliferating interchange of media and sense modalities that interacted, fused, and blended into a coherent, if complex, continuum: a multimodal system of sensation and mediation, a sensory apparatus defined by its functional multimodality (a term designating a composite operation consisting of several perceptual and communicative resources, multiple sensory and semiotic modalities of transmission, and manifold material modes of mediation – either intersensorially *fused into* each other or multisensorially *combined with* each other).[26]

The defining property of this aesthetic, medial, and sensory syncretism, it should be added, was not the lack of ability to make and recognise distinctions between diverse phenomena due to some flaw in a critical attitude. It represented rather a deliberate (if not necessarily always conscious) co-operation of various forms of experience based on an all-encompassing sense of media inclusion and sense integration: a synthesising and synaesthetic sensibility – a preference for consonant and concomitant sensation. If we follow Eco, it expressed an "integrated sensibility […] within a unitary scheme of values – […] an integrated culture whose value systems are related to one another by mutual implication. […] Medieval taste was concerned neither with the autonomy of art nor the autonomy of nature. […] Life appeared as something wholly integrated".[27] The historical voices cited in the preceding pages abstained from discriminating, separating, and isolating mutually exclusive categories, not because they could not, but because it would apparently have been a reductive simplification of the enriching complexities of sensory and extra-sensory experience. Their 'project' was not to distil the reified essence and proper particularities of self-sufficient media, but to grasp a more wide-ranging truth in their structural interrelations, experiential overlaps, and fundamental compatibility at a deeper level. The mutual incorporation of moral and sensory values was not so much a philosophical problem as a social and perceptual practice. Without trying to unduly idealise or exaggerate the praised "concept of integration"[28] into a smooth harmonisation elevated above ideological tensions, cultural contrasts, or socio-historical differences, the chapters that follow each take on a central feature of the integrated perception and mediation of life in the Middle Ages.

Mediation and Mediators

Before our immersion into medieval matters, we should, however, make one final clarification – or rather, integration or saturation – which was also eventually recognised by the group behind this book. As the research project evolved from the described premises, it became increasingly clear to the group that *mediation* was indeed a central principle of medieval perception, integral to the function of its internal and external faculties. While the modern category of 'media' involves the risk of a certain entrapment within contemporary notions of representation and communication, the broader concept of 'mediation' may be more appropriate in relation to historical understanding of such transmissions. Nowadays, media in the most elemental and general sense are taken to be codified systems of communication transmitting – through representational techniques and semantic codification – some sort of information, meaning, or message between two parties, each of whom is usually human. In the medieval tradition on the other hand, mediation also entailed something else, implying a more inclusive and far-reaching conception of exchange and transference more akin to the transgressive embodiment of presence observed in cult texts and images. As noted by Richard McBrien, mediation is one of the constituent principles of universal Catholicism, including medieval Christendom. It is the corollary of a sacramental world-view, where the perceptible, the material, the tangible, the worldly, and the mundane always possess a latent potential for actualising and manifesting the imperceptible, the immaterial, the intangible, the otherworldly, or the divine, revealing itself in either space or time. What lies beyond the senses can nevertheless become available to perception and realise itself for the earthly percipient through the mediation of sensory apparitions and intermediaries: persons, beings, places, sites, events, acts, rituals, words, visions, bodies, objects, media, matter etc.[29] Sacramentality in this very expansive sense is a vital axiom to Catholic culture, religion, practice, and inevitably perception. It entails an acute sensibility for the power of all sorts of material vehicles and 'media' to reproduce and substantiate – or even transubstantiate – featured things, values, and virtues in order to make them present to the senses. The mediated experience is a productive and real experience – not just a second order signification or re-presentation. Far from just reproducing their content, the intermediate signs themselves produce and substantiate what they signify.

All sensory reality, both animate and inanimate, is potentially the instrument and mediator of an ineffable presence, realised in – or through the means of – this perceptible world. Sensory matter nurtures the ability to convey extra-sensory matter, mediating both physical and metaphysical entities, powers, and presences into a discernible form.

From this point of view, the 'medium' may be considered a channel, vessel, or instrument – an intermediary vehicle or body – for transferring an *efficacious message* (e.g. prayer, blessing, act of consecration, oath, legal announcement), *quality* (e.g. healing power, divine grace, holiness), or *substance* (e.g. the sacrament, spiritual or bodily presence, the Word of God incarnate in some shape of mediator or mediatrix). This kind of transport or transmission transcends signification and requires a much more substantial mediation between two parties, amounting to incarnation and embodiment. The medium itself may be a non-representational artefact or material, even a physical person, living or dead, and not merely a symbolic technology of representation. First and foremost, this is the case with Christ, the archetypal mediator of Christianity communicating the natures of God and man, and hence a paradigmatic model for a Christian media culture saturated with mediators at all levels, from human flesh and bones to Holy Spirit. The culture of immanent incarnation and sensory concretisation (rather than abstract and transcendent signification) constitutes a contagious matrix of mediation where media are empowered and animated by the very thing or entity they transmit. In the conflation of thing and sign, the mediated property or presence itself cannot be wholly distinguished from the medium carrying it or (re)presenting it. This ontological transfer is most notable, but in no way exceptional, in the instituted sacraments, whose exchange of substance – body in bread or wine, spirit in oil or water – would not be possible within our more prohibitive and restricted conceptualisation of media today. By way of exemplification, the mediation of sanctity and miracle-working power in saintly bones also conflate symbol with reality, the dead sign of the saint perceived as instrumental to the living thing signified, endowed with his or her actual presence. The little piece of stuff in the metal receptacle is not only a token of sanctity; it *is* the saint – not just a revered reference to some bygone personage, but a concrete relic of him or her, which actively participates in the production of his sacred presence and the execution of his thaumaturgical deeds. Similarly, other instruments of sensory mediation – staged consumption of food and alcohol, enacted celebrations, processions, pronouncements, scriptures, figures, plays, and so on – were not simply signs, but relics and partakers of what they represented; not merely significative reproductions of a given reality, but also instruments for production, construction, and codification of that very reality.

For a more thorough discussion, exemplification, and saturation of these matters, the reader must now turn to the subsequent sections of the palpable body of writing in her hand. One chapter discusses principles of representation, another addresses instances of incarnation and medieval materiality, a third evokes the mechanisms and mediations of memory. One chapter reviews remediation, while others deal with the sensory operations of sacraments and rituals, all of which were each in their own way underpinned by this potent potential for mediation, itself contributing to the enthralling realities it communicated. Whether in practices of consumption, devotion, or sanctity – explored in other chapters – multisensory performance produced social and cultural forms of incarnation and embodied presence; whether in the perceptual environment or in liturgical space – examined in other chapters again – a constellation of multiple mediations ingrained the experience of sensory saturation and embedded it deep in the history of medieval sensation. This process required the institution of a suitable paradigm of perception enabling the senses to apprehend such saturating mediations and access their mediated matter. As a whole the volume may be seen as an attempt to describe and understand this sensorial paradigm in a representative variety of its principal domains and functions. In the following chapter, a critical definition of medieval perception is proposed in the shape of a historical sense model, termed: *hagiosensorium*. The 'sacred sensorium' indicates a perceptual system aimed at sensing the property of holiness in its multimodal manifestations across the whole range of the sensory continuum. It describes an apt and purposeful organisation of the culturally construed apparatus of perception, empowered to grasp, confirm, enliven, and authenticate the incarnation of divine phenomena, thereby also taking part in the sensory sanction and sanctification of those phenomena. While some chapters apply the hagiosensorial perspective to their particular field of investigation, showing the many facets of its culture and history, others emphasise secular sensation and mundane media, often structured in similar ways. They all have in common an interest in the integrated, hybrid, and pluriform character of past perception and mediation. To study the saturated sensorium is to open up a privileged window into the cultural history of the multiple Middle Ages: the 'Multi Media Ages.'

Notes

1   According to Hans Ulrich Gumbrecht's entry in *Geschichtliche Grundbegriffe* on the historical concept of modernity, the "Epochenbezeichnung Mittelalter" had its "Lateinische Erstbelege" in *media tempestas* (1469), *media aetas* (1518), and *medium aevum* (1604); Gumbrecht 2004, p. 98. The 'Middle Ages' is an early modern concept, in other words, whereas 'modernus' and 'modernitas' are medieval notions. This just goes to show the epochal relativity of these very terms and makes it possible to suggest redefinitions and reinterpretations like the one undertaken here.

2   As the reader will observe, the material chosen for exemplification is often of Scandinavian origin, but neither exclusively nor necessarily so, since it has been elected for its representative value to the more general topics dealt with, e.g. sensory consumption, devotion, or remediation.

3   Boëthius: *De institutione musica*, I, 2; Tatarkiewicz 1970, pp. 81 f., 87; de Bruyne 1946, vol. I, p. 12 f.; de Bruyne 1969, p. 49 ff.

4   Tatarkiewicz 1970, p. 81.

5   Aurelianus: *Musica disciplina*; quoted from de Bruyne 1969, p. 54; de Bruyne 1946, vol. I, p. 308 f. See also the excerpt in Tatarkiewicz 1970, p. 133.

6   "[…] consonantia ergo habetur in omni creatura", according to Otloh of St. Emmeram (c. 1010-1070); quoted by de Bruyne 1946, vol. II, p. 109; de Bruyne 1969, p. 55.

7   Boëthius: *De institutione musica*, I, 34; Tatarkiewicz 1970, pp. 81, 87.

8   Iacobus of Liège: *Speculum musicae*; Tatarkiewicz 1970, p. 133.

9   Robert Grosseteste: *De artibus liberalibus*; Tatarkiewicz 1970, p. 132.

10 Roger Bacon: *Opus maius*, III, 232; Tatarkiewicz 1970, p. 137.

11 John Cotton: *De musica*; quoted from de Bruyne 1969, p. 193. See also de Bruyne 1946, vol. II, p. 123 ff.

12 Guido of Arezzo: *Micrologus*, XIV, "On the tropes and on the power of music"; a significant topos quoted by both de Bruyne 1946, vol. II, p. 126, and Tatarkiewicz 1970, pp. 128, 137. The edition of the treatise by Babb & Palisca 1978 offers a slightly different translation of the passage (p. 69 f.), although informed by a less suggestive understanding of its multimodal implications.

13 See the subsequent chapter in this volume on the medieval *Sensorium* and its Aristotelian foundations, treated in a section on the historical 'Intersensorium'.

14 de Bruyne 1969, p. 53. See in addition the chapter on *Remediation* in this volume.

15 See Faulstich 1996, p. 31, for an initial discussion of the term.

16 Tatarkiewicz 1970, p. 131.

17 Guido of Arezzo: *Micrologus*, XVII, "That anything that is spoken can be made into music"; Babb & Palisca 1978, p. 74.

18 Assunto 1982, pp. 32, 132, fig. 18, commenting on the "objektiv-materialistische Auffassung der Schönheit" common to both medieval works of art, words, written pages, sculpture, painting, and buildings.

19 A phrase borrowed from Pentcheva 2010, p. 1. See also below.

20 As in a telling case reported by Beda Venerabilis (672-735) in his *Ecclesiastical History of the*

English People (*Historia ecclesiastica gentis Anglorum*, I, 1; Colgrave & Mynors 1992, p. 20 f.). See also a number of examples of physical texts applied to the body as magic amulets, for instance Gospel books, recorded by Skemer 2006.

21 For a treatment of concrete medieval examples or reports of such pictorial activity in animated imagery, see for instance Freedberg 1989; Bynum 2011; or Hans Henrik Lohfert Jørgensen: **23** "The Image as *Contact Medium* – Mediation, Multimodality, and Haptics in Medieval Imagery", *Medieval Iconography, Means and Methods for the Interpretation of Medieval Images*, ed. Lena Liepe, Oslo (forthcoming).

22 See the subsequent chapter for further definition and discussion of the integrated sensorium as a historical paradigm of perception.

23 Pentcheva 2010, p. 2 (my emphasis). She introduces her objective with a lament relevant to the purpose of the present book: "Medieval objects were offered to the senses, their rich surfaces teasing the desire to touch, to smell, to taste, and to experience them in space. Treated as art, displayed in clinical and transparent glass cases, they lose their wider sensorial dimension and submit to our regime of the eye. The textured surfaces, flattened by the even electric lights, deflate to reveal a dead, immobile, taxidermised image" (p. 1). See also Pentcheva 2006, p. 631 f.

24 Pentcheva 2006, pp. 631, 651; including a pertinent discussion of possible definitions of synaesthesia with respect to the sensual experience of "the display and performance of the Byzantine mixed-media icon."

25 Pentcheva 2010, pp. 1-2.

26 Recent multimodality research has proved very rewarding both within (inter-)sensorial anthropology (e.g. Howes 2009A; Howes 2006), media and intermedia studies (e.g. Elleström 2010; Mitchell 2005), and the interdisciplinary investigation into semiotic resources or modes of extraverbal communication (e.g. Jewitt 2009). If we leave aside the different theoretical ramifications of these positions, they can be synthesised into a rough working definition of multimodality like the one here proposed.

27 Eco 1986, pp. 15-16.

28 See Eco 1986, p. 15, defining *integration* as a model of explanation and discussing the "integration of values [that] makes it difficult for us to understand nowadays the absence in medieval times of a distinction between beauty and utility or goodness."

29 McBrien 1994, pp. 9-17, 262-264, 787-790 & 1196-1201. Mediation is closely related to the general principles of sacramentality and communion: "The special configuration of these three principles within Catholicism constitutes its distinctiveness. It is a tradition that sees God in all things [as] actual or potential carriers of divine presence (sacramentality), using the human, the material, and the finite (mediation), to bring about the unity of humankind (communion). [...] These principles, at once philosophical and theological, have shaped, and continue to shape, Catholicism's Christology, ecclesiology, sacramental theology, canon law, spirituality, Mariology, theological anthropology, moral theology, liturgy, social doctrine, and the whole realm of art and aesthetics."

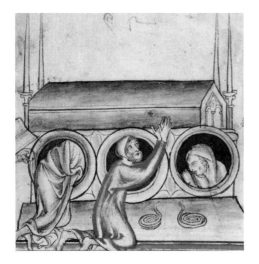

[**SENSORIUM**] The first chapter sets out to explore central assets of the medieval sensorium, comprehended as a paradigmatic model of perception that was to be followed, embraced, incorporated, or contested. Generalising in scope, perspective, and material, it employs early medieval miracles as well as high medieval perceptual theory and late medieval cult practices to present the distinguishing properties and principles of medieval perception. A new concept of this pervasive paradigm of perception is introduced: the *hagiosensorium*. The senses, it is claimed, were organised in a hagiosensorial matrix of experience, a sensory system aimed at sensing the holy, but also at authenticating and sanctifying holy sense experiences thus obtained. For the sacred to become an authentic experience it needed sensory mediation. This mediation of the senses was orchestrated through a multisensory repertoire of props, instrumental to medieval perception in general and to holy perception in particular. Because of their common purpose and goal, the multiple modalities of the hagiosensorium could be bent into each other, fused, and integrated in ever new ways. Consequently, the perceptual apparatus also constituted an *intersensorium,* integrating all available sense modalities in a multisensory synthesis of perceptual domains, exemplified by the notion of a unifying 'common sense'.

SENSORIUM

A Model for Medieval Perception

[Hans Henrik Lohfert Jørgensen]

Introduction to the Saturated Senses

This chapter provides an overall introduction to the saturated senses in their histori-cal existence, function, and state of being. It asks how *the saturated sensorium* came into being in its historically grounded reality and ideality: How did the purported saturation of the senses occur in a historical perspective? How were the medieval senses established, arranged, and practised as a social sense system? How did the senses work and operate in their particular cultural operation? How did they perform their tasks, fulfil their designated functions, and realise their perceived realities? In trying to answer these operative questions, I will explore central assets of the medie-val sensorium, comprehended as a customary model of perception that was to be followed, embraced, incorporated, or indeed contested by past percipients. General-ising in scope, perspective, and material, the chapter employs early medieval miracles as well as high medieval perceptual theory and late medieval cult practices to present the distinguishing properties and principles of medieval perception. A new concept of this saturating system of sensation is introduced, defined, and discussed: the *hagiosensorium*. Cutting across the finer geographical and chronological differences, this sweeping concept is used to describe a constitutional feature of 'medieval' modes of sensory experience, focused on an operative principle they often had in common, instead of on their functional variance and diversity.

The senses, I claim, operated within a *hagiosensorial matrix* of experience, a per-ceptual organisation aimed at sensing the holy and at authenticating and sanctifying holy sense experiences thus obtained. For the sacred to become an authentic experi-ence it needed sensory mediation. For the senses to become saturated with sanctity they needed not only an internal cultivation and idealisation of modes of perception but also an external framework provided by sensory instruments and media in the widest meaning. In order to be recognised and enter the sphere of human perception, holiness depended on mediation *for* the senses, mediation *by* the senses, and – ultimately – mediation *of* the senses. This multi-layered mediation of the sensorium was orchestrated through a multisensory repertoire of props instrumental to medieval perception in general and to holy perception in particular. The crucial issue of mediation and instrumentalisation is addressed in the latter parts of the chapter attending to the prosthetic enactment and support of sacred sensation as well as the ensuing codification of the senses.

This formative process of codification, however, also implies another underlying precondition of past perception, which has to be considered first. Because of their joint purpose and goal, the multiple modalities of the saturated sensorium influenced, informed, and sustained one another in mutual interchanges and transactions. The respective senses saturated each other and absorbed impulses from one another. Sensory modes could merge, assimilate, and blend into each other in ever-new ways, leading to ever-new exchanges and crossovers. Consequently, the continuous and flexible apparatus of perception also formed what we may label an *intersensorium*, which integrated all available sense modalities in a multisensory synthesis of perceptual domains. Before establishing this continuity, though, we must initially assess the historical standard or pattern of perception that allows us to speak of such a thing – or construct – as 'the medieval sensorium' in the first place.

The Medieval Sensorium: A Paradigm of Perception

Recently, some very interesting and noteworthy research has been done on the medieval sensorium and its greater historical outline, duly recognised as an important articulation of cultural history.[1] The present exposition of the subject distinguishes itself from these efforts by presenting the medieval senses, not one by one or according to a specific context or body of sources. Rather, historical sensation is apprehended within a different conceptual scope, the purpose of which is to provide a general model that is able to describe past sense experiences, at the same time both from the outside (the critical, constructivist stance) and from the inside (the experiential, phenomenological stance). The aim of this generalisation and its admittedly quite undiscriminating, perhaps even stereotypical conception of the Middle Ages, is to understand more fully and with greater nuance and depth how sensory reality came into being for the senses and how it in reality affected its historical percipients. The human senses are not simply natural, biological, and physical – given as an intrinsic and unmediated property of our embodied being – but are also fundamentally cultural, social, and historical – mediated by changing ideological frameworks and contexts of use. In dealing with "the sociality of the senses and sensations", David Howes, an influential exponent of sensorial anthropology, "highlights the fact that the senses are constructed and lived differently in different societies and periods. The perceptual is cultural and political".[2]

In the following, I will consider a particular policy of perception, a construction of the medieval sensorium, which produced not only distinctive sensual experiences but also distinctive ways of organising sensation and setting up the senses. Despite their function as embodied and material systems of communication, the medieval senses were culturally shaped and attuned to sensing, and thus confirming and legitimising, a particular world-view. Ultimately, this normative and paradigmatic mode of perception produced the medieval world for the senses, mediating all bodily experience through its sensorial ideology. The ongoing process of Christianisation was very much a process of fashioning, modelling, and structuring the senses of the faithful, furnishing their apparatus of observation with suitable capabilities and desired sensitivities. Ideally, to be a Christian was also to perceive and observe in a specific manner and thus to share a certain sense of things.

In her "Foundations for an anthropology of the senses", Constance Classen introduces the useful notion of the sensory model or paradigm considered as a socio-historical formation often imbued with religious significance:

> [P]erception is fashioned by culture. [...] an odour may signify sanctity or sin, political power or social exclusion. Together, these sensory meanings and values form the *sensory model* espoused by a society, according to which the members of that society 'make sense' of the world, or translate sensory perceptions and concepts into a particular 'worldview'. There will likely be challenges to this model from within the society, persons and groups who differ on certain sensory values, yet this model will provide the basic perceptual paradigm to be followed or resisted.[3]

In other words, the sensorial framework of medieval Christian culture was a basic model, which everyone had to face, either adopting and internalising it, or actively rejecting it. It was possible to maintain alternative or competing perceptual orientations, for instance those deemed profane, licentious, or heterodox, but at the cost of having such sensory practices codified negatively – or even eschatologically – by the prevailing Christian judgement.

Whereas such apocryphal practices may at times have been more transient, pluralistic, and poly-directional, the canonical way of seeing and feeling things was structurally Christocentric. Even sensory experiences, which at a first glance may seem to have belonged to primarily secular domains of medieval culture, such as food consumption, sexuality, or courtly behaviour, could be measured against, and hence understood through, the ethics of religious experience and Christ-like sensory conduct. Even systems of sensory representation stemming from other areas of life, such as romantic literature or popular ballads – both considered in upcoming chapters of the present volume – shared structures, spaces, or modes of expression recognisably paralleled in the religious sphere. In this integration of cultural values,[4] the Christian sensorium was fundamentally structured and formed by the urge to identify and apprehend the signs of God's presence in this world, or of the vicarious authorities representing Him on earth.

The religious idea of monotheism (i.e. convergence and centrality of the divine), modified and conditioned by the common belief in God's incarnation (i.e. immanence of the divine), are the essential preconditions for organising perception around the incarnate manifestations of a different, higher state of being – that is, the holy. While inserted 'in' this sense world, the sacred is also perceived as being founded by and focused at something 'other' than it – a perceptually pluriform, yet ontologically convergent quality showing itself in prominent persons, places, occasions, and things.[5] As noted by Richard McBrien, one of the constituent principles of universal Catholicism is a sacramental world-view, where the physical, the material, the visible, and the tangible always harbours a possibility for manifesting the metaphysical, the immaterial, the invisible, or the ineffable, communicating itself through the means of this temporal world. All reality, both animate and inanimate, is at least potentially the bearer of God's presence – a potential, which is not necessarily realised in actual fact though. Sacramentality, in this very expansive sense, is a qualifying precondition for the ability of sensory matter to mediate and convey what lies beyond the senses. On the level of sensory experience, this basic principle corresponds to a certain feeling of things: a general sensibility – whether actualised in a given sensory situation or not – for perceiving "the divine in the human, the infinite in the finite, the spiritual in the material, the transcendent in the immanent, the eternal in the historical".[6]

In this manner, certain 'centres of immanence' are located and sanctified as privileged goals or objects for the senses where a special presence can be felt, either in space or in time: churches, shrines, and other buildings or demarcated sites of worship; altars, graves, and a range of relics exposed as the focal points of such spaces; a variety of liturgical feasts, celebrations, and Masses producing presence; sacraments conceived as God's real presence and self-revelation, or as mysteries of faith, channels of grace, and efficacious rituals, as well as the consecrated objects resulting from such cultic actions; pious processions and performances, evocative enactments and diverse sorts of spectacle invoking and animating the holy; tabernacles, monstrances, ostensoria, cult images, sacred books, amulets, and many other media embodying or transmitting divine power; and last but not least a choice of material substances such as holy water, blessed salt, fragrant oil, sweet chrism, and savoury sacramentals consecrated by prayer, ceremonially scented, and used in rites to anoint the very sense organs of Christians, or "Christs" (meaning "anointed", in the odoriferous phrases of St. Cyril of Jerusalem).[7] The sacred centre ramifies and branches into a plethora of perceptible forms in order to meet worshippers and their senses in different places and at different levels of attention. Thus, the sensual world is experienced as a locus for the inherent nearness of sanctity in select hotspots distinguished by their sensory quality. The extrasensory incarnates itself in the senses, the transcendent becomes immanent, and as a consequence of this belief, holiness takes on a sensory appearance addressed to, and hence conditioned by, human perception. Indeed, the sacred may simply be defined as the extrasensory materialising itself or appearing in the sensory. It is a property of perception precisely because it both depends upon and purports to transcend the senses.[8]

Institution of the Christian Senses

Accordingly, the Christian sensorium is 'hagiocentric', that is, centred on the odour, sight, and sound of sanctity, extracted from the sensual continuum and foregrounded, sometimes even monumentalised or reified. Select perceptions are evoked from the continuum to be cultivated, objectified, and experienced in a more or less fixed Gestalt, perceptually identifiable as the sacred. Even when identifying an experience as unholy and off-centre, the senses assert the same monistic scheme and the same underlying convergence in order to pass their judgement over the percepts in question. At the end, there is a unified cause determining the sensorial value of any perception: its beauty, its truth, and its moral implications. The perceptual system converges upon the signs of Christ, whether manifest or underlying, whether present or represented. In the very act of perceiving, the faithful perform a kind of 'cognitive credo'.

It is not just a question of making believers look *at* Christ, but of making them look at everything else *through* Christ, installing a particular perspective on the world and its appearances. Christ was a way of seeing and sensing. The Son of Man became a filter or matrix in Man's eye and ear. This matrix was implied in an oft quoted dictum in 2 Corinthians 2:14-16, typical of the suggestive sensuality induced to communicate faith. Here, Paul exploited the long-established Biblical use of fragrant metaphors to state that "we are to God the aroma of Christ", *Christi bonus odor*. When filtered through the appropriate scheme, the pleasing perfumes of bodily ointment were made to evoke God's Spirit pouring out grace over the faithful, who received His presence in an aromatic offering of sacrifice, sacraments, and gospel: Christ perceived in good smell.

The divine presence opened and released the devout senses – as in St. Cyril's elaboration of Paul in the context of "Holy Baptism and the Mystical Chrism":

> For as the Bread of the Eucharist, after the invocation of the Holy Ghost, is mere bread no longer, but the Body of Christ, so also this holy ointment is Christ's gift of grace [...] applied to thy forehead and thy other senses; [...] on your ears; that ye might receive the ears which are quick to hear the Divine Mysteries, [...] on the nostrils; that receiving the sacred ointment ye may say, *We are to God a sweet savour of Christ, in them that are saved.*[9]

In order for the baptised to become "Christs", their very senses were chrismated and christened, anointed with the gracious unction of the life-giving Spirit (later to be singled out in the West as a separate sacrament of confirmation or chrismation). In their ritual opening, their aperture or *apertio*, the sanctified senses were marked by the sign of the cross to become Christ-like. Eventually, baptismal exorcism also came to involve a whole series of oral and olfactory exchanges such as breathing on the face (*exsufflatio*), putting salt on the tongue, and smearing saliva on ears and nose, following Mark 7:33-34: "Ephphatha, that is, Be opened!"[10] Thus, the Christian sensorium was instituted by an expressive sequence of opening rites that conveyed the sense of a new beginning of perception – an institution of sensorial salvation, enacted individually, but firmly rooted in the social regulation of sensation. Within this sensorial community that so acclaimed the sacramentality of odour, to smell good was to be good (soon leaving behind a certain early Christian reluctance to perfumed practices such as incense).[11] Conversely, the devil's stench was made out to be an anti-Christian reek of suffocating sulphur, thus establishing an olfaction-based scale of good and evil conditions, a deodorant eschatology of aromas. Still, despite this totalising system of fragrances, it was ultimately the percipient's own moral and sensorial disposition that determined whether the Saviour's presence was smelled as the sweet "odor vitae" of everlasting life or the perishable "odor mortis" associated with death and disease.[12] To sense the Saviour – and sense Him right – was eventually also to be saved.

31

Hagiosensorium

Consequently, I propose the term 'hagiosensorium' to designate this medieval paradigm of perception and its corresponding model of the senses (from Greek: 'hagios', *holy*, and Latin: 'sensus', *sense*). This concept indicates a pervasive principle of historical sensation, which was – in the manner of an ideal or standard – to be realised, practised, and negotiated at different levels and with varying success by members of the Christian society, assimilated by many, while opposed by others. As a sensorial concept, it conveys a dual meaning, denoting the 'sacred senses' as well as the 'sensing of the sacred'. Of course, these two dimensions of the medieval sensorium were intimately related and interdependent, perception of the holy effecting and requiring holy perception. When the perceptual apparatus was cultivated to grasp the inherent holiness of things, as a consequence, the sensory system was itself influenced and shaped by the holy percepts of its apprehension. A sensorially committed defender of icons, John of Damascus (675-749), knew this very well when he spoke of "the approach through the senses":

> When we set up an image of Christ in any place, we appeal to the senses, and indeed we sanctify the sense of sight, which is the highest among the perceptive senses, just as by sacred speech we sanctify the sense of hearing. [...] what the word is to hearing, the image is to sight.[13]

Gazing at Christ, or at just a perceptual representative of Christ, would Christianise the gaze itself. According to John, the sacred image induced sacred seeing and the spoken word inflamed sacred hearing. Sanctity had a contagious effect upon the medieval senses. The striving for sanctification was apparently a common or shared condition that underpinned various channels within and across the socio-religious sensorium. Listening to the Word of God installed a holy listener and looking at the portrait of God produced a godly onlooker. In some sense, view and viewer, percept and percipient, mirrored one another, or converged towards doing so. This reciprocal interaction between sanctified senses and sensed sanctity was precisely what constituted the ideal hagiosensorium. Visual, aural, and presumably also other sense impulses exerted a compelling appeal strong enough to become a vehicle of a mutually engaging transmission of holiness.

In other words, the experience of sanctity would reside both in *what* is perceived – the object of the hagiosensorium – and in *how* it is perceived – in the subject of the hagiosensorium. Hagiosensorial perception implies the subject's mode of sensing (e.g. godly vision) as well as an objective and purpose for the senses (e.g. vision of God). The process of sensory sanctification runs both ways between these dialectically connected positions. Indeed, as a prerequisite to sensing an object as sacred, the subject must also accept and adopt a sacred manner of sensation. Beatific eyes see beatitude, hallowed hands handle holiness, sanctified senses produce sanctity. When the Damascene promotes the experience that "material things are endued with a divine power" and when he venerates material objects, among others "the wood of the blessed cross, […] as being full of the grace of God, […] as being overshadowed by the grace of the Holy Spirit", then he also implies his and his fellow believers' ability to sense in the matter this holy quality, tacitly yet knowingly assuming the sacred sensibility of the recipient in question.[14] If "the material becomes partaker of grace […] by faith", as he claims, then conversely the gracious aptitude for sensing it becomes a distinguishing feature of true believers, or true sensors, so to speak. In this ontological construction of the holy, the two dimensions – sanctified object and sanctified subject – presuppose, qualify, and reinforce one another mutually, convincingly knit together.

In fact, John's contagious engagement in holy perception is akin to media scholar James Carey's definition of an aspect of communication, which is not primarily concerned with the transmission of information (as in secularised, modern perception), but rather with the ritual effect of communion and sharing between the parties of communication. In the ritual view of communication, the archetypal form of which is the sacred ceremony, a sense of participation and community is created, "that operates to provide not information but confirmation".[15] Similarly, the hagiosensorial experience approaches a ritual exchange, a mutual sharing of the holy quality transmitted and perceived. In this reciprocity, the sacred and its sacralised observer confirm each other, joined in a sensory communion of sanctity, a bond of graceful perception affirming the status of both percept and perceiver. The result is an encompassing naturalisation of the sacred as something that is really there because it can be felt (when sense impressions confirm sanctity), and vice versa, something that can be felt because it is really there (when sanctity confirms sense impressions). This is the reason why the sacred appeared a wholly 'natural' and undisputable phe-
nomenon to medieval observers such as John, a part of sensory reality to be counted with and taken in by the senses. Hagiosensorium and holy reality proved each other in a tight tautology that secured the holy experience a true existence in the natural order of things.

33

Senses of Sanctity

One model example of this may stand for many others: the cult of holy relics as it was experienced at St. Peter's grave in Rome by the late sixth century. In his eight "Books of Miracles", Gregory of Tours (539-594) recorded an array of wondrous ex-periences comprising all the senses – sacred sights, sounds, touches, tastes, and smells, usually interconnected and combined. In discussing the faith in miraculous incidents of sense perception "and of the so-called credulity of medieval people", Aron Gurevich maintains that the common confirmation of sacred objects and inter-ventions was not due to a lack in critical attitudes towards sensory information: "But the border between the likely and the unlikely did not lie where it does today. Con-fidence in the possibility of the miraculous was exceptionally strong, since it re-sponded to [...] the proper order of things. Faith did not oppose fact, but embraced a circle sufficiently wide to include facts".[16] He rightly assigns to the holiness of miracles a pivotal position in the analysis 'from within' of the logics of belief and perception of medieval popular culture. Noting that the ecclesiastic Gregory, a lead-ing prelate, did not distance himself neither from the thaumaturgical conception of sanctity nor from its visual and perceptible expressions, Gurevich goes on to demon-strate "[...] the lengthy prevalence, to the very end of the Middle Ages, of the popu-lar stereotype of the [wonderworking] saint found at the beginning of the period. [...] Belief in a saint's magical properties (expressed in venerating relics and expect-ing miracles from him) was characteristic of all medieval people, from commoner to pope – this was an integral part of medieval mentality".[17]

Accordingly, the copious miracles spanning the whole medieval period are a good place to look for general patterns of perception. Widely disseminated, told and retold yet again, these paradigmatic miracle tales were perhaps as influential as the Christian cult and its formative rites in choreographing sensory practices.[18] Their exemplary accounts of 'archetypical' sense experiences and occurrences configured the senses by acting as models of what to perceive (such as holy power) and how to perceive it (through powerful interventions in ordinary sensory matter). Through their propagation and dissemination, they helped codify the hagiosensorium and shape medieval worshippers' belief in the sensory manifestations of the sacred.

At Peter's shrine, itself a prominent model, Gregory of Tours reported such an emblematic manifestation of sanctity. He related how a pilgrim might insert his head through a small window into the dark shaft of the *confessio* to feel the virtue of the apostle's presence ("virtus apostolica"). Next, the visitor could lower a piece of cloth ("palliolum") on to the tomb, which was not itself within immediate reach. The true devotee would pray most earnestly, keep vigil, and fast in order to prepare duly for the awe-inspiring encounter with the holy. This ritual preparation was typical of the careful measures taken to ensure that receivers, which were about to approach and sense the sacred, were themselves in a blissful state free of sin that would facilitate their solemn contact with the saintly remains. Then, finally, occurred the materially mediated transfer that communicated the spiritual and sensorial communion of dead and living:

> Extraordinary to report! If the man's faith is strong, when the piece of cloth is raised from the tomb it will be so soaked with divine power [*divina virtute*] that it will weigh much more than it weighed previously; and the man who raised [the cloth] then knows that by its good favour [*gratia*] he has received what he requested.[19]

As a perceptible token of sanctity, the *brandeum* – i.e. cloth or contact relic – grew in weight and became considerably heavier because it had absorbed the miraculous power of the holy grave and had become saturated with grace. With Peter's material body encased at a sensory distance, virtually out of sight and out of reach at the bottom of the dark pit, the pilgrim would instead use the projected fabric as an extension of his senses – a vicarious "extension of man", if we apply Marshall McLuhan's definition of media – to establish hagiosensorial contact.[20] Through this tactile 'medium', the devotee would feel the apostolic presence when it soaked the cloth, saturated the air, and transcended the threshold between the tangible and the intangible. Generally, when absorptive objects, such as textiles or liquids, were placed in the vicinity of powerful saints they were apt to grow in spiritual density, which would also affect them physically and sensually.[21] But, as Gregory ensured, we are told this objective sanctification only occurred through the subjective communication with the devoted recipient whose own faith and spiritual disposition was a prerequisite to the sacred transmission.

In another instruction of how to perceive sanctity, the bishop of Tours related that a miracle-working crystal – due to its Trinitarian powers – would only come out bright and clear if adored by a righteous beholder free from sin, whereas it would blacken and appear all opaque to the sinful, denying its clarity to the unworthy: "The gem wonderfully distinguishes between innocent and guilty, since it is black for one but clear for another".[22] Thus, the colour-changing stone acted as a moral mirror reflecting both its divine maker and its human receiver, whose own character was exposed by the sensitive jewel. On the one hand it influenced and improved those engaging sensorially with it, for instance by effecting physical cures for the ill and heavenly protection for adorers, on the other hand its appearance to the senses was itself directly influenced by the current state of the onlooker. In hagiosensorial perception, objective appearance was conditioned by subjective disposition; not only because subjects perceived differently, but also because objects actually changed according to their percipients. Sensory reality mediated holiness in a profound interdependence of the sacred and the sensor.

To sum up, the *sensory impact* on cult objects, manifest in the change of shade, brilliance, weight, or other perceptual features, attested to the *sacred impact*, the presence of virtue, grace, or power: sense impressions confirmed sanctity. But at the same time it was the believed *sacred transformation* of an object – its 'transubstantiation' – that verified the, otherwise unbelievable, *sensory transformation* and lent perceptual credibility to the supposedly transformed object: sanctity confirmed sense impressions. Himself expecting the sacred saturation of the cloth he lowered to touch St. Peter, the pilgrim really did feel it to become heavier in his hand and somehow different of texture. Even something as fundamental as the sense of weight proves to be a historical and cultural experience. Notwithstanding our modern, metric notion of weight-perception as relatively stable, this was not the case in the medieval sensorium, which possessed both an instrument and an explanation for a kind of experience to which we are less sensitive.[23] Likewise, precious stones do change dramatically in material and visual appearance. Within a hagiosensorial model of perception these fluctuations of clarity and obscurity, shade and hue, may well be explained by moral variations. Gregory's instructions taught people how to perceive such variations within the adequate paradigm. Providing his striking examples with a sensory exegesis of physical phenomena, he offered a 'miracle manual' of perceptual experience. His writings, along with others of the genre, contributed to cultivating, conventionalising, and canonising the hagiosensorium – and to making the material world a possible place for hagiosensorial manifestations.

This of course neither meant that all perceptual change without a direct and apparent cause was automatically and naïvely taken as a sign of holiness, nor that sanctity necessarily had to reveal itself to the senses in this particular way. But it did take part in creating a sensibility for sacred interference with the world of the senses, a world-view allowing for otherworldly intrusions, which conferred upon all sensory matter an inherent potential for divine intervention and incarnation, even if this latent possibility was not actualised in most perceptual situations. The hagiosensorium formed a matrix for everyday perception, not because of sensing the sacred everywhere and in everything, but because of nurturing the potentiality for its incarnation and immanence in select perceptions: the ordinary as an occasion for the extraordinary, the sensory as an occasion for the extrasensory.

In conclusion, we modern critics of historical sense constructions may accept the sacred as phenomenologically real and authentic to medieval observers, not in spite of, but exactly because of being produced by (or in the process of) their very observation of it. However precarious or volatile that construction may seem to us, the sacred came to be an undeniable reality by manifesting itself to the senses for authentication. Sanctification took place in the senses and for the senses. By investing sensory reality with sanctity and infusing it with sacred experience, at least potentially, the hagiosensorium created that very reality. It was precisely because Gregory, John, Cyril, and their fellow 'constructors' in themselves contributed to creating a sacred reality that they could take it for granted and safely assume its real, objective existence. In order to embrace this objective sense experience, the faithful would themselves have to endow it with hagiosensorial values, which would then seem all the more real and convincing because they were founded in the perceiving subject. The living experience of the hagiosensorial subject animated, vitalised, and sustained the life of the hagiosensorial object. Holy sense perception enacted and gave life to the holy – and the holy responded by being there and being real (or becoming real). *"Mirum dictu* – Extraordinary to report!"

Intersensorium

All of the medieval senses were involved in hagiosensorial perception, and often at the same time. The sacred was a common objective, unifying the senses in a basically multisensory experience entertained by all accessible means. Contact with the sacred took place in all possible ways and by all possible channels of sensory communication and mediation. In perceptual theory, the classical Aristotelian division and com-
partmentalisation of the sensorium into a somewhat reductive and bureaucratic five sense-model may have been rehearsed often enough,[24] but in lived sensory practices – like the ones described by Gregory of Tours – the senses interacted, overlapped, and combined into a rich and abundant whole.

In reality, sense domains could not be separated that easily and in order to explain the totality of sensory experience, even the most systematic categorisations had to take these overlaps into consideration. Right from the outset the scholastic theory of discrete and exclusive *sensibilia propria* (or *sensibilia particularia*), the proper sensibles particular to each of the senses, had to be modified and complemented by the much more inclusive notion of *sensibilia communia* or common sensibles – that is, universal categories of human perception grasped by a general sensibility integrating all the senses.[25] This intersensorial cohesion of shared physical qualities integral to objects in space, synthesised by the so-called *sensus communis* or 'common sense', established a communal middle ground of all bodily sensation, a unifying confluence of perceptual modalities.

Augustine (354-430) believed all the senses to be analogous and share a similar structure,[26] and he even added an integrational inner sense, *sensus interior*, superior to the five individual senses, whose perceptions it gathered, processed, and judged.[27] Later commentators on the synthetic processes and dimensions of sense perception would refer to both Augustine and Aristotle. Thomas Aquinas (1225-1274), elaborating on 'the Philosopher's' understanding of the *sensus communis*, held that all physical sensation is based on a common root and principle ("communis radix et principium"), which engenders the distinct senses, so that all perceptual power, information, and stimulation express this general principle.[28] The notion of a conjoint origin and common root of the whole range of diverse senses, also propagated by Alexander of Hales (-1245) and Bonaventure (1217-1274) among others,[29] reflects a fundamental feeling that the perceptual faculties were deeply interconnected and intertwined, and only at the surface differentiated into what appear to be 'individual' modalities. The more or less separate organs of sense perception could only perform their function through the synthesis of the common sense, the central processor and communicator of the whole sensory system at the intersection of external and internal faculties.

Bonaventure, in summarising the sensory theology of his day, acknowledged the compound and composite character of perception but at the same time stressed its ability to lead to underlying spiritual principles:

> [W]e are led to contemplate God in all the creatures that enter our mind through the bodily senses [*per corporales sensus*]. […] man has five senses like so many doors [*portas*] through which the knowledge of all that exists in the sensible world enters into his soul. […] So the simple bodies, as well as the compounds resulting from their combination [*corpora composita* or *mixta*], enter through these doors. Our senses do not perceive only the proper sensibles, that is, light, sound, odor, taste, and the four elemental qualities identified by touch; they also perceive the common sensibles, that is, number, size, shape, rest, and motion. […] when, through the five senses, we perceive the motion of bodies, we arrive, as from effect to cause, at the existence of the spiritual principles that move them.[30]

In order to grasp the divine cause that enables the compound bodies of the sensible world to move, we need all the senses. From the first cause or mover, God, pours a flow of power ("virtus"), filtered down through the mixed substances of the perceptible world to ensure the movable operation of natural things, which offer their mixtures to the complex human sensorium. "Taking perceptible things as a mirror [*speculum sensibilium*], we see God in them" – and because these things are often conglomerate, so is perception.[31] The sensorial system mirrors the complexities of God's creation, whose fundamental motion is contemplated among the common sensibles.

Beyond the imagined boundaries of abstract sensory learning, this coherence of the perceptual experience may also have influenced, or at least paralleled, the perception of sacred 'bodies'. Cult objects, however diverse, shared the quality of holiness as a 'common' or synthetic feature presenting itself to more (or all) of the senses. As a multisensory feature addressing an integrated sensorium, sanctity – if perceptibly present in an object – seems to have been apprehended not unlike a sort of common sensible of a spiritual and holy class. Since the sacred transcended the threshold between the sensory and the extrasensory, it was also open to transgressions of the construed borders between the individual senses. Crossing the limits of the tangible and the intangible opened an expanded continuum, which – due to their greater or lesser tangibility, material concretion, and sensory saturation – the physical senses could slide right into. The hagiosensorium was an *intersensorium:* an integration of sense modalities braided into a complex and coherent whole.

When subjected to closer scrutiny, even the specialised and particular approaches of the seemingly pure, individual senses consisted of impure blends of perceptual modalities. The senses were not practised as isolated, autonomous, and reified channels of perceptual information transmitting the purely visual, the exclusively auditory, the wholly tactile, the solely olfactory, or the neatly gustatory, but as dynamic interchanges of combined and co-operating perceptual functions. However satisfactory the five sense-framework of *visus, auditus, tactus, olfactus,* and *gustus* may have seemed at a conceptual level, it was an abstraction of the mutual embeddedness and messy convolutions of actual experiences. Thus, medieval observers recognised that some senses, even the most basic ones, were of unclear definition or that they spilled over into each other in their way of recording and interpreting sense impressions.

The heterogeneous, and yet elementary, sense of touch suffered an especially ambiguous status within the overall system, because of its uneven conglomeration of palpable sensibles. In the light of the Aristotelian categorisation, touchable *sensibilia* encompassed material qualities such as weight, texture, surface, solidity, sharpness, humidity, temperature – "and many other things", according to Richard of Fournival (1201-1260).[32] On the one hand an uncertainty remained as to whether touch was indeed a single or multiple sense, casting severe doubt upon the question of its proper definition.[33] Thomas Aquinas discussed "whether there are several senses of touch or only one", concluding that "formally speaking [as opposed to "substantially"] the sense of touch is not one sense, but several".[34] On the other hand tactile perception held a fundamental position in the sensorium, necessary to the general workings of the sensory apparatus and somehow present in all sense perception. The *doctor communis* endorsed Aristotle's view that without the sense of touch there can be no other senses and that tactility is closely aligned with the *sensus communis.* Arguing that one general, all-embracing sense faculty is needed to compare sensations such as whiteness and sweetness or blackness and bitterness, "indeed any one sense-object and another", Thomas appointed touch the most likely faculty for this synthetic function because it originates in an intersensorial condition prior to the particularity of the senses:

[…] touch, the first sense, the root and ground, as it were, of the other senses, the one which entitles a living thing to be called sensitive. [T]ouch […] as the common ground of the senses, as that which lies nearest to the root of them all, the common sense itself.[35]

Touching is communal, not only because it physically unites the subject and the object of touch, but also because the haptic is rooted in a deeper level of sensation beyond the differentiation of individual modes of perception. This intersensorial character of touch, felt to be a basic component of all the senses in their mutual kinship, was also corroborated by the encyclopedist Bartholomeus Anglicus (-1272) who explained how the tactile underpinned all the other senses by imprinting its feeling in them.[36] The opinion that all sense experience ultimately stems from the feeling capacity of skin and flesh is in fact not unknown to modern perceptual theory. For instance, anthropologist Ashley Montagu contributes to a near-mythical construction of the skin as the haptic foundation of perception:

> The skin […] is the oldest and the most sensitive of our organs, our first medium of communication. […] Touch is the parent of our eyes, ears, nose, and mouth. It is the sense which became differentiated into the others, a fact that seems to be recognized in the age-old evaluation of touch as 'the mother of the senses'.[37]

In the medieval evaluation of haptics, the presumably archaic nature and parenthood of touch was perhaps best expressed in its interrelations with the sense of taste, considered a particular form of touch since the object of taste perception is also touchable.[38] Thomas reproduced the Aristotelian observation that there is touch in the tongue, which feels all kinds of tangible objects as well as savours because the tasteable is a sort of tangible, i.e. discerned by touch. Making clear that "taste is a kind of touch", he assessed the conditions under which touch and taste, though two in principle, would seem to be one and the same sense: "Obviously then, the pleasures afforded by food and drink, in so far as these are things perceptible and drinkable, accompany taste inasmuch as it is a kind of touch […] a species of touch. For the drinkable is common to touch and taste".[39] In this intimate relationship, the gustatory exercised an intersensorial function precisely due to "the manifold sensations of touch", the root sense that was "the foundation of all the others".[40] It *felt* good to eat and drink. Savoury consumption activated the intersensorium and exposed the multisensory dimensions inherent in corporeal and perceptual processes.[41]

Sweet Synthesis of the Senses

This sensorial intricacy caused repeated crossovers between the – in reality not that 'individual' – senses. It affected the rather diffuse sense of smell too, the perceptible categories of which (such as sweetness) depended on or coincided with those of taste.[42] Due to the vaporous nature of its *sensibilia*, smelling with the nose could also convey spiritual things and qualities ("vel odor vel spiritus"), as observed in the *Etymologies* of Isidore of Seville (560-636) and later followed by others.[43] Not surprisingly, then, the sweet-smelling odour of sanctity exhibited a tendency to cross the presumed boundaries of tangible perception and merge into the expanded intersensorial continuum. In the words of Woolgar, noting the association between fragrance and holiness, "smell, like all other aspects of sensory perception in the Middle Ages, was charged with moral and spiritual dimensions". He goes on to quote a highly aromatic account of the marvellous (yet perceptible) effusion of sweetness condensed in the air after the burial of a saintly man of God named Godric (-1172):

> Indeed the air of Heaven in all the surrounding woods became honeyed, because the trees and branches, wood and leaves, fruits and green places had appeared to be filled and moistened by a mellifluous dew from Heaven, which taste, look, savour, touch, substance and odoriferous vapour they retained for two whole months. Many [...] were accustomed to extract the liquid honey with their fingers and to taste it.

In making the most of the age-old notion of honey as heavenly dew, Godric's scented sanctity liquefied into "a mellifluous sacrifice to God, which was openly shown to all on earth".[44] When the saint's holy soul and deodorising spirit ascended through the absorbent air it left behind an otherworldly perfume and flavour of the sacred, literally a taste of Heaven. The syrupy condensation of divine olfaction offered an intense multisensory experience of God's presence, abundantly spilling over the (really not that) 'separate' sensory channels and flowing around the whole intersensorium. Truly worthy of the multifaceted hagiosensorium, this tasty holiness of dense dew, materialised vapours, and liquid tactility engaged a fluid range of perceptual faculties seeking for God's scent across the whole register of possible sense experiences. It was centuries ago since St. Cyril's "Mystical Chrism" had baptised and opened the Christian senses, but these were certainly still open to "the sweet aroma of Christ" and its lavish *effluvium* into the plentiful profusion of holy perception.

41

Admittedly, the Platonic or Augustinian-minded reader may be more accustomed to having the medieval sensorium organised around the noble sense of sight, hovering above – or representing – the rest of the senses. Yet, even to look or gaze at something was nevertheless also equivalent to making physical contact with it. In the different optical theories inherited from Antiquity, the perceptual acts of seeing and touching were not as distinct and isolated from one another as the strict modern division between the senses of contact and the senses of distance would have us believe.[45] Seeing was understood as a way of touching the object of vision with the visual rays projected from the eyes like beams or sticks. Augustine himself expressed this haptic quality of vision quite tangibly when, in *De trinitate*, he stated that the optical rays emitted by the bodily eyes reach out to touch or make us touch ("tangunt", "tangimus") whatever body we apprehend: "We see bodies through the eyes of the body, because […] the rays shine forth through those eyes and touch whatever we discern".[46]

Thus, the inherent tactility of vision amounted to a contact stimulus: a sensorial confluence of sight and touch, optics and haptics. This fusion of the sense of greatest distance and the sense of greatest proximity, bridging the whole range of the sensorium, was indeed constituent of hagiosensorial perception. It allowed a sanctifying contact with the sacred in various perceptual situations where the holy percept was either close by or further away – for example, when gazing and praying at a powerful image as opposed to kissing and touching it, or when contemplating the powers of the exposed sacrament of the Eucharist as opposed to receiving its grace by oral consumption and communion.[47] The hagiosensorium conflated different sensorial approaches and modalities into the common goal of sacred experience, whatever means they used and whatever perceptual distances they mediated. The hagiosensorium made purposeful use of the intersensorium as its medium of sensation – communicating, accessing, and producing the sacred at the interchange of senses near and far, touchable and visible, worldly and otherworldly.

Mediation of the Sacred
Mediation of the Senses

In order to fully understand medieval perception we need to consider yet another dimension of the hagiosensorium: its implied mediation of the senses. The edifying spiritual and moral properties of sacred sensation should not lead us to assume that it was essentially given as a more direct, unaided, or indeed unmediated mode of perception – quite on the contrary. "The human sensorium has always been mediated [...] enhanced by our technologies and extended prosthetically", claims a recent essay on *the mediated sensorium:* "[...] our senses are instrumentalised: we are joined to the sensory tools we have made".[48] Likewise, medieval techniques and modes of mediation used perceptual props for their material transference of sensory values and percepts. The technologies and prostheses of the hagiosensorium were indeed instrumental to authenticate holy perception and encode the senses with corresponding beliefs. Manifold mediations of the sensory contact with the sacred (or, alternatively, the profane) instructed the faithful in how, why, and where to seek contact with the special (or ordinary) objects of perception, which were to be sensed as holy and empowered (or not). Media in a very broad sense took part in generating a sacramental bond between the physical and the sacred, not just as an abstract idea or notion of 'incarnation', but as an acute feeling of materiality embodied in concrete sense experiences.[49] This feeling of 'immanence', itself a kind of divine mediation, was very much a product of the devices and contrivances used to engender a distinguished perceptual presence in the midst of the physical surroundings. Cultic and sensory tools, devotional and informational instruments, helped embed the sensuous expectations of holiness in tangible experiences.

Alongside sacramentality, *mediation* is in fact one of the founding principles of Catholic culture and religion, according to Richard McBrien, of course also including medieval Christendom. "God is disclosed mediately, not immediately".[50] The encounter with God must necessarily be a mediated experience, realised through some sanctified medium or other. In the end, the sacred sensorium was both the target and the locus of this sanctifying mediation. The communication of divine presence through sensory intermediaries was really a corollary of the sacramental world-view where the perceptible could always be used as an instrument for revealing the imperceptible. Any kind of sensory matter could be made to mediate, animate, and reproduce higher values and presences. But one must not forget that sacred mediation was a complex process operating on several mutually interacting levels. It had a dual purpose in relation to the senses and their object. The transmission simultaneously worked two ways and had the double effect of mediating *sanctity for the senses* (on the level of the perceptual object), while also mediating *the senses for sanctity* (on the level of the perceptual subject). Material mediation gave sensory shape to the sacred, but it also gave a sensible shape to holy perception, casting its stimuli into recognisable patterns of sacred experience (or, alternatively, the lack thereof). Sensory mediation of the sacred necessarily entailed sacred mediation of the senses.

On the one hand, mediators – be it artefacts, events, or persons – cast holiness into a perceptible form enabling it to be apprehended by the saturated sensorium. On the other hand, those same mediators structured the sensorium with perceptual coordinates and preferences, prescribing the proper direction, content, and mode of apprehension. Within the hagiosensorial matrix, the medium was the very point of perception where the sanctified object and the sanctified subject were knit together and woven into each other. Thus, the pilgrim's cloth reaching out for the thaumaturgical tomb was a medium in a twofold sense, as we have already seen, both as an extension of the human hand grasping for contact with the holy grave and as a means of communication from the saintly corpse sharing its sanctity through this vehicle of contact. Facing the fundamental obstacle that the immediate perception of its ultimate object was not possible, the hagiosensorium had to avail itself of mediation at all functional levels. In addition, to complicate things even further, the senses needed to be mediated in their function as *recipient* of sanctity as well as *producer* of sanctity. At either level and in either function, perception was mediatised and operated by extrinsic mechanisms of mediation.

Before turning to a few cases to demonstrate and substantiate this, let me corroborate the assertion by pointing to a parallel argument by David Morgan about sensory mediation as "the medium of belief". In *The Sacred Gaze*, Morgan sets out to explore "[t]he mediation of belief that goes to the heart of belief as a historical phenomenon." Confirming that "belief is mediated", he looks into the visual and material culture of religion as "the physical domain of belief": "A sacred gaze is the manner in which a way of seeing invests an image, a viewer, or an act of viewing with spiritual significance. […] visual practice alongside images themselves, insofar as religion happens visually, constitute the visual medium of belief." Inquiring into the operation of vision as a religious act, he investigates "[…] how religious belief takes shape in the history of visual media. How is visual piety, visual belief, a function of its mediation? […] A medium – whether it is words, food, or looking at pictures – is where belief happens".[51] Against the long tradition of medieval cult imagery, we may confidently accept this ocular mediation of belief, which certainly helped shape both conceptions and perceptions of faith, that is, both "orthodoxy" and "orthopraxy", in Morgan's words. For that reason, let us now take a look at images as sensory instruments and props of perception.

Props of Perception

Images represented the tenets of faith ('orthodoxy'), but they also enacted the ritual and sensorial practices performed by believers engaged in worship with all of their senses ('orthopraxy'). Altarpieces and cult figures pictured events, persons, and objects of worship, often in tandem with the material or liturgical presence of the depicted bodies or objects, thus sustaining their visual and cultic appearance to worshippers. Crucifixes and portable pictures exerted an irresistible tactile appeal to be touched, held, lifted, carried around, and worn on the body by compassionate beholders who identified with the imminently touchable body of Christ. Scented icons were surrounded by or themselves emitted a flowery smell to be associated with the odour of sanctity by olfactory observers who might relate this effusion of precious perfume to the sweet fragrance known to have been given forth by the sacred wood of the holy cross itself.[52] Osculatories or 'Kußbilder' invited the ceremonial kisses of priest and congregation, and made them feel as if they were paying tribute to Jesus by mouth.[53] Exuding pictures encountered in miracles, visions, or real life could discharge a holy *effluvium* that sometimes solicited oral response, even the tasty drinking of images.[54] Cult statues and effigies awaited to be spoken to by devotees and readily returned an audible answer, as if it was a conversation with the enshrined saint him- or herself, acting as a living agent of communication, a multisensory 'medium of belief'.[55]

In this way, pictures invited sensory and spiritual exchange as the locus of a two-way communication of faith, a mediatised 'Augenkommunion'. Visions and theophanies would materialise in brilliant mosaics, in colourful wall paintings, and in luminous stained glass in order to illuminate the spectator's own gaze with the visionary power supposedly required to receive such otherworldly sights. As prostheses of vision, pictures mediated the sacred gaze by defining its holy percept as well as the appropriate perceptual mode for addressing it (such as awe, veneration, illumination, or compassion). By framing, staging, and exposing the object of cult, images directed the viewer's gaze at the holy, just as they directed and instructed the sensory and spiritual attention to be paid to it. They were an effective instrument for the hagiosensorial exchange between the viewer and the viewed, a sort of 'fenestella' or viewing frame with a built-in focus and scopic structure ready to implant itself in the beholder's eye. On the one hand, through their selection and mediation of sensory information, images fixated, enhanced, and sanctified the exhibited entity, endowing it with the hieratic qualities of a sacrosanct object or being. On the other hand, by

45

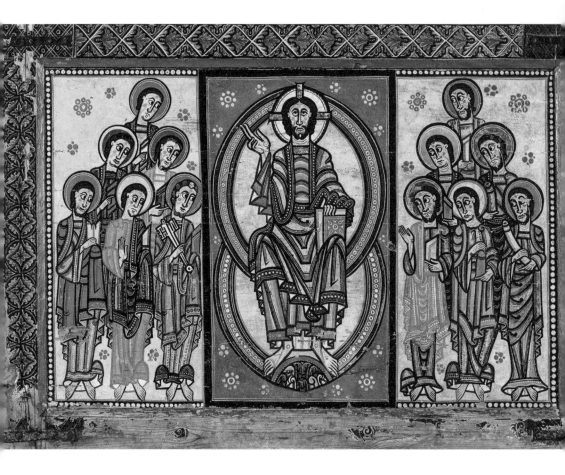

[III. 1] Codification of sight in early medieval imagery: allowing the worshipping viewer a heavenly vision of a prophetic revelation and monumental theophany, Christ in Majesty commands a retinue of reverent apostles, enthroned in his radiant mandorla on an altar frontal from La Seu d'Urgell (late eleventh or early twelfth century, Museu Nacional d'Art de Catalunya, Barcelona). Confronted with the stern symmetry, authoritative frontality, severe stylisation of forms, and hierarchical perspective of the tremendous sovereign, the illuminated gaze approaches in courtly awe and God-fearing respect to let divine glory and power shine upon it. © MNAC, Barcelona.

presupposing the gifted ability of holy seeing, holy touching, and holy smelling, they installed in their viewer those very perceptual properties. The material medium of images produced sacred senses – and thus paved the way for the perceptual medium of the senses to produce sanctity.

According to Marx Wartofsky, philosopher of representation, the human sense of sight is a cultural and historical product of the constructive activity of making pictures: "[…] vision is an artifact, produced by means of other artifacts – for example, by pictures." It is actually the image that teaches its spectator how to see, presenting him with a sensory schedule or matrix intended to exercise the culture's cognitive and perceptual preferences in the act of seeing. Images instruct our perception and inform our view of the visual world, constituted by how we choose to represent it:

> The plasticity of the visual system […] is an historically variable mode of perception, which changes with changes in our modes of representation. […] modes of picturing change, with changes in form of our social, technological, and intellectual praxis; representation has a history, and thus, in coming to adopt different modes of representation, we literally change our visual world. Human vision is an artifact created and changed by the modes of picturing […] – that is, we *see* by way of our picturing. […] representational pictures are *didactic* artifacts. They teach us to see: they guide our vision.[56]

Without images, no vision. Without media, no senses. Without props, no perception. This could of course be further elaborated and qualified, for instance by considering medieval codes of pictorial representation in their changing reflection of the contemporary world-view: The aristocratic and hieratic solemnity of early medieval imagery organised in a majestic visual hierarchy of cosmic proportions, suitable for instituting a far-sighted and revelatory mode of perception through an abstract symbolic codification of sight [ill. 1]. Or, as opposed to this awe-inspiring prophetic outlook, the material realism, physical delicacy, and emotional intimacy of late medieval views devoted to an engaging and nearby world – a concrete sensual world visualised and given shape by images encoded with passion and compassion, images investing the gaze with personal involvement and perceptual empathy, images inspiring cultic animation and sensation [ill. 2].[57]

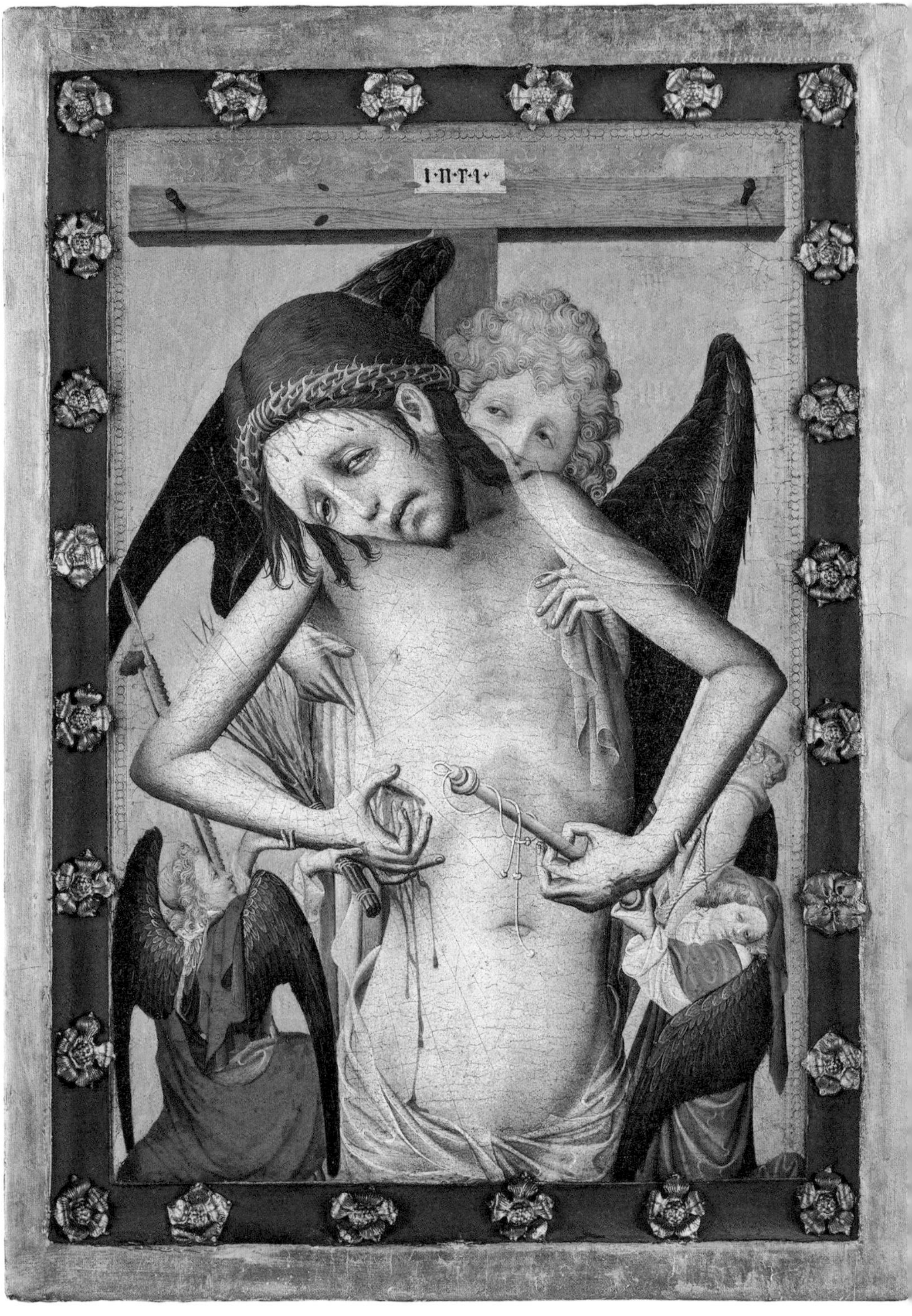
I·N·T·I·

[**III. 2**] Codification of sight in late medieval imagery: presented to the susceptible eyes of the onlooker by angels, Meister Francke's *Man of Sorrows* (c. 1420-1430, Museum der bildenden Künste, Leipzig) invites a tender, empathetic, personally involved and identifying gaze, an individualised and sensitised sense of sight, embodying other modes of pious perception as well in a suggestive sensory and corporeal concretisation – feeling the touchable texture and fragile vulnerability of Christ's soft skin, tasting the Saviour's bleeding sacramental body as a Eucharistic substance, smelling the blossoming beauty and fragrant love of 'rosa mystica' in the gilded metal roses, and hearing the vocalisation of the holy name of Jesus in the three letters "IHS" repeated in the tooling of the gold background like a kind of 'acoustic mandorla' (according to Michael Camille). © bpk – Bildagentur für Kunst, Kultur und Geschichte, Berlin.

Instrumentalisation of Perception

The point to be made here is more general and pervasive though: that the medieval sensorium always depended on mediation. The historical plasticity of perception applied to other sensory domains as well, mutually exchanging and integrating strategies of representation and mediation. A historical class of power images empowered the historical viewer and produced powerful vision, equipping eye and mind with the hagiosensorial disposition needed to authenticate and animate such images in their multisensory materiality, beyond sight alone (as in the above mentioned examples of more-than-visual reception of diverse picture types). Similarly, other types of sensory artefacts acted as 'didactic' guides for their recipient, implying their own propositions and properties of perception through their particular mode of sense mediation. The mediatised operations of the senses thrived on both representational and non-representational modes of mediation across the whole sensorial spectrum. Even a cult item that was not a 'medium' in the conventional communicative sense could instigate cultic perception and contribute to the construction of the hagiosensorium. In spite of being himself the ultimate source of the perceptual experience of holiness, the percipient was certainly aided and guided in his efforts by the sensory objects and media available to him. In the following, we shall see how such utensils and materials encoded, facilitated, and augmented the hagiosensorial experience.

In the case of cultic vision this may perhaps best be shown by reviewing a variety of liturgical or paraliturgical devices designed to offer sacred sense experiences to believers' eyes; or to be contested by doubting unbelievers, who would then be deemed unworthy and unable to really see. Most emphatically, at least during the late Middle Ages, the sight of *corpus Christi*, the sacramental body of Christ, was promoted by implements of exposition like the 'monstrance' – a designation deriving from the Latin *monstrare:* to 'show' [ill. 3]. This demonstrative tool was really a kind of 'scope', a piece of exhibition machinery, visually and materially staged as a holy apparition in order to suggest the ritual theophany of its Eucharistic content. Ceremonially exhibited on the altar, in processions, or in translucent tabernacles augmenting and celebrating its glorious visuality, it enacted a kind of perceptual transubstantiation or consecration: a sensory ostentation of extrasensory substance, substantiating the higher reality of the exhibit. No longer taking the shape of a sealed shrine, this innermost house of God featured an angelic architecture emblematic of the whole 'stage' of the Gothic Church displaying its means of heavenly salvation. Thus, unlike earlier types of receptacle, the monstrance equipped the exposed sacrament with an insistent visibility that demonstrated the *real presence* it embodied by adorning, framing, and contextualising the consecrated host as a divine spectacle to be looked at in reverence and devotion.

The transparent cylinder of the monstrance acted as a sort of sacred looking glass – a 'hagioscope' – proposing an intense and consuming mode of visual inspection, a devouring ocular consumption of the edible wafer with oral and tactile undertones. It furnished a potential viewer with a particular gaze at a particular object. It *made* the faithful look. Not only that, it made them look in a certain way – craving for the sanctified sight of and sensorial contact with the corporeally present Lord. As an instrument of vision, the scenic showcase fabricated the holy gaze *for* the spectator: a dedicated focus enhanced and intensified by the host-shaped glass or crystal in the centre. It worked like a lens, an optical and spiritual magnifying glass telescoping visual attention on to the specular body in focus. This sacramental viewing mechanism instrumentalised seeing, in order to invest the eyes with a pious ability to see the sacred, even in a lowly piece of bread – in itself not very spectacular or sensually appealing. Had the humble wafer not been so grandiosely paraded to eager onlookers seeking sensory manifestation of God's presence, it might have remained merely bread in their perception of it. As the very medium of visualisation, the ostensorium tutored the mediated gaze and coached it to perform the sanctifying transubstantiation in the very act of looking, holy seeing hence creating holy reality.

Indeed, this is why the visualisation was so comprehensive. During the sacrificial celebration of Mass, the whole church – comprising the physical shrine, the solemn ecclesiastical enactment, the celebrant elevating host and chalice, the carved and gilt

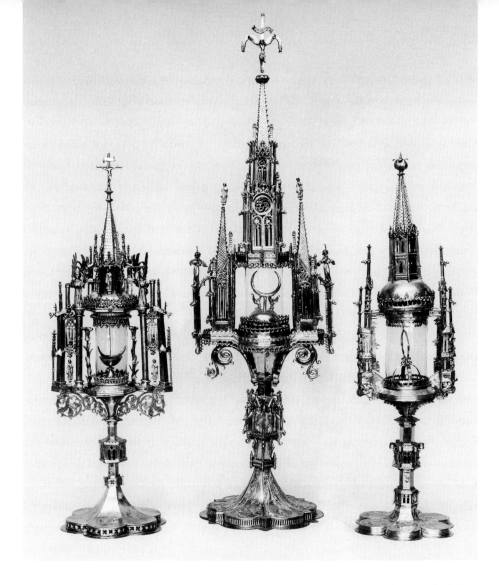

[III. 3] Ennobling carnal vision through the sacramental *Expositio:* three typical, late medieval *monstrances* for the consecrated host, mounted in a glass cylinder surrounded by precious ornaments and imagery in order to enhance the visual spectacle and satisfy the longing gazes of the faithful (all of gilded brass, 64-90,5 cm high, fourteenth-fifteenth centuries, The National Museum of Denmark, Copenhagen, inv. 10475, 10476, 10477). The cultic and optic instrument transubstantiated the sight of bread into the sight of God and mediated it to the senses in a digestible material form. Passionate devotees wanted to see ever more of their incarnate Lord – more body, more display, more visibility, more palpable presence. This apparatus of sacred scopophilia enabled them to behold the immaterial in the material, the extrasensory in the sensory, the immediate in the mediate. License: Creative Commons Attribution 2.5 – http://samlinger.natmus.dk/DMR/168604.

altar picturing Christ's body, the lavish liturgical vestments, the sacramental acces-
sories, the ringing of the *Sanctus* bell, the ceremonial effusion of incense, the acolyte
lighting the *elevation* candle – all participated in the multisensory mediation of
Christ's visible apparition at the very moment of consecration. This magnificent
apparatus of display taught late medieval worshippers the sensorial economy of
'spiritual communion': instead of actually eating and imbibing the meal of the
Eucharist, they should stare devoutly at the elevated body and blood of Christ, hoping for their visual reception – the *manducatio per visum* ('eating / chewing by sight')
– to emulate and attain a taste of the graces of oral communion – the *manducatio per
gustum* ('eating / chewing by taste').[58] The visual mediation and mastication of God's
body assimilated gustatory perception, tasteful digestion, and bodily incorporation
in a nourishing 'communion of the senses'.

Again, we are reminded of James Carey's portrayal of the ritual dimension of
communication, providing the community with a sense of participation, communion, and mutual confirmation.[59] The naked host itself could actually not communicate and transmit much sensory information, but when it was displayed as the con-
sumable *corpus Christi* it offered percipients a feeling of corporeal and social unity
with the Christian society understood to be the mystical body of Christ and the
Church. Through the prolific act of sacramental seeing, virtuous viewers were somehow united with the wholesome object of their holy sight, whose showing and viewing were meant to convince the congregation of the true reality of the transubstantiated body, and hence the whole construction of sanctity it confirmed and authorised.

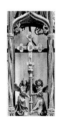

[III. 4] A holy 'hagioscope' processing the pilgrim's pious experience of
the scoped substance: Tilman Riemenschneider's *Heiligblutaltar*, Jakobs-
kirche, Rothenburg ob der Tauber, limewood and fir (1499-1505). Just one
little inconspicuous drop of the assumed blood of Christ is microscoped
and enlarged into this 11 metre high altarpiece, encased as a sacred
specimen in a reliquary crystal in the exalted superstructure. The mighty
mediator itself undertakes the visualised institution of the Eucharist: "hic est sanguis
meus". Towards the end of the Middle Ages, the material mediation of sanctity acquired telescopic proportions, as if the sensory actualisation of holiness required ever
more sumptuous instruments to convince recipients and consecrate their senses.
Photo: Achim Bednorz.

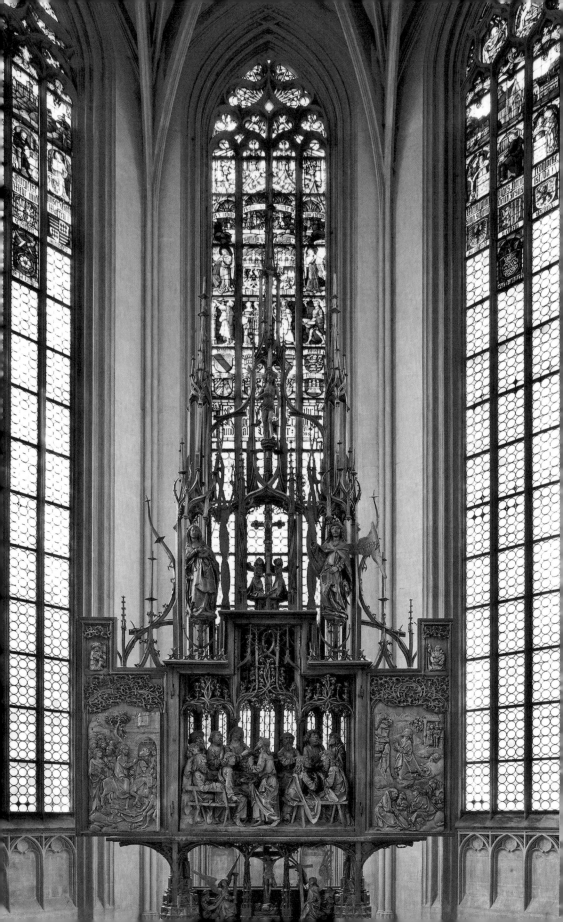

A Choreography of Holy Touch

Bread, bone, stone, wood, cloth, liquid – all these, perceptually somewhat meagre carriers of sanctity, were in need of enriching sensory mediation and confirmation to become vehicles of holiness. Therefore, a repertoire of ostentatious receptacles gradually developed, comprising – besides golden monstrances – also anthropomorphic, gem-encrusted reliquaries with *oculus* openings for the saintly bones, crystalline see-through containers, shimmering translucent ostensories, transparent openwork tabernacles, diaphanous tomb arrangements, glazed architectural shrines, and ever-loftier altars with built-in spaces for figural and liturgical vessels [ill. 4]. One such sensory extravagance would be the showcase architecture of Sainte-Chapelle, the 'Holy Chapel' of Louis IX (1226-1270), consecrated in 1248 to assure the Parisian public that his sumptuously staged collection of passion relics had in reality acquired the true crown of thorns, symbolic of his sacred rule [ill. 5].[60] Spectacular and eye-catching as these contraptions were, their exhibition of sacred material did not appeal exclusively to visual reception. Other modes of sensory contact were also addressed in the mediation of hagiosensorial experience. From time to time haptic impulses of sacred touch and tactility were seemingly manufactured in 'touching devices' designed to grab the holy and handle it in palpable ways. Indeed, the instrumentalisation of touch could be very persistent and suggestive when it directed the faithful to engage bodily and materially with tangible objects of cult.

The most instructive example of this is perhaps the so-called *foramina*, waist-size 'portholes' cut into the casing around a venerated sarcophagus or tomb. Through these openings, pilgrims were allowed to put their hands and head into the shrine or even crawl into the structure with most of or their whole body so that they could kiss and touch the coffin inside. Sometimes the apertures were formed as niches that

[III. 5] A magnificent apparatus of display, itself magnifying the displayed exhibit into a holy reality: the upper chapel of Sainte-Chapelle, Île de la Cité, Paris (consecrated 1248, and later restored). In this shimmering, translucent space of exposition, the palatine shrine of Louis IX featured ostentatiously staged appearances of the recently acquired crown of thorns, paraded by prelates or the priestly king, himself crowned as a *vicarius Christi*. The monumental reliquary *made* the monumental relic, that is, made it become real and genuine to the heavenly king's earthly followers. Photo: Achim Bednorz.

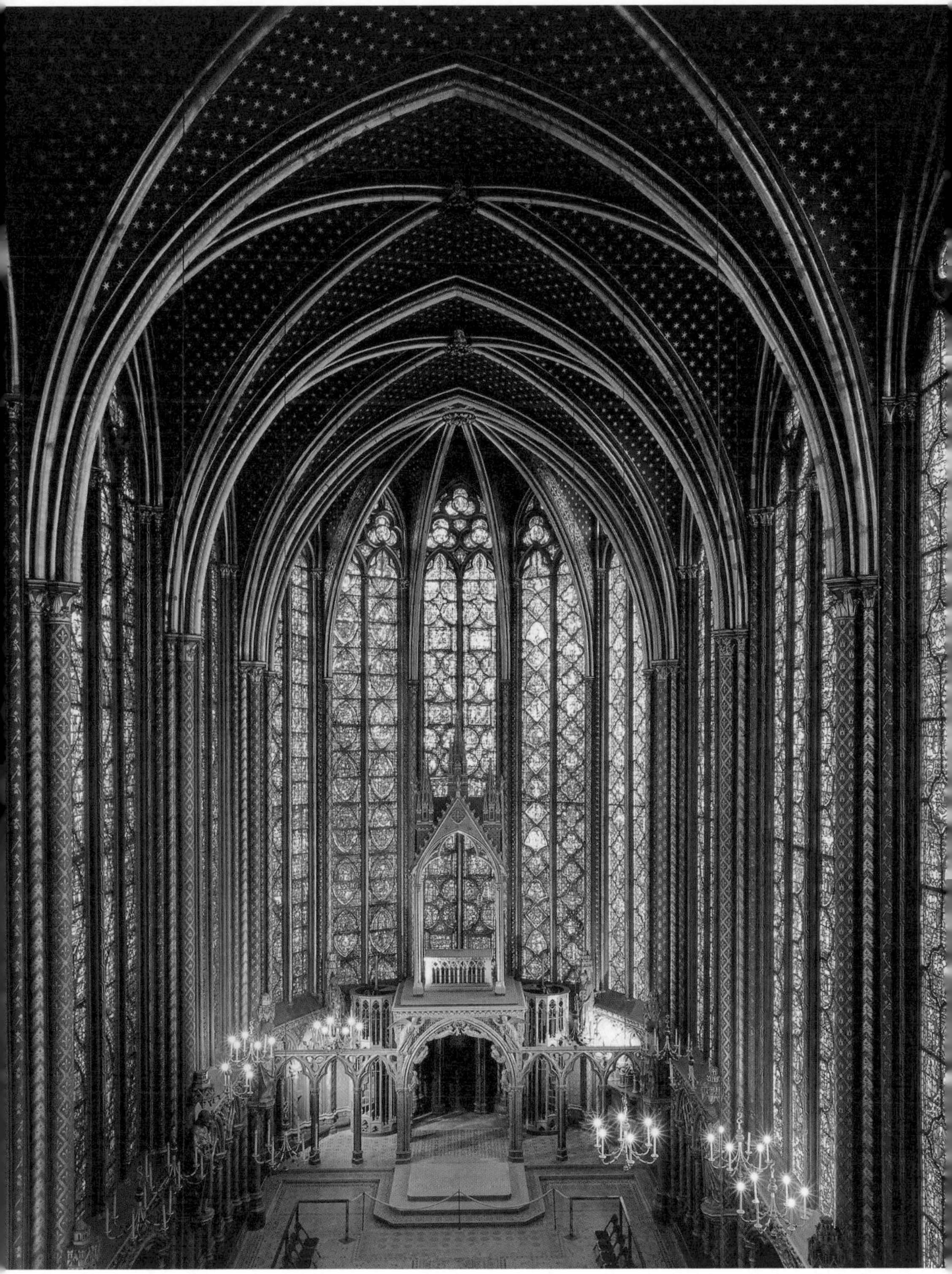

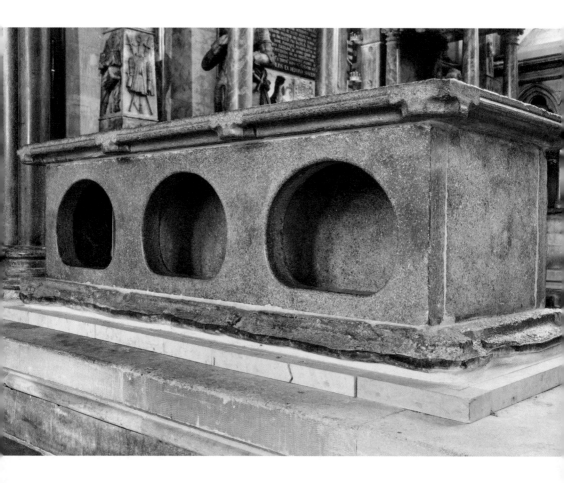

[III. 6] A highly haptic remedy for revitalising paralysed sensory organs through the staging of intimate contact with the vital corpse of a saint in the making, able to make the blind see, the deaf hear, the paralytic hand feel, the insane and insensible come to their senses again: Purbeck marble shrine of St. Osmund, Bishop of Old Sarum, who died in 1099 and was later translated to the present site in the Trinity Chapel at Salisbury Cathedral (late twelfth or early thirteenth century, originally with eight shafts framing the *foramina* or *fenestellae* into the structure covering the coffin). In the historical course of reported events, it may actually seem that the material monument made (i.e. enacted) the corporeal cult, which made (i.e. produced) the holy miracles, which then made (i.e. fabricated) the saint, only canonised as late as 1457 after many miraculous occurrences at the tomb. Photo: John Crook.

made it viable for visitors to lodge themselves in the monument with the aim of being as near to the miracle-working corpse as possible or of falling into a curative sleep while their sore limbs absorbed the physical contact with the inner core of the powerful shrine.[61] With body against body, skin against sepulchre, such tactile practices enacted a choreography of holy touch shaped by the layout of the tomb. The pierced outer shell did not really offer protection of the grave, but on the contrary drew attention to it, invited a cult of touching, and instigated intimate contact with the holy remains harboured right inside, above, or under the dramaturgical holes. At the reputed tomb of St. Osmund in Salisbury Cathedral from the late twelfth or early thirteenth century, the slab inside the openings – arguably the lid under which the would-be saint resided – shows patterns and traces of wearing from repeated tactile, manual, and oral encounters with generations of faithful.[62] The portholes are of an organic, subround shape that may correspond to a cross section of the human body on its way through this channel of contact [ill. 6]. The monument itself advertises its corporeal usage and program of haptics. The arrangement is literally an instrument for sensing the sacred: an apparatus for haptic experience. Relatively simple in visual terms, yet curiously fascinating, so much more appealing is the embedded intersensorial plea for ritual interaction with the monument. It is a staging of ritualised touch that gives physical directions regarding what is to be done by a fervent supplicant approaching the venerable place. The believer only has to step in (or crawl in) and play the assigned part of the 'sense ritual' – as if the appropriate way of feeling and touching has already been laid out for him and merely awaits his corporeal realisation.

The Christian prototype for this enticing structure was an eleventh-century staging of the rock-cut 'Tomb of Christ' in the church of the Holy Sepulchre at Jerusalem, enthusiastically revered by hosts of medieval pilgrims, such as the German monk Theoderic visiting around 1172: "In the side [the sepulchre] has three round holes through which travellers give the kisses they have for so long desired to give to the stones on which the Lord lay".[63] Mediating the corporeal contact with the Saviour's historical body, "the holy stone" was perceived as permeated with the bygone presence of *corpus Christi*, saturated with sacrifice, passion, and resurrection. No wonder that devotees so fervently desired to lay their own limbs on the substituting rock relic, a perceptual *Leerstelle* dense with projected feelings of an absent substance. No wonder that the 'pious peepholes' made percipients want to touch and behold the inspirited stone – and, on the other hand, that it seemingly itself desired to be saturated with devout prayers, touches, and kisses, impressed upon it by pil-

[**III. 7**] Consuming a corpse, feeling a funeral, inhabiting a grave: no less than four miniatures in a manuscript of *La Estoire de Seint Aedward le Rei,* attributed to Matthew Paris, show suppliants crawling into or lying inside the venerated "tumbe", accessed through *foramina* (fol. 29v, 30r, 33r, 36r; *Life of St. Edward the Confessor,* executed around 1255, Cambridge University Library, MS Ee.3.59). Three physical and mystical bodies convene in an exchange of meaning, power, and substance, mediated by the transgressive portholes corporeally connecting king and followers: 1.) *corpus Christi,* the body of the heavenly king incarnate – 2.) the body of the saintly king on earth, himself a *vicarius Christi* buried in a similar fashion – 3.) the body of their earthly believers, voluntarily 'entombed' with their sovereign's holy corpse.

grims' living organic bodies. Following this desirable model of shrine, represented in standard iconography of the Resurrection, saintly graves with *foramina* (most often three on the side) proliferated in Western Christendom from the twelfth century onwards.[64] Death and absence was exchanged for the sensory presence condensed into the stone, a compellingly tactile and textured material, enigmatic and suggestive in its untouchable core of unapproachable solidity, yet also absorbent of sacred memory and holiness, receptive to the warmth of stroking hands and caressing lips.

A corresponding palpable practice is also documented in miniatures and stained glass showing prostrate pilgrims at (or inside) such funeral shrines, kneeling, supplicating, and acting out the bodily postures of devotion through the evocative portholes. This dramaturgy of desirous touch may apparently be performed while the holy body in question is still displayed, censed, and celebrated; while the entombed saint's miracles are read aloud, inspiring miraculous re-enactments to take place; while the faithful are queuing up for their moment of thaumaturgical touch; or while some other paraliturgical activity is undertaken at the scenic burial site [ill. 7].[65] Sometimes the suppliants even seem to emulate the enshrined corpse – their prostration and remedial redemption ultimately an imitation of the dead and risen Christ himself. Staged in all the sensory scenery surrounding the sarcophagus, the deadly contraption amounts to an enactment of the hagiosensorium, an instrumentalisation of the sense of sanctity. It offers a pre-designed matrix of experience to the pilgrim of the sepulchre, the pilgrim of the sensorium, incorporating a medieval model of touch in its material structure. When mediated by this instrument of tactility, contact becomes a sacred activity – an act of faith. As it fabricates and builds up the touching

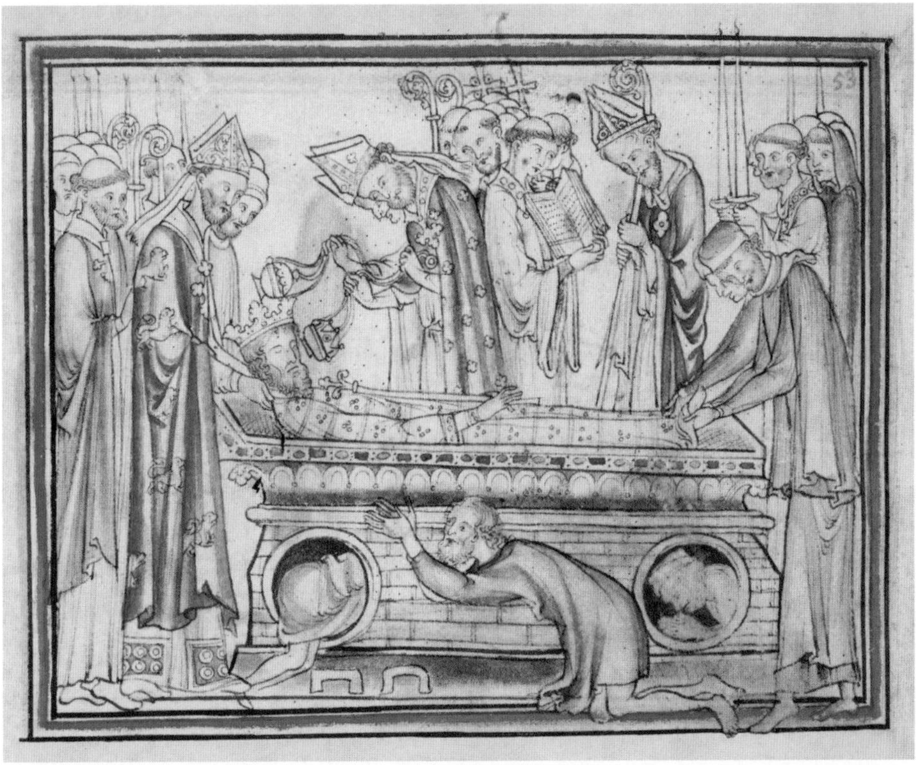

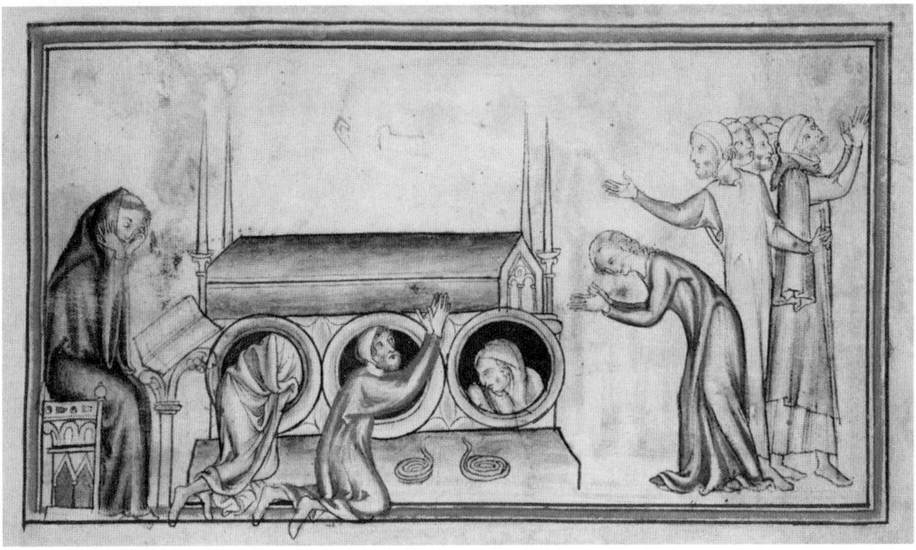

experience, the charismatic contrivance contributes to the Christianisation of the senses. It is a mechanism for feeling in a faithful way, a 'medium of belief'. The rather mechanical character of this physical machinery of perception certainly does not prevent it from producing divine and cultic sensations. On the contrary, it is the very mediation of the senses that makes them holy and sanctifies the sensory world. The cult of sacred touch relies on a touch of technology.

On occasion, this 'systematic' sanctification of the senses is concretised and confirmed by miracles, typically cures, that affect the sense organs and restore perception of the healed recipient – not unlike the ceremonial opening of the senses in baptismal exorcism, which takes its cue from Christ's miraculous healing of (and by) the senses.[66] While blindness (as in John 9:1-41) and deafness (as in Mark 7:32-35) may have often been the object of such tactile treatments and their symbolical reinstatement of the ability to hear and see the truth, other sense impairments too could be resolved by saintly intervention. At St. Hugh's much revered resting place in Lincoln Cathedral, a woman named Iveta, according to Gerald of Wales, had been cured of paralysis in her hand by placing herself "in medio foramine tumbae", thus presumably becoming able to feel and act once again with the dead limb after it had been somehow in touch with the departed saint's vigorous and vivacious limbs – touch curing touch, as it were.[67] At St. Osmund's purported sarcophagus in Salisbury, the frater Gervasius Brode reported how a "furiosus" named Thomas was brought forward to the tomb because of his ailment, chained with his hands bound in iron manacles. This 'Loony Tom' put his tied hands into the *foramina* ("posuit manus suas maniculatas ferro ligatas in foraminibus sepulcri") while bystanders prayed and appealed to God and Osmund, hence ritualising the moment of sacred contact. When after a while he extracted his hands – extraordinary to report – they were freed of the heavy chains and his sanity recovered.[68]

The renown of this manual miracle soon spread, carried by the "publica vox et fama", that is, it became a motive of popular belief and veneration, a model of a 'hands in hole' cult, which would excite the sensory and spiritual expectations of others who put their limbs into the able apertures in the hope of remedy.[69] The contact with Osmund's physical remains had proved to transfer the saint's powers to the faithful touching him, or more precisely, touching the material mediation of his presence for palpable perception. The channels in the tangible medium of the tomb fitted the hands and bodies of believers and presented their sensitive skin with a haptic interface to the faith, a mediation of sensory access capable of creating miracles. The deed of freeing a manacled man's hands dramatised that the percipient's own sense of touch was released by the sacred touch of the saint, symbolically liberating the very organ of tactile sensations (i.e. the hands) from its burdening chains. Unbound by human 'illness', the freed hands could grasp holy experiences of a higher order and reach for divine contact. Cured of his furious madness, the emancipated toucher recovered his common sense, his feeling of things and touch of reason, so to speak. Casting off the ailing bounds, tactility was unleashed for a higher purpose.

61

Woolgar, who admittedly only deals very briefly with the phenomenon, suggests that *foramina* "were constructed […] to allow pilgrims to get even closer to the relics".[70] Indeed, it may seem so, but had that been the case, the pierced outer casing around or over the contained coffin could just as well have been wholly omitted. Rather, the 'double shell' arrangement of such shrines emphasised the mediation of holy contact, opening the tomb for the senses precisely by inserting an extra layer between them and the saintly remains. This materialisation of perceptual proximity added a porous shell to be transgressed only by a special sensory effort on the part of the pilgrim. In other words, the transgressive holes were constructed to provide the sacralising mediation that allowed visitors the *experience* of getting even closer to the relics. The inviting cavities framed the sacred feeling and condensed it into a holy kind of touch, fit for the transference of power and exchange of beneficence. They staged the hagiosensorial experience by making contact a special and privileged achievement, a tangible transgression. The hallowed holes required and produced a mediated sensorium. Here, hallowed hands handled holiness exactly *because* they were guided by the channeling niches to do so and to feel so. When the remnants of the saintly body could only be reached by corporeally crossing this sensory barrier, the relics were apt to be perceived as powerful objects with an impact so potent and intense that it equalled receiving a little share of the charismatic corpse – of its mediated virtues, that is. The material intermediary intensified perception into a physically and spiritually exalted mode imbued with an aura of sanctity. In the reciprocity inherent in the hagiosensorium, material mediation was at the same time both an instrument of sensory sanctification and a communication of it.

Props of Transmission

Accordingly, the sensory sanctification of relics in turn required sensory mediation and communication. Dry and hollow bones were perceptually authenticated, enlivened, and saturated with divine power, their dead stuff animated into tangible spirit by media of transmission and presentation. If no one had cared to enshrine, encase, and expose a poor piece of bone for sacred sensing, it would have remained mere bone and would not have been blessed with virtues of curative efficacy. It did not become a relic until it was conceived and perceived as one. It needed to be announced through a medium (verbal, visual, or physical) to implore the solicited response. Hence, a whole series of mediations could be involved to gradually transmit the perceived powers from the perceptible body of a saint to the perceptive body of a beholder. Cultic corpses were believed to pass on their sacred presence via burial places, shrines, monuments, or crypts in which they were entombed and localised; reliquaries, caskets, altars, retables, or other containers in which their relics were identified and presented; sculptures, effigies, or figures in which their relics were encapsulated and re-presented; vestments, cloths, or other fabrics in which their relics were dressed and shrouded; blessed water, wine, or oil in which their relics were soaked and washed; as well as other physical objects placed in the vicinity of their graves or adjacent to their remains.[71]

All of these transmitters were assumed to be permeated by the outpourings of holiness that they themselves contributed to establishing and realising. At the end of the line, the sacred radiation was to reach its destined reception (and realisation) in the pilgrim who would look at the diffused saintly presence through a *fenestella* or an *oculus*, touch it through *foramina*, drink it as a liquid of an *ampulla*, or feel its palpable mediation in a *brandeum* or contact relic – as reported by Gregory of Tours at St. Peter's grave. Whether it was Peter's sixth-century grave cloth or Osmund's twelfth- or thirteenth-century marble tomb, this 'strategy' of inserting physical intermediaries as extra layers or secondary vehicles of mediation was widely used throughout the Middle Ages for the sensory encounter with the holy. Whether a projecting textile or a framing stone, they mediated the touch of the grave, which in turn mediated the touch of the saint. The very notion of 'secondary relics' implies a mediation of the sensory contact between the percept and the percipient. These 'intermediate relics' handed on, it was believed, the contact with the sacred with which they themselves had been in contact. They shared and distributed the sanctity of which they themselves had acquired a share.[72]

In this way, a whole chain of mediations could be established that would gradually transmit the prophylactic benefits from the supposed source, typically a dead person, to a living recipient, sometimes distanced from one another by hundreds of years or thousands of miles. To overcome the chasm between saint and believer, spatial as well as temporal, ontological as well as physical, their mutual engagement needed sensory mediation, relics being the prominent, but not the only, channel for this exchange [ill. 8]. One after another, the secondary media of sense communication could chain up and accumulate their production of sanctity. It was as if the sweet-smelling corpse was more of an object of cult than the living saint, the fragmentary relic more tangible and tactile as an object of cult than the corpse as a whole, the reliquary more visible and appealing as an object of cult than the relic it had once contained, the ampoules of water in which the reliquary had been washed more miraculous and efficacious as an object of cult than the reliquary itself. In the words of pope Gregory the Great (540-604), who played a crucial role in the manufacture and distribution of so-called *sanctuaria*, portable relics sanctified by contact, "[…] how is it that as a rule, even the martyrs in their care for us do not grant the same favours through their bodily remains as they do through their other relics? We find them so often performing more outstanding miracles away from their burial places".[73] Remarkably, the props of transmission served to strengthen and intensify the favourable impulse transmitted.

Through this process of sensory saturation, perceptual proximity could be mediated over a distance. The power of a distant shrine or relic could be compressed into a few drops of potion to be ingested orally, hence being not just near, but also inside the recipient's body. This was the case, for instance, in the chain of sacred contacts established when people at Poitiers had their fevers cured by drinking a sip of water in which a small robe had been washed that was formerly used in Jerusalem to wrap around the holy cross onto which Christ's body itself had been attached – thus communicating the Saviour's body from the East to the sick body in the West via wood, textile, and liquid, a sequence of materials becoming gradually more and more like the body.[74] Each time a saint's miraculous virtues were mediated they seemed, not to fade, but to become stronger and denser, simply because they were produced in the very process of mediation (and its reception). Apparently, sanctity was apt to be accumulated, densified, and concretised in tangible mediators of easy distribution and access, such as cloth or fluids, distinguished by their highly touchable appeal to the senses and the skin. When transported, the force of thaumaturgy would saturate and sanctify the media of transportation, reifying these as compact and concrete targets for sacred perception. Indeed, sensory mediations of holiness, far from just transferring some pre-existing holy power, contributed to its perceived existence. Contact relics derived from the sacred substance they had touched, it would seem, but in effect it was their mediation of contact that was responsible for promoting the notion of such a substance worthy of touch in the first place. It was the medium that sanctified the message. It was the purposeful touch that sanctified the otherwise

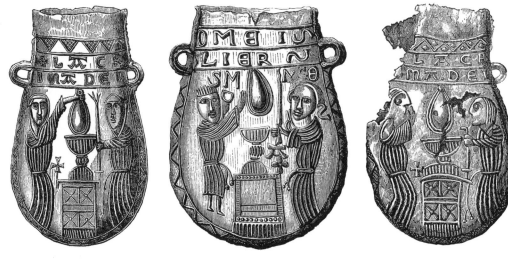

[**III. 8**] A string of material media chained up to communicate the healing powers of "Lacrima Dei", the holy tear of Christ (John 11:35): thirteenth and fourteenth century pilgrim ampullae of *Sainte Larme* from Vendôme, showing the venerated tear relic and mediating physical contact with it through a series of sensory intermediaries (66-71 mm, drawings after Arthur Forgeais). In a fluid mediation of holiness, the tear-shaped reliquary of rock crystal, itself inserted in layers of precious casing, was submerged into a large chalice filled with water from a holy well underneath or near the altar, drops of which would be poured into small pewter receptacles for pilgrims, to be drunk as a potion, rubbed on the skin as a lotion, or applied to the sensory organs as a gracious ointment.

ordinary material of the relic – and it was the purposeful mediation that sanctified the otherwise ordinary touch of the relic. Media were integral to the sensory experience of sanctity, and hence to the hagiosensorium.

That the senses were in reality thematised as a central issue within the miracle cult so characteristic of the Middle Ages, may be finally adduced by quoting another exemplary tale of Gregory of Tours – one that also demonstrates his own material belief in a synthetic sense of sanctity. In the town of Dijon, at the shrine of the local martyr Benignus, the saint's followers came to have their organ of sight healed through an intersensorial communion of sensory motives and materials:

> Many people pour wine and cider into the depressions that were made on top of the stone to which Benignus' feet were affixed with molten lead. Then, once eyes afflicted with inflammation or some other sores are soaked [with this liquid], immediately the illness leaves and they are healed. I certainly experienced this. For when my eyes were severely inflamed, I was touched with this holy ointment and immediately lost the pain.[75]

The physical pain of the martyr's suffering was grasped by a tactile impression in the holy stone, the power of which could be felt by the means of a tasty fluid. This was, however, not consumed orally but was instead used as a remedy to touch and anoint the painful eyes. Benignus' benign suffering relieved the hurting beholder's malign ailment through a sequence of sensory intermediaries that passed from the martyr's feet, via stone, liquid, and hands, to the recipient's eyes. The fluid mediation entailed an intersensorial integration of the powers and organs of several senses, and Gregory hardly even bothered to distinguish them as such. In this liquidity of the sensorium, stimuli flowed freely from one sense capacity to another. The virtues of martyrdom seem to have liquefied in a flexible fusion of the senses, the holiness of which dissolved conceptual distinctions between different perceptual domains. Because of their common purpose and goal, the perceptual modalities of the hagiosensorium could be bent into each other, fused, and integrated in ever new ways. In the productive dynamics of this multisensory union, we find the true 'common sense' of the Middle Ages.

Notes

1   E.g. Palazzo 2014; Palazzo 2012; Baert 2013; Baert 2011; Classen 2012; Pentcheva 2011; Pentcheva 2010; Schleif 2010; Nichols, Kablitz & Calhoun 2008; Smith 2008; Woolgar 2006; Harvey 2006; Jütte 2005; James 2004; Tellkamp 1999; Sears 1993.

2   Howes 2005, p. 322.

3   Classen 1997, p. 401 f.; also quoted by Howes 2005.

4   Eco 1986, pp. 15-16, and Webb 2008, p. 267, are among the many who have commented on this integration of medieval value systems, which also applied to sensory and aesthetic properties. See in addition the introduction to this volume for the concept of integration.

5   For further discussion of the possible definitions of "the holy"/"the sacred" and of the intricate relations between the subject and the object of the holy experience, see Eliade 1957; Laugerud 2003, p. 111 ff.; Colpe 2005; Oxtoby 2005 (also reviewing earlier literature on the sense of the 'numinous' as a fundamental element in religion).

6   McBrien 1994, pp. 9-10, 787-788, 1196-1199. See also the introduction to this volume on McBrien's principles of sacramentality, mediation, and communion, applied to the general endeavour of the book.

7   Cyril of Jerusalem (315-386): *On the Mysteries*, III, 1-6, "On Chrism"; 1893, pp. 384-387. On the materiality of sacramentals, "impregnated with a physical power that it conveyed to those who touched or consumed it", see Bynum 2011, pp. 229, 147 f., 160 ff.

8   To paraphrase the considerations of Kristin B. Aavitsland in the present volume, on "the paradox of sense perception", recipients of the sacred perceive something that according to the Christian matrix of perception is something else, i.e. a medium for it.

9   Cyril of Jerusalem: *On the Mysteries*, III, 3-4; 1893, p. 386 f., providing a different translation of 2 Cor. 2:15.

10   Spinks 2006, p. 110 f.; Johnson 2007, p. 222 f.

11   Smith 2008, p. 62 f., concluding: "By the mid-fifth century, Christianity had reconstituted the meaning of smells and their religious significance so that they took on meanings beyond sensuality and paganism".

12   Harvey 2006, p. 19 (*Scenting Salvation*), commenting on 2 Corinthians 2:14-16, the text that "more than any other scriptural passage provided the ancient Christian paradigms for considering the experience of smell".

13   John of Damascus: *Oratio I*, quoted from Bryer & Herrin 1977, p. 183. In his treatise *On the Divine Images*, I, 17, John voiced a similar opinion: "We use all our senses to produce worthy images of [God] and we sanctify the noblest of the senses which is sight." See also James 2004, p. 529 ff., who employs this passage and others from the treatise to argue a composite picture of the senses, providing a "bridge between the physical and the spiritual: everyone 'knew' that the smell of incense indicated holiness, that touching an icon was touching a saint, that the image of Christ meant that Christ was there. [...] By using all the senses, the worshipper – who was viewer, listener, smeller, toucher, taster, all at once – was transported into a visionary world beyond objects, to the point where the ontological differences [were] erased. [...] the interplay of the five senses around the object opened its audience to a fuller perception of its meaning and purpose.

[…] the whole sensory continuum allowed the believer to pass beyond the physical realm to the spiritual."

14 John of Damascus: *Oratio II*, reproduced in an *Anthology of Texts in Translation*, by Bryer & Herrin 1977, p. 183 f.

15 Carey 2009, p. 15.

16 Gurevich 1990, pp. 54-55.

17 Gurevich 1990, pp. 75-77, 39 ff. See also the discussion of concepts of sanctity in Brian Patrick McGuire's chapter in the present volume.

18 See also the remarks of Dahlerup 1998, pp. 260-261, on the rhetorical and performative function of miracles, mentioning as the prime example the *Libri miraculorum* of Gregory of Tours, the greatest miracle collection from the Middle Ages.

19 Gregory of Tours: *Glory of the Martyrs*, 1988, p. 46; *De gloria martyrum*, XXVII; Migne: *Patrologia Latina*, 1849, vol. LXXI, col. 729. See also Thacker 2002, p. 18; Toynbee & Ward Perkins 1956, pp. 212 f., 234.

20 McLuhan 1997. See also Jørgensen 2010, p. 171.

21 Finucane 1977, p. 26, offers a pertinent formulation of this hagiosensorial mediation: "Relics emitted a kind of holy radioactivity which bombarded everything in the area. [Their] beneficent aura […] affected cloths placed nearby, water or wine which washed them, dust which settled on them, fragments of the tomb which enclosed them, gems or rings which touched them, the entire church which surrounded them, and of course the hopeful suppliants who approached to kiss, touch, pray before and gaze upon them."

22 Gregory of Tours: *Glory of the Martyrs*, 1988, p. 34.

23 Correspondingly, the long exegetic tradition of the Book of Wisdom 11:20 made weight (as well as number and measure) an indicator of the divine. See for instance Bonaventure: *Itinerarium Mentis in Deum*, I, 11; *The Journey of the Mind to God*, Bonaventure 1960, p. 13, which, though of a much later date, construes the weight of perceptible things as a sensorial indication of the point towards which they tend, in the end meaning God.

24 Aristotle: *De anima*, "On the soul", followed in this respect by Augustine, Avicenna, Averroës, Albertus Magnus, Bonaventure, Thomas Aquinas, and others. For a brief survey, see Jütte 2005, pp. 38, 46 ff., 55.

25 E.g. Thomas Aquinas: *Sentencia Libri De Anima*, II, 13; *Commentary on Aristotle's De Anima*, Thomas Aquinas 1994, p. 124 f. See also Tellkamp 1999, p. 160 ff. The distinction in fact goes back to Aristotle's *De anima*, quoted extensively by Thomas in his commentary – and briefly by Jütte 2005, p. 39.

26 Augustine: *De trinitate*, XI, 1, 1; *On the Trinity*, 1998, p. 144: "It is not necessary, that we should inquire of all these five senses about that which we seek. For that which one of them declares to us, holds also good in the rest". See also Tellkamp 1999, p. 26.

27 E.g. Augustine: *De civitate Dei*, XI, 27; *Confessiones*, I, 20. See Wolfson 1935, p. 71; Jütte 2005, p. 46.

28 Thomas Aquinas: *Summa Theologica*, I, q. 78, 4, ad 1; *Sentencia Libri De Anima*, II, 27. See Tellkamp 1999, p. 191 f.; Th. Dewender: "Sensus communis, II. Mittelalter", *Historisches Wörter-buch der Philosophie*, vol. IX, col. 634-639.

29 Dewender: "Sensus communis", col. 636.

30 Bonaventure: *Itinerarium Mentis in Deum*, II, 1-3; *The Journey of the Mind to God*, Bonaventure 1960, pp. 18-20. This passage is discussed in greater detail in Laura Katrine Skinnebach's chapter on *Devotion* in the present volume.

31 Bonaventure: *Itinerarium Mentis in Deum*, II, 1; *The Journey of the Mind to God*, Bonaventure 1960, p. 18.

32 Quoted by Sears 1993, p. 23.

33 Sears 1993, p. 24.

34 Thomas Aquinas: *Sentencia Libri De Anima*, II, 22 (on "Touch: One Sense or Many?"); *Commentary on Aristotle's De Anima*, Thomas Aquinas 1994, p. 162 f.

35 Thomas Aquinas: *Sentencia Libri De Anima*, III, 3; *Commentary on Aristotle's De Anima*, Thomas Aquinas 1994, p. 187. See also Jütte 2005, p. 42.

36 Woolgar 2006, p. 29, quoting from *De proprietatibus rerum*.

37 Montagu 1986, p. 3. This passage has often been quoted by Pallasmaa 2005 and others who advocate an architecture of the senses through a return to the haptic properties of the skin.

38 Jütte 2005, p. 41; Sears 1993, p. 24.

39 Thomas Aquinas: *Sentencia Libri De Anima*, II, 21; *Commentary on Aristotle's De Anima*, Thomas Aquinas 1994, pp. 158, 159 f.

40 Thomas Aquinas: *Sentencia Libri De Anima*, II, 22; *Commentary on Aristotle's De Anima*, Thomas Aquinas 1994, pp. 161, 164.

41 See also Jette Linaa's chapter on *Consumption* in the present volume.

42 Consider the intersensorial ambiguity of olfactory and gustatory terms such as 'aroma', 'flavour', and 'savour'.

43 Isidore of Seville: *Etymologiae*, XI, 1, 47. See Woolgar 2006, p. 14.

44 Citations from Woolgar 2006, p. 118, quoting Reginald of Durham: *Libellus de vita et miraculis S. Godrici*. Woolgar collects several noteworthy sources for and examples of reported manifesta-tions of the odour of sanctity, but omits to treat their apparent multi- and intersensory dimen-sions.

45 Lindberg 1976, pp. 2-11. See also the considerations of Montagu 1986, p. 310 ff., on "the tactile quality of vision", i.e. a subconscious tactile base of the visual world, mostly repressed and ne-glected in the distinction between the established categories of distance senses and proximity senses sustained by modern Western civilisation.

46 Augustine: *De trinitate*, IX, 3, 3; *On the Trinity*, 1998, p. 127. See also IX, 6, 11; p. 130.

47 Dumoutet 1926. See also the considerations on multisensory imagery, sacramental viewing, and Eucharistic perception in the following paragraphs.

48 Jones 2006, pp. 5, 8, 17, assessing the current sensory situation (separation, bureaucratisation, and channeling of the senses) in a far-reaching historical perspective.

49　See Bynum 2011 for a further discussion of the tensions and potentialities embedded in "Christian materiality", exemplified by late medieval conceptions of sacred matter.

50　McBrien 1994, pp. 263, 11-12, 1196-1199.

51　Morgan 2005, pp. 3, 6, 8. For a different, but certainly related, definition of cultic vision and sacred seeing, see Jørgensen 2003; Jørgensen 2004.

52　Jacobus de Voragine: *Legenda Aurea*, CXXXVII, The Exaltation of the Holy Cross; *The Golden Legend*, 1993, vol. II, pp. 168, 170. See also Woolgar 2006, p. 120 f.

53　See for instance Hamburger 1998, p. 330 f.

54　A characteristically ardent case being that of Margarethe Ebner (1291-1351), dominican mystic of Medingen in Bavaria, who saw herself imbibing the blood of Christ's heart wound gushed forth by an embracing crucifix; Arnulf 2008, p. 110 f. See also Bynum 2011, p. 21.

55　According to Kamerick 2002, p. 59, "[…] animated images perform on multiple levels. The images' movements and speech naturally inspire wonder and deference […] implicitly refer[ing] to and deriv[ing] authority from the most significant medieval precedent for animated images – the crucifix in the church of San Damiano from which St. Francis of Assisi heard the voice ordering him to rebuild the house of God."

56　Wartofsky 1979, pp. 272, 273, 274, 282.

57　See for instance Bynum 2011, p. 37 ff. featuring several examples.

58　Dumoutet 1926, pp. 18-21, discusses the respective positions on the issue of several scholastic theologians, and concludes: "On peut dire que le parallèle entre la 'visio' et la 'manducatio' de l'Hostie était un lieu commun de la scolastique du XIIIe siècle". See also Browe 1967, treating various forms of Eucharistic worship of the elevated or exposed host. Spiritual favours, such as indulgence gained from paying honour and devotion to the raised sacrament, also imply beholding the body of the Saviour and reflect a belief in the gracious powers of cultic vision. In the context of spiritual communion at the moment of consecration, Rubin 1991, pp. 63-64, 150, notes a "growing appreciation of the quasi-sacramental value of gazing at the present Christ", resulting in "[…] widespread understandings entertained by the laity that gazing was as good as reception [of the Eucharist proper]."

59　Carey 2009, p. 12 ff., makes the crucial distinction between the idea of communication as a transmission of information over distance (e.g. sensory signals and information) or as a ritual sharing of beliefs in time (e.g. sensory beliefs and world-view). See also above.

60　See Cohen 2008 for a convincing discussion and description of the public function of display exerted by the Sainte-Chapelle in Paris, including architecture, liturgy, processions, and indulgences, which "[…] publicized the king's new relics to all the faithful in the kingdom and invited the people to celebrate the feasts at the Sainte-Chapelle" (p. 869).

61　As recorded at Lincoln by Gerald of Wales and at Canterbury by Benedict of Peterborough, who recounted that a certain Ælward of Selling managed to entomb himself by climbing into Thomas à Becket's old shrine in the crypt and lying directly on top of the encased coffin, thus emulating the dead body immediately below him; – see Crook 2011, pp. 195, 197. Crook treats the historical, archaeological, and art historical documentation of several other English examples of extant or lost tomb-shrines with *foramina*. Finucane 1977, pp. 27, 123, pl. 4-7, gives as prominent examples the shrine of Edward the Confessor at Westminster, the first tomb of Becket at Canterbury, and the enigmatic burial monument attributed to St. Osmund in the Trinity Chapel at Salisbury.

62 "This slab is indeed considerably worn, by generations of kissing, touching, and perhaps scratching away of the friable shells of which the Purbeck marble is composed", according to Crook 2011, p. 203.

63 Quoted by Crook 2011, p. 192, along with other pilgrims reporting from Jerusalem between the twelfth and fifteenth centuries.

64 Crook 2011, p. 194, explaining how the three portholes became an iconographic shorthand for Christ's tomb in numerous depictions.

65 Contemporary illustrations of pilgrims' dramatised behaviour – eagerly pressing their bodies through the apertures of the sepulchre in search for the physical proximity of the saint – are reproduced by Finucane 1977, pl. 4; Wall 1905, p. 225 f.; Crook 2011, p. 188 ff., pl. 7.3; Blick & Tekippe 2005, vol. II, fig. 209. At Canterbury Cathedral, early thirteenth-century stained glass in the Trinity Chapel many times depict the oval openings in the first shrine of St. Thomas, through one of which King Henry II allegedly thrust his head and shoulders when he received the scourge in public penance – surely a quite tactile experience of faith. The repentant king was rewarded with a flask of 'water of St. Thomas' containing Becket's diluted blood, a token of his physical, oral, and haptic communion with the saint's slain body.

66 See above on the *Ephphatha*-rite.

67 Gerald of Wales: *Legend of St. Hugh*, XV; quoted by Crook 2011, p. 195; – see also p. 220 ff. for a treatment of the long lost shrine.

68 Quoted from documents for the commission into the sanctity of St. Osmund; Malden 1901, pp. 77-78.

69 For Osmund's shrine, cult, cures, and miracles in general, see Crook 2011, pp. 197-204, 280-281.

70 Woolgar 2006, p. 42. See also Crook 2011, p. 191 ff. for a more detailed and nuanced discussion of *foramina's* possible functions of protection versus limited access, yet without paying much attention to the sensory and spiritual effect of their ritualised manifestation and mediation of the grave.

71 See also note 21 above.

72 See Thacker 2002, p. 17 ff., recounting early medieval opinions about how a sanctified *brandeum* would bleed when cut in order to confirm its status and corporeal identity with the primary relics of the saint from whom it stemmed.

73 Gregory the Great: *Dialogi*, II, 38; quoted by Thacker 2002, p. 19. See also Classen 2012, p. 35 ff.

74 Gregory of Tours: *Glory of the Martyrs*, 1988, p. 26; *De gloria martyrum*, V. Similar liquidations of relics' powers recur throughout the Middle Ages.

75 Gregory of Tours: *Glory of the Martyrs*, 1988, p. 75 f.; *De gloria martyrum*, L.

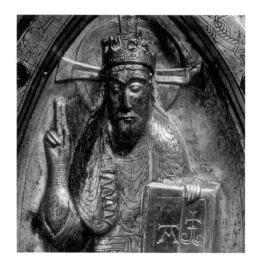

72

[**INCARNATION**] This chapter argues that the dogma of God's incarnation in human flesh is a fundamental precondition for medieval thinking about the senses, the purposes of perception, and the potential for mediation. The argument, however, centres not so much on theology and philosophy as on religious and cultural practice. Here the focus will be on the Eucharist and the sacramental celebration of Christ's redemptive death in the Holy Mass. The mediation of Christ in the Eucharist establishes the purpose, but also the limitations, of the medieval sensorium. This paradoxical mediation of an invisible and immaterial God through visible, tangible, and edible matter is not only the centre of Christian cult and belief, but may also be conceived of as a demonstration of the fundamental conditions of sensory perception in medieval culture. Furthermore, this chapter addresses the visual and material framing of the Eucharist, in order to explore how the paradoxical nature of perception and mediation is reflected upon and communicated. It argues that a certain type of altar decoration, especially from the Romanesque period, exhibits formal and rhetorical features that articulate the paradox involved in sensing and mediating the divine.

INCARNATION

Paradoxes of Perception and Mediation in Medieval Liturgical Art

[Kristin Bliksrud Aavitsland]

The Paradox of Perception

The senses are far from unproblematic and univocal in medieval outlooks on human life and human cognition. Texts and images testify to diverse and even diverging views on the status of sensual media, and on the limitations and potential danger of sensual perception. Thus, the issue of the medieval sensorium remained one of contradictions, negotiations, and conflicts. Notwithstanding the many learned controversies about the relationship between the senses and reason, and competing epistemological models, the sensorium of medieval Christendom was rarely conceived of as neutral. Contrary to an empiricist conception of the senses, which has shaped modern science and the sensorium of modernity, medieval thinkers did not consider sensual perception as passive reception of information about the external world. The medieval sensorium was basically teleological, targeted at the perception of the holy – it was hagiocentric, as Hans Henrik Lohfert Jørgensen has put it.[1] Since God was the ultimate end of this medieval hagiosensorium, deviation from this end – undirected sensualism – was considered dangerous. Senses astray had missed not only their target, but also the very purpose of human existence. This is the first precondition for medieval sensing. The second complicates the matter: although focussing on its goal, the hagiosensorium was inherently feeble and incomplete. Perception of the sacred remained unfulfilled, piecemeal, and dim, as the true glory of God was unrevealed and inconceivable in this world. As Augustine, Dionysius the Aeropagite (Pseudo-Dionysius), Anselm of Canterbury, and a whole range of their companions on the theological *via negativa* suggest: the boggling mind's only refuge in any attempt to contemplate God's nature was the dissimilar similarities of the sensuous world. In other words: the target of perception was imperceptible.[2]

This tension between the ultimate goal of perception and the deficiency of the senses is a recurring and problematic issue in medieval philosophy, which was treated in numerous theological tracts.[3] In this context I want to present less theoretical genres, in which the same problem is addressed verbally as well as visually. To begin with, I shall present a concise and pedagogic exposition of the issue as it is found in a vernacular treatise on the art of hunting. This work, composed in Normandy between 1350 and 1380, seems purely secular at a first glance. It survives in about thirty manuscripts, and some scholars connect it to the aristocrat Henri de Férrières. It is known as *Les livres du roy Modus et de la royne Ratio*, and takes the form of a dialogue.[4] King Modus and Queen Ratio are personifications of 'practice' and 'theory', although their names also give associations to the concepts of 'moderation' and 'reason'. They instruct a group of courtiers on hunting techniques, different types of game, snares and traps, the handling of weapons, and the use of hounds and falcons. The courtiers pose questions and the king replies as far as practical matters are concerned. However, he leaves it to his queen to instruct in theoretical issues. The text therefore proves multi-layered, as medieval literature of the didactic genre usually is. Queen Ratio employs the hunting instructions as a pretext for lessons in theology and morals. Being asked how it is possible that the deer sees through the hunter's tricks and avoids the traps set up for it, while the hound is able to catch the deer, the Queen responds that this is due to very acute senses of the animals. One should not be surprised, she maintains, that animals have keener senses than man. Man is himself guilty of having a weak and imperfect sensory apparatus. Originally God gave Adam, the first "beste humaine", a set of perfect senses, because he was determined to perceive the glory of God. At that time the mute beasts, who neither had a soul nor a concept of their Creator, naturally stood below man with respect to the acuteness of perception and insight into the wisdom of God. Queen Ratio and King Modus – reason and moderation – were sent to Earth by the Lord in order to lead man's will towards good. Man chose to neglect both reason and moderation however, wherefore he is blinded by the world and the devil. He has in other words lost track of his sacred destination. Hence, his senses have grown dull, and he is not able to perceive God anymore. So deep is man's fall and so hurt his faculties that even the soul-less beasts surpass him greatly with regard to sensory perception.[5]

Queen Ratio takes the impressive acuteness of the deer and hound's senses as a pretext to remind her audience that human senses were meant to be even sharper.

Her exposition gives the text on hunting methods a surprising twist, revealing the metaphysical implications of man's dull senses. Rhetorically original and innovative, the text nevertheless presents a representative outlook on sensory perception in medieval culture. It contains two fundamental predicates for the medieval sensorium. First: the one and only legitimate purpose of sensory perception is the recognition of God. Second: because of the Fall of Man, human senses are corrupted and have lost their potential to experience the glory of God. Together, these two ideas constitute the medieval paradox of perception: the noble purpose of sensation is incompatible with the corrupted state of man's sensory apparatus. Thus, the senses are likely to be remedies for Man's salvation as well as for his damnation.

However, Christian soteriology suggests an eschatological solution of the paradox of perception. Christ's redemptory sacrifice of his own human body and the glorious resurrection of the same, allows his adherents to wait for their own bodily resurrection at the end of time. This belief implies the hope for a fulfilled perception of God in the future. The afflicted Job, realising that his body was bound to be worm food, still knew prophetically that: "yet in my flesh shall I see God" (Job 19:26).[6] In this future act of incarnate viewing, the acuteness of his senses will be restored to their pre-lapsarian state. As St. Paul puts it: "For now we see through a glass, darkly; but then face to face" (1 Cor 13:12).[7]

According to the above argument, the medieval sensorium develops in the course of salvation history. The quality and potential of the senses are determined by its principal events: the fall of man, the incarnation and sacrifice of Christ, and the resurrection to eternal life at the end of time. Thus what conditions medieval sensual perception is: 1) that the true end of perception is God; 2) that this end is unattainable, since the senses were corrupted by the Fall of Man; but 3) thanks to Christ's salvific sacrifice and triumph over death, the resurrection of the flesh will restore the senses. In due time – or rather, beyond time – they will fulfil their end: to perceive the glory of God. This trifold and procedural comprehension of the senses remains stable from the early to the late Middle Ages, and forms a common denominator for the many and often contradictory opinions about the status and limits of sensual perception.

The Paradox Unfolded

The medieval paradox of perception – that the ends and means of perception are mutually incompatible – is conceived of as temporary and will be solved when salvation history has reached its end. During Man's earthly existence, however, his sensory apparatus might, instead of distracting him and leading him astray, guide him towards his destination and increase his knowledge about God, although by imperfect and insufficient means. Sense perceptions of the natural world might carry messages about its Creator. Mediation of the sacred manifested itself in two possible ways: as likeness or as presence.[8]

Likeness is a prerequisite for allegory. Scholars have often characterised medieval intellectual culture, and especially that of the twelfth and thirteenth centuries, as dominated by an allegorical understanding of the perceptible world.[9] The properties of nature – the looks, sounds, smells, and textures of plants, animals, stones, and minerals – were construed allegorically as representations of the qualities of God and his relation to Man, of faith and its mysteries, of moral behaviour. By analogy, the perceptible world became didactic as the Cistercian Alain of Lille declares in his twelfth-century edifying poem: "The whole of the created world is a book, a picture and a mirror for us to decode".[10] The various colours of different species of doves taught about the different offices and gifts of grace in the church; the sound of the rooster every morning reminded of the Christian obligation to watch and pray; and the comforting warmth that the flock of chicks found under the wings of the hen mirrored Christ's love and care for his church.[11] Via a detour of allegorical interpretation of analogous properties, the material world could reflect God indirectly – "through a glass, darkly". Perceptible matter pointed to the transcendent God as signposts along the pilgrim's track. In this way, allegory became an epistemological crutch to help the shortcomings of Man's feeble and dull sensorium.

However, at certain points, holiness was mediated in ways that exceeded the principle of allegory. At these points, matter did not simply gesture towards the divine. Rather, it enclosed holiness in itself: in these "centres of immanence", the celestial mysteriously resided in an earthly form.[12] When faced with shrines of saints, wonder-working images or relics, and above all the consecrated Host, the human senses did not receive knowledge of the sacred by analogy or likeness, but by disparity, and hence – paradoxically – as presence. In these places, bare matter contained the holy. Thus, something could be experienced that was both more than and fundamentally different from what could be learnt from the senses. Whenever the medieval hagiosensorium came into touch with 'holy stuff', this paradox of mediation came into play. A true paradox, the merging of the transcendent with the immanent, of earth with heaven, was not conceived of as a compromise or reconciliation. On the contrary, the integrity of either part was not violated, but remained intact.[13]

The elevation of select samples of matter to act as media for the holy was not always unquestionable. It caused much controversy during the high and late Middle Ages. Far from all relics proved to be authentic. Many alleged wonders worked by images, sculptures, relics, and Eucharistic wafers were met with theological scepticism and distrust from ecclesiastical authorities. However, the very conviction that matter could paradoxically embody the holy lay at the heart of Christian orthodoxy. Nobody questioned the dogma of the Incarnation without accusation of heresy. So, notwithstanding the many problematic occurrences of 'holy stuff', the very principle of mediating sacredness in matter went right into the core of Christian faith: When the infinite, invisible, and incomprehensible Word of God was made flesh, matter was dignified and became worthy of mediating the divine. Thus, the Incarnation fundamentally conditioned the relationship between the creator and his creation – between God, man, and nature. To describe the centrality of the Incarnation of Christ to medieval societies Jean-Claude Schmitt states that: "The Incarnation [was] not only a particular dogma, but a whole way of thinking that made its imprint on all Christian representations and practices".[14] But the Incarnation not only made its imprint on medieval representations and practices, it also affected Christian anthropology and the human sensorium in a fundamental way. Christ could be heard, seen, smelled, tasted, and touched. God had become available to human senses: historically as the man Jesus of Nazareth, sacramentally as Eucharistic bread and wine, but also mystically as the members of his Church, dead and living. Conditioned by the mystery of Christ, the senses were aimed at Christ.

Framing the Eucharist

It comes as no surprise then that the paradoxes of perception and mediation were particularly acute during the liturgical celebration of Christ's sacrifice. The Eucharist was – and still is – a paradoxical staging of a non-perceptible reality communicated to the faithful through all five senses. The sparkling vessels and decorations of the altar stimulate sight as the chant and ringing of bells stimulate hearing. The incense that consecrates the altar and the Eucharistic species saturates the olfactory sense, and the consumption of the Body of Christ is perceived through both taste and tactile sense. Admittedly, the saturation of the senses during the Eucharist was differentiated along social lines of division. Through most of the Middle Ages, the Holy Communion was but rarely distributed to the general congregation. Chancel screens with squints and openings of different kinds conditioned visual access to the chancel and the consecrated Host.[15] But everyone could hear the tolling bell signalling the moment of transubstantiation, and everyone could smell the consecrating incense. As Hiltrud Westermann-Angerhausen remarks, the smell of incense was probably the most democratic experience of the Sacrament in the twelfth century.[16]

Although exclusive, the strictly formalised and carefully directed performance of the Eucharistic liturgy can be interpreted as a manifestation of the paradox of sensory perception. The celebrant perceives something that – according to Christian doctrine – is something else, out of reach from his corrupted, human senses: He watches, smells, touches and tastes God himself. In a certain sense, the Eucharist is a staged deception. This is expressed by St. Thomas Aquinas in his celebrated hymn *Adoro te devote:* "Visus, tactus, gustus in te fallitur"; "Seeing, touching, tasting are in thee (i.e. Christ) deceived".[17] Yet the Church insisted that the Eucharist should be consumed *sensualiter*, through the senses.[18] This point became especially important for the theologians who, during the last half of the eleventh century and the first half of the twelfth, put much energy into rejecting Berengar of Tours' doubts about the substantial transformation of bread and wine on the altar. Their argument seems to be that sensual perception of the Eucharist is, paradoxically, *necessary because* it is imperfect and insufficient.

It is noteworthy that during this period, in the aftermath of rejecting Berengar (1059) and before the doctrine of transubstantiation was finally settled at the fourth Lateran council (1215), objects surrounding and serving the Eucharist were designed in a conspicuously 'sensual' way. Book covers, altar crosses, censers, chalices, reliquaries, altar frontals, and retables exhibit their material substance in an almost insistent manner during the Romanesque period. The brilliant surfaces, sumptuous materials, and rich ornamentation not only appeal to the eye, they also display tactile or haptic qualities. Metals, ivory, enamels, and stones of different colours and transparency were employed to form figures, figure scenes, and ornaments, saturating the senses with their sumptuousness and brilliance.[19] In most cases, the materials seem to have been chosen to resemble or imitate what they depict and hence invite allegorisation. The bright radiance of noble metals imitated the celestial glory of God, the sparkling variety of coloured precious stones was thought to simulate the multitude of Christian virtues.[20] Some altar frontals were adorned with gems or polished rock crystals set against pieces of coloured parchment. This was done in order to imitate different coloured precious stones that according to the description in Rev. 21 bejewelled the heavenly Jerusalem [ill. 9].

In this way, through their similitude with the celestial glory as far as the corrupted human senses were able to imagine it, the materials became allegories. Sur-

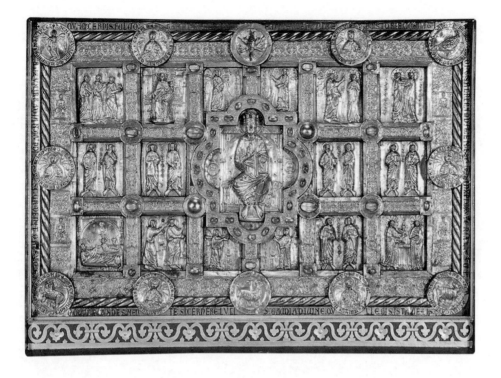

[III. 9] Altar frontal, Stadil Church, Western Jutland, Denmark.
Photo: The National Museum of Denmark, Copenhagen.

rounding the mystery of the Eucharist, the shining metals and bright stones of the retables, frontals, chalices, and censers pointed towards the future dissolution of the paradox of perception, when glory was to be perceived incorruptibly and without mediation. The likeness between spiritual and material glory was didactic and prompted allegory.

The material splendour of Romanesque *ornamenta ecclesiae* simultaneously displayed another strategy of representing the holy, however. Framing the Eucharist, the most prominent 'centre of immanence' in medieval culture, the altar decorations were also designed to demonstrate the paradox of mediation – to reveal their inherent and fundamental inability to represent the glory of God. For even if the materials were in the service of representation and ornamentation, their material qualities were not disguised. The Romanesque *ornamenta ecclesiae* were designed in a way that emphasises and clarifies the materials as such.[21] The glow of enamels, the transparency of rock crystals, the hardness of stone, the whiteness and smoothness of ivory, the

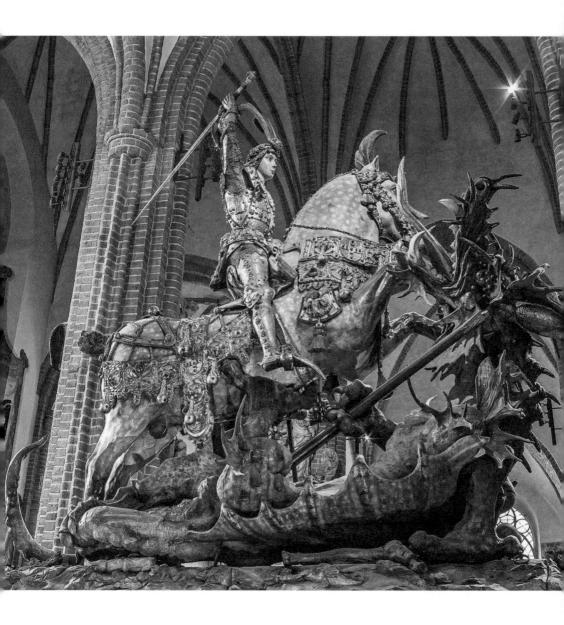

[**Ill. 10**] Bernt Notke: St. George and the Dragon. Stockholm, Storkyrkan.
Photo: Kristin Bliksrud Aavitsland.

brilliance of gold and silver do not primarily represent the spiritual realities of the transcendental world. Rather, the materials ostensively expose their very materiality. Representation and exposition of material splendour coexist in these works, but rarely correlate. This is a sensorial strategy that is alien to other periods and other sensory paradigms, such as the Late Medieval or the Baroque. In ecclesiastical art of the fifteenth to seventeenth century, materials tended to be employed in order to evoke illusion. Hence they subordinate their true materiality to represent other matter. Hard marble may allude to soft human skin, gilt and painted wood may allude to floating brocades – and, as in Bernt Notke's monumental group of St. George in Storkyrkan, Stockholm (1489): elk's horns may represent the imagined bristling spikes on the body of a dragon [ill. 10].[22]

Contrary to such illusionism, Romanesque representations do not strive for mimesis – rather the contrary. By their explicit materiality, the pictures and objects insist on their status as artefacts and appear to human senses in a phenomenological manner. Hence they enable figuration that, paradoxically, transcends the perceptible. Jean-Claude Bonne has described this quality of Romanesque liturgical art as *choséité*, thing-ness. According to Bonne, *la choséité* is constitutive for the paradoxical representation of the transcendental by the material.[23] In a manner similar to the Eucharistic bread and wine, the vessels and the altar decoration demonstrate the paradox of sensory perception precisely because of their *choséité*, their material substance. Perceivable matter is absolutely necessary, yet totally insufficient to reach the end of medieval perception: knowledge of God. Demonstrations of how this paradox unfolds are found in a spectacular group of Scandinavian metal altar frontals from the twelfth and early thirteenth centuries. Produced to embellish the Eucharistic table, these wooden frontals and retables, usually called 'golden altars', are covered with embossed, fire-gilt copperplates with repoussé reliefs.[24] The main image of most of these frontals is the Maiestas Domini: Christ enthroned as cosmic ruler in celestial glory. A mid-twelfth-century altar frontal from Broddertorp Church in Sweden offers one example [ill. 11].

According to standard iconographical conventions, the figure of Christ is surrounded by an almond-shaped aureole, a mandorla. As a pictorial sign, the mandorla indicates that what is represented within it, is a theophany or a revelation of the transcendent God – a manifestation of the holy beyond time and space.[25] The framing of the transcendent is emphasised by the fact that the mandorla's gilding is more burnished than any other area of the altar frontal's gilt surface and lacks, as the only part, brown varnish ornamentation. As a result, it stands out as the only completely

82   golden and light-reflecting field. Simultaneously, the material design seems to contradict the illusion of theophany and transcendental vision. The heavy frame of the aureole suggests solid weight rather than spherical lightness. Hardness, another tactile quality of metal, is articulated by the engraved ornamentation along the mandorla's brim. Moreover, the image accentuates its own materiality by the fact that the four angels surrounding the mandorla actually carry it and try to lift it by a rope that runs along the brim. Indeed, the mandorla is represented as a kind of technical device. The two angels at the lower end are represented as if they struggle to lift it, knees bended, digging their heels in, and pulling upwards. The angels are purely spiritual beings; hence their physical effort is conceptually absurd, as is the material heaviness and hardness of the celestial vision. The pictorial design as well as the treatment of the metal surface underscore that the vision is but a physical, man-made image.[26] In this way, the image demonstrates the defiance of matter as medium for the holy. Although God is materially present at the altar above the image, perceptible to all senses in bread and wine, he is still beyond the reach of the human corrupted sensorium.

"The pure in heart"

So far, I have argued that by the means of eye-catching material splendour, the Romanesque *ornamenta ecclesiae* display the paradoxes of perception and mediation, and simultaneously anticipate their future dissolution. Another equally conspicuous feature in Romanesque ecclesiastical art is the persistent use of inscriptions. The liturgical epigraphy on altar frontals, retables, reliquaries, censers, and altar crosses consists of carefully composed verses that comment on the significance of the pictures adorning the object or the entire object itself. Being verbal arguments, the inscriptions belong to a fundamentally different medium than the mute, yet highly ostensive and significant materiality of liturgical art. Conventionally, we tend to conceive of text as the more potent medium and consequently read the inscriptions on liturgical objects and altar decoration as exhaustive explanations to the objects' iconographical meaning or liturgical function. The written word validates the correct interpretation, so to speak. However, I would argue that in Romanesque liturgical

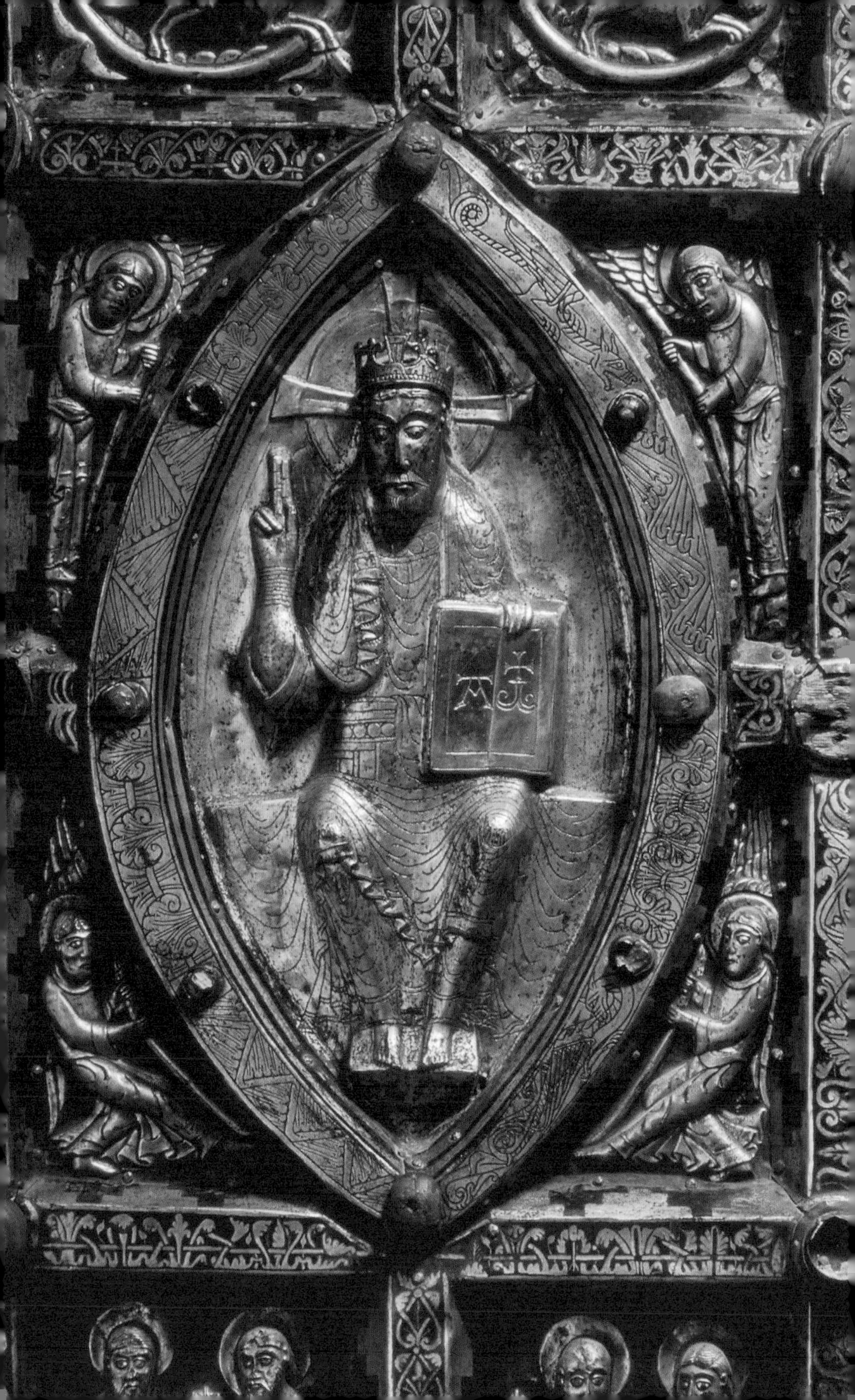

art, the inscriptions are subordinate to the materiality of the objects they inscribe. In perceiving these objects, their *choséité* clearly subdues the power of the written word.

The inscriptions testify to this subordination through their form as well as their content. I shall illustrate this through some examples drawn from the body of gilt metal altars from Scandinavia mentioned above. Although younger than comparable pieces elsewhere in Europe, the Scandinavian altars are highly representative of pre-Gothic altar decoration. An initial and striking feature of the inscriptions on these altars is the enhancement of individual letters. A keen appreciation of the purely visual qualities of script certainly lies behind their design. The letters are embossed in some inscriptions, whereas in others they are painted on the copperplates with gilding or brown varnish. In all the altars the script is clearly monumentalised, in some of them variously ornate. Visual enhancement seems in fact to take precedence over legibility. This is especially striking in the longer verse inscriptions along the frames of the frontals and retables.[27] This does little to facilitate reading as it instead constricts it. Although some inscriptions have small crosses beginning a new sentence, but also periods and dots separating words, the epigraphy offers no clue as to where the verses begin or end. On some altars, such as the one from Lisbjerg, the words all run together. Unlike the way in which script is displayed in contemporary manuscripts, where the disposition of the text is visualised through decorated or otherwise clearly accentuated initials, punctuation, and paragraphs, the inscriptions on the altars reveal neither grammatical nor poetic structure visually. No attempt is made to match the length of the verses to the length of the frames. Rather than displaying the verbal structure, the sequence of letters exhibits one continuous border in which the script assumes an ornamental, even iconic status in its own right. The display of script appears to be as significant as the script itself. The viewer is thus invited to enjoy what he sees before reflecting on what he reads.

"The image of the word delivers its own powerful message quite distinct from the spoken counterpart", Leslie Webster states in a study of inscriptions on Anglo-Saxon artefacts.[28] This stresses the point that, in medieval culture, any display of ornate writing indirectly contains an allusion to the Incarnation of Christ – the Word of God made visible. This allusion becomes very explicit in the golden altars by virtue of their proximity to the table where the Eucharist is celebrated. Liturgical relations between the Incarnation of Christ on the one hand and the celebration of the Eucharist on the other have a long tradition in medieval theology, and became increasingly important during the twelfth century in the wake of Gregorian reform.[29] For example, according to Peter Damian (c. 1007-1072), the mystery of Christ's incarnation is repeated every time the rite of the Eucharist is celebrated, making the invisible God present in the Eucharistic species (the Body and Blood of Christ) to the human senses.[30] Thus, due to their strong aesthetic aspect, the inscriptions seem to enforce this cultic reality in a purely visual manner. No matter what its content, the ornate script *represents* the *logos* incarnate.

The ornate design of the letters implies a 'materialisation' of the script. Commenting upon the mysteries of faith and salvation that are mediated through the sacraments, the ornate inscriptions display tangible and perceptible realities as much as abstract ideas. Thus, the written word on the altars submits to the *choséité*, which remains – phenomenologically and by analogy – the foremost medium of cultic meaning.

This idea can also be traced in the content of some of the inscriptions. The frame of the celebrated altar from Stadil Church in Western Jutland, dated c. 1225, carries an inscription, which reflects the contrast between verbal argument and visual perception [ill. 9]. Three distiches running along the four sides of the frame read:

+ QVAM CERNIS FULUO TABULAM SPLENDORE
NITENTE(M) PL(U)S NITET YSTORIE COGNITIONE SACRE
PANDIT ENIM CHR(IST)I MYSTERIA QVE SUP(ER) AURVM
IRRADIANT MVNDIS CORDE NITORE SVO
ERGO FIDE MVNDES MENTE(M) SI CERNERE LVCIS
GAUDIA DIUINE QVI LEGIS ISTA UELIS

You see this panel shining with golden splendour, but even more it shines through the knowledge it spreads of the sacred history. For it reveals to those pure in heart the mysteries of Christ, whose own lustre outshines gold. Thus, you who read by means of that (panel), purify your mind by faith if you want to behold the joys of the divine light.[31]

The inscription is appellative, directly addressing the reader or observer. The argument concerns what the reader is seeing and ought to see in his/her contemplation of the frontal.[32] In this text, contrasts and similarities between material and spiritual light, material and spiritual splendour, and the physical and mental eye come into play. As the Stadil frontal is one of the most spectacular of the extant Scandinavian altars, insistent on its own material sumptuousness, these juxtaposed concepts are especially suggestive. The verb "cernere" is used for both kinds of seeing. In the first distich it refers to the physical perception of the panel (*cernis tabulam* / "you see this panel"); in the third, however, it refers to the spiritual perception of the joys of heaven (*si cernere lucis gaudia divine velis* / "if you want to behold the joys", etc).

The Stadil inscription may be and certainly has been read as a warning against materialism. In that respect it is related to Abbot Suger's famous inscription on the bronze doors of St. Denis. It may however also be read as a kind of meta-comment on perception and cognition. The reader is reminded that the true splendour of the golden tablet does not derive from the brilliant materials it is made of, but from "the knowledge it spreads of the sacred history" ("nitet ystorie cognitione sacre"). This can hardly refer to anything but the reliefs depicting scenes from Christ's childhood, i.e. the pictures ('historiae') of the frontal. Thus, an interpretation of the inscription may be that the altar's perceptible splendour is analogous with the radiance of knowledge revealing the mysteries of Christ ("Christi mysteria") mediated in the images. On the other hand, the inscription itself is given the humble function to direct the gaze of the viewer. Thus the 'historiae' – in the sense of the Biblical accounts, physical representations of them, as well as mental images stored in the memory of the spectators – are the primary carrier of meaning for those who are pure in heart ("mundis corde"). Here, the Beatitudes from the Sermon of the Mount is clearly alluded to: "Beati mundo corde quoniam ipsi Deum videbunt" – "Blessed are the pure in heart, for they shall see God" (Matt 5:8). In other words, perception of the holy is clearly conditioned.

The Stadil inscription indicates that for the devout, the mysteries of Christ are perceptible in the object they have before their eyes. A few medieval commentators, especially those who were in favour of the monastic reform movement associated with Cluny, shared this view. If we are to believe the chronicler of the abbey of St. Benigne in Dijon, the zealous monastic reformer and celebrated church architect William of Volpiano (962-1031) may have been one of them. Indeed William was appointed abbot at St. Benigne after his stay at Cluny. During his abbacy, he commissioned extensive rebuilding and decoration of the abbatial church. Describing the marvels of William's new constructions, the chronicler states: "It is not futile that the form and subtlety of his work of art are demonstrated by letters for those who are less educated, because many aspects of the work are endowed with mystical meaning, which should be attributed more to divine inspiration than to the ability of the craftsman."[33] One century later, in a far more celebrated and often-quoted text, Abbot Suger of St. Denis promotes a similar idea.[34] It is striking that these two abbots, who were both initiators of large-scale building projects and patrons of ecclesiastical art, stress the visuality and materiality of images as the primary bearer of meaning. This meaning is of a mystical kind however; hidden from unlearned men, who need explicatory inscriptions to 'read' the images properly. The Stadil inscription indicates a similar assumption: the inscription is auxiliary, while the images communicate the divine mysteries *sensualiter* – for those pure in heart.

Against this background, the sensory perception of the objects surrounding the Eucharist is not only a question of phenomenological appearance, of *choséité*, but also of anticipation. The bodily perception prompted by the staging of the Eucharist is paralleled by a spiritual perception. This is because man possesses an intact sensorium of the soul in tandem with the corrupted sensorium of the body. Guided by faith, the spiritual senses foresee a state in which the paradoxes of perception and mediation is dissolved: the bliss of perfected bodily perception of God 'face to face' awaiting the righteous after their resurrection. For the inner senses, the Holy Mass is in itself an anticipation of the realisation of the Kingdom of God at history's end. Thus, the strictly directed and carefully staged sensory experience of the Eucharist and its surroundings may be interpreted as a prolepsis, a performed anticipation of the sensory experience of God awaiting his faithful. In this way, as faith-guided sensuality, the *hagiosensorium* may be sensitive to the material mediation of the holy.

Dignifying the Senses

In the beginning of this chapter I used a vernacular French text from the fourteenth century to shed light on the paradox of perception in medieval culture. I will close the chapter by turning to another Old-French text, this time from the twelfth century. This is done to expose the issue of faith-guided sensuality. About 1120, the Anglo-Norman poet Philippe de Thaün wrote a versified bestiary, a collection of descriptions of animals interpreted allegorically according to the idea that the created world is part of God's revelation to man (as referred to above).[35] In the middle of Philippe's interpretation of the industrious ant, there is an interpolation reflecting the preconditions for good and true sensory perception – as opposed to sensuality led astray. This meta-comment on how to use the senses properly is moulded on Jesus' parable about the wise and foolish virgins waiting to meet the groom (Matt 25:1-13). The rhetorical structuring is done to facilitate remembering, but also to indicate the range of the issue's importance, as the parable concerns the eschatological Kingdom of God. For, as Philippe's explanation shows, wrong use of the senses indeed has fatal eschatological consequences. Philippe construes the five virgins as the five senses.

Their virginity points to chastity or, perhaps more precisely, control and restraint. Furthermore, their burning lamps filled with oil stand for the soul filled with Christian faith, burning with fire that is the Spirit of God. The five wise virgins bring their lamps into the wedding, where they are most welcome – which is to say that they shall come safely to the judgement and will meet God in majesty and be united with him. But the foolish virgins with their empty lamps are not let in.[36] They must stay outside, because they do not bring anything with them: "Les foles n'i entrerent, ki nent n'i aporterent". Carrying nothing in their lamps, that is their souls, they are empty, worthless, and good for nothing. The lesson to be learned is that undirected sensuality with no guidance from the light of faith leads to nowhere.

Any study of medieval senses must acknowledge the intimate and yet paradoxical relation between the perceptible and the transcendent in medieval culture. This relation is conditioned by the Incarnation of Christ, which is repeated liturgically and mystically in celebration of the Eucharist. In a certain sense, the Eucharist dignifies the senses and makes them exceed their own capacity. In my opinion, this is the fundamental condition of medieval sensory perception, making it integrated, 'intermedial', and 'intersensorial' in a way that postmodern 'intermedial' culture is not. Fuelled by rapidly changing technological innovations, the postmodern insight that 'all media are mixed media' has influenced contemporary culture to the extent that the distinctions between separate art forms, media types, and cognitive strategies seem useless and irrelevant. This situation has indeed prompted a scholarly interest in sensory paradigms beyond modernity – this very book being a case in point. However, the intermedia of medieval culture rest on a premise that is not shared by postmodernism: all media and all perceptions, secondary and imperfect as they are, await the replacement of the perfect perception of absolute reality.

Notes

1   See Hans Henrik Lohfert Jørgensen's chapter on the medieval *Sensorium* in this volume. For a discussion of the content of the holy, see Brian Patrick McGuire's chapter on *Sanctity*.

2   Anselm of Canterbury, *Proslogion* (1077-78), ch. XVI, 1982, p. 43. For the negative theology of Pseudo-Dionysius, see Jones 1996. A general survey of negative theology in the Western tradition is found in McGinn 1992 & 1995.

3   As demonstrated in the essays collected in Nichols, Kablitz & Calhoun 2008.

4   Edited by Tilander 1932.

5   Aavitsland 2012, pp. 218-219.

6   "[…] in carne mea videbo Deum". See Brian Patrick McGuire's chapter on *Sanctity* in this volume.

7   "Videmus nunc per speculum in aenigmate; tunc autem facie ad faciem."

8   The English title of Hans Belting's pivotal study on the premodern religious image, *Likeness and presence*, reflects this doubleness; Belting 1997.

9   Chenu 1997, pp. 34-38.

10   "Omnis mundi creatura / quasi liber et pictura / nobis est et speculum." Alain of Lille, *Rhytmus alter, quo graphice natura hominis fluxa et caduca depingitur*, PL, vol. CCX, col. 579.

11   Morini 1996, p. 238; Aavitsland 2007, pp. 82-84.

12   See Hans Henrik Lohfert Jørgensen's chapter on the sensorium in the present volume.

13   See Caroline Walker Bynum's discussion of the nature of the paradox in relation to Christian materiality in the Middle Ages, Bynum 2011, p. 158.

14   "L'Incarnation n'est pas seulement un dogme particulier, mais toute une forme de pensée qui a imprimé sa marque à toutes les représentations et à toutes les pratiques caractéristiques du christianisme", Schmitt 2004, p. 278. Translation by author.

15   Duffy 2005, pp. 97-98.

16   Westermann-Angerhausen 2011, p. 230.

17   Moser & Anderson 1993.

18   Ferrari 2006, p. 268.

19   Bagnoli 2010.

20   Honorius Augustodunensis, *Gemma animae*; Suger, *De rebus in administratione*. See also Raff 1994, p. 17.

21   Kessler 2004, p. 19.

22   Liepe (in press).

23   Bonne 1996; Aavitsland 2007; Bynum 2011.

24   Nørlund 1968. An internationally published general survey of the Scandinavian golden altar frontals and retables is still lacking, and most literature about this group of ecclesiastical art is published in Scandinavian languages. Among the internationally available studies are Braun 1924, vol. II, pp. 90-108, Nørlund 1930, Norn 1990, Kaspersen 2006, Liepe 2006, Sonne de Torrens 2006, Thunø 2006, Aavitsland 2008 & 2011.

25   Jørgensen 2004, p. 26.

26   Aavitsland 2007, pp. 87-88.

27 For a discussion of the visual appearances of the inscriptions of the Scandinavian altars, see Aavitsland 2011.

28 Webster 2005, p. 21.

29 See Van Dijk 2006 for this idea in the early Middle Ages. For the twelfth century in particular, see references in Wirth 1999, pp. 195-200.

30 "Illud siquidem corpus Christi quod beatissima Virgo genuit, quod in gremio fovit, quod fasciis cinxit, quod maternal cura nutrivit, illud, inquam, absque ulla dubietate, non aliud, nunc de sacro altari percepimus, et eius sanguinem in sacramentum nostrae redemptionis haurimus", Peter Damiani, *Sermones*, CCCM, vol. 57, p. 267.

31 My translation varies a little, but not substantially from that found in Nørlund 1968 & Thunø 2006.

32 For a more thorough analysis of the inscription, see Dahl 1971, Norn 1990, & Aavitsland 2011.

33 "Cujus artificiosi operis forma et subtilias non inaniter quibusque minus edoctis ostenditur per litteras: quoniam multa in eo videntur mystico sensu facta, que magis divine inspirationi quam alicujus debent deputa[r]i peritie magistri", *Chronicon Sancti Benigni Divionensis*, Mortet 1911, p. 27. The chronicle is dated to c. 1060. While Wilhelm Schlink interprets "ostenditur per litteras" as a reference to the chronicle itself, Robert Favreau argues that the expression refers to architectural inscriptions; see Schlink 1978, p. 172 & Favreau 1997, p. 192. In any event, the author regards written text as an explicatory service "for those less educated" (quibusque minus edoctis), for those unable to interpret the meaning manifest in the visual and spatial artwork.

34 Suger 1979.

35 Morini 1996, p. 105.

36 "Ke ceo dit Escripture, .v. virgines, par figure/ E.v. lampes pleners de olie e de lumers/ A unes noces alerent, ardantes les porterent/ .V. foles en i out, en lur lampes nent n'i out/ Iceles i entrerent ki pleners les porterent/ Li mari les cunut, à joie les receut/ Les foles n'i entrerent, ki nent n'i aporterent/ Ceo est grant signefiance, aiez en remembrance./ Par cinc virgines entent cinc sens veraiement/ Veer, oir, parler, tucher, & odurer/ E la virginité demustre casteet/ E ki ceo averat, as noces ben vendrat/ Ceo est al jugement vendrat securement/ U li mariz serat ki les granz duns durat/ Iceo ert Dampne-Deu ki ert en majesté./ E le lamppe signefie aneme en ceste vie/ Le olie, Christiented; le fu, le Spirit de Dé", Morini 1996, pp. 158-160.

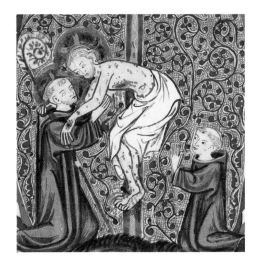

92

[**SANCTITY**] This chapter considers the life and influence of the Cistercian abbot Bernard of Clairvaux (1090-1153) and how he embodied and reflected the concept of sanctity in the medieval Christian tradition. Bernard inherited the sanctity of the Desert Fathers of Late Antiquity, but he also added to this tradition through his use of the senses. In the desert the senses had been denied, for the desert dweller tried to separate him- or herself from every sensual impression. Bernard claimed to follow the same path, but the stories that circulated about him – both before and after his death – convey his life and sanctity in terms of touch and embraces. These sensual encounters are very much in harmony with a Cistercian love of place and celebration of friendship. At the same time Bernard was successful in communicating his spiritual-sensual experiences, as can be seen in the near avalanche of miracles that came from his activity once he left his monastery and began travelling about in what we now call France and Italy. The Cistercian talent for mediation of the monastic life to a new generation of men and, later, women is a product of Bernard's person and ability to communicate. He succeeded in communicating various forms of sensuality as manifestations of holiness. In so doing he altered the monastic tradition, which until the twelfth century had looked upon asceticism as the single way to sanctity. In Bernard's sensuality we find also his spirituality.

SANCTITY

The Saint and the Senses:
The Case of Bernard of Clairvaux

[Brian Patrick McGuire]

The Concept and Origins of Sanctity

Medieval civilisation, the culture of Western Europe from about 500 to 1500, concentrated on one great goal, the pursuit of the holy. The word is formidable but the meaning can be captured in the Old English root *hal*, meaning sound, happy, or whole. Old English writers used the term in translating the Latin sacer or *sanctus*. We can add the dictionary definition of spiritually perfect or pure, untainted by evil or sin, and so regarded with or deserving deep respect, awe, reverence, or adoration.[1]

Every single time the Latin mass was recited in the medieval world, the priest called upon the congregation to invoke the holiness that emanates from the godhead: *Sanctus, sanctus, sanctus. Dominus Deus Sabaoth. Pleni sunt caeli et terra gloria tua. Hosanna in excelsis*: Holy, holy, holy. Lord God of hosts. Heaven and earth are full of your glory. Hosanna in the highest.

The word *sanctus* belongs to Roman civilisation, the foundation of the Middle Ages, and is found in Cicero in describing good and upright men.[2] The infinitive is *sancire*, to render sacred, and so *sanctus* was originally a past participle, but it became an adjective; that which is sacred or holy, and finally a noun, the holy person. In the Christian Church the term was attached to men and women who were considered especially blessed by divine grace and living in the presence of God, where they shared with each other in the *lumen gloriae*: the light of glory that comes from the beatific vision.[3] The saints were *beati*, meaning not just blessed but downright happy, for they who had been God's friends in this life were privileged to share with him his eternal life and joy.

Sanctity or holiness is thus a state of being by which the person becomes whole and realises his or her God-given potentialities as these are conveyed in the bestowal of divine grace. This definition may sound abstract, but if we add the fact that body and soul are united as a whole in Christian belief, both in this life and after the resurrection, then sanctity manifests itself in sensual ways. The saint is never a disembodied soul that leaves behind the bodily dimension: the saint rejoices. As we hear in Händel's Messiah: "in my flesh shall I see God," which is taken, remarkably not from the New Testament, but from the Book of Job (19:26).

In his or her life the saint embodies and reflects the concept of sanctity. As we shall see with Bernard, the fact of sanctity can easily be connected with the senses. The saint makes use of sight, taste, touch, and even smell, in order to relate everything in his or her existence in accord with the presence of God. Asceticism does not destroy the senses: like grace, it perfects them, in linking the senses to the Creator who is the foundation and source of all that is, visible and invisible.

In allowing the growth of a cult of saints from the first Christian centuries, the Church emphasised that in showing respect for what we are as bodies, we become complete human persons. Thus, the suffering of the first saints, the martyrs, was not emphasised out of a sadistic enjoyment of blood and body parts, but in the belief that the pain of these men and women was a witness to their belief in Christ, the first martyr.[4] When the time of the martyrs was over in the fourth century, a new kind of saint emerged: the confessor. This kind of person witnessed the truth of Christianity through the actions of his life and death. The best-known confessor-saint of Late Antiquity, Martin of Tours, became a model of charity for the centuries to come. On a freezing winter's day he cut his cloak in half in order to share it with a beggar. In a dream that night he saw that the beggar was Christ himself.[5] The point was thus made that in giving up part of one's possessions, one shared oneself with Jesus and became one with him. Martin, who at this point in his life was not even Christian, was on the way to becoming a saint, a person who in body and soul was linked to God.

In the lives written about saints, hagiography, we are often told about how the saint denies himself the enjoyment of sensual objects. If we turn to the stories written about Bernard of Clairvaux as a case in point, we hear how – when he was in his novice year at Cîteaux – he failed to notice that the room where he slept had three windows. He thought it had one, for he apparently never actually looked up at the windows. Bernard's first biographer, William of Saint Thierry, also claims that he left the novitiate without ever realising that the building had a ribbed vaulting in the ceiling. William concludes: "[...] he had put to death all sense of curiosity, and so he perceived nothing of this kind".[6] The biographer explains that Bernard's memory was otherwise engaged, so he failed to notice.

William saw memory as the point of departure for all sensing, an interesting point of view that suggests the depths of his own insight as perhaps the leading monastic theologian of the twelfth century.[7] To understand William's point of view, it is necessary to go back to the Desert Fathers in the transition period between Antiquity and the Middle Ages. Here we find fierce and even fanatical men who felt they had escaped from the sensual pleasures of Roman city life and shed the outer layers of civilisation in order to find peace and meaning in the wilderness.[8]

The desert also contained women who had abandoned their previous lives. One of them, Syncletica, was asked "if to have nothing is a perfect good?" Her answer was that this is "a great good for those who are able. For those who can endure it endure suffering in the flesh, but they have quiet of soul".[9] Suffering is part of the desert way, because it is an imitation of Christ and his suffering. But there is a difference: Jesus was said to have fasted for a short time in the desert and then to have begun his public life, where he enjoyed eating with his apostles. The desert fathers and mothers prolonged the stay in the desert into a way of life, even if they at times did interrupt their fasts in order to look after the needs of guests.

Syncletica promised "quiet of soul", but many of the desert dwellers came to experience inner turbulence, uncertainty about their way of life, sexual temptation, and the assaults of demons. The response to these trials was to control the senses by ridding one's life of everything but the presence of God. As abbot Alois said, "Unless a man shall say in his heart, 'I alone and God are in this world', he shall not find quiet".[10] This sentence perhaps summarises the ethos of the Desert Fathers, seeking God by reducing daily life to the bare essentials. These included manual labour, whose products such as baskets had to be sold in nearby villages, and prayer, at all hours of the day and night.

The Fathers lived on the fringes of agricultural society and, as the historian of Late Antiquity Peter Brown has shown, the holy man could become a central person in village life.[11] Precisely because he was set apart from the passions of other men, he could be consulted when the villagers were in disagreement. The Father became a spiritual guide and councilor, and thus in danger of losing his status set apart from the rest of humanity. But so long as he maintained the *ascesis* or discipline of body and soul, he was considered to be in contact with truth and meaning, a genuine resource for village society at a time when Roman government was breaking down. The function of the ascetics gathered in the desert of Scete, south of Alexandria, is described as "to give courage to those who were besieged by any passion and who struggled in travail with themselves that they might come to good".[12]

This characterisation of the Desert Fathers makes it clear that they were descendants of Stoicism, which also tried to make it possible for its practitioners to minimise human passions in what is called *apatheia*.[13] This goal does not mean the crushing of human emotions, but it does require their limitation and subjugation, so that there is room for intellectual endeavor, meditation and, for the Christian Stoic, the desire for God. This concentration can mean forgetting physical acts because of the intensity of one's meditation: "It was said of the abbot John that he was once plaiting palm-leaves to make two baskets, and used them all in one basket but knew it not until he reached the wall. For his mind was taken up with the contemplation of God".[14]

This ethos is more than the 'absent-minded professor' syndrome. The Desert Father sought actively to cut back on sense impressions, as in the case of an abbot Silvanus, who lived on Mount Sinai. He was asked why he covered his face with a hood when he watered his garden. His answer was that he wanted to avoid letting his eyes "see the trees and my mind be taken up with looking upon them and cease from its task".[15] It is important to notice that Silvanus did not condemn the trees or see them as products of the devil. Such a dualistic view of the world is not characteristic of desert wisdom. What Silvanus and his fellow hermits aimed for was to be able to concentrate on one thing, the pursuit of the presence of God, and thus to remove themselves from other concerns.

The Desert Myth and the Cistercians

The early Cistercians in the twelfth century felt that they in many ways had chosen to recreate the lives of the Desert Fathers.[16] They knew that their predecessors had not remained hermits for long, but had begun to form settlements where they supported each other in a common way of life. They also knew that Benedict, the founder of monasticism in Western Europe, had begun his life as a hermit, but had been convinced by other ascetics to let them join him. When Benedict wrote his Rule, which became the foundation for monastic life in the West, he conceded that life in seclusion is more commendable, but he added that only a few can handle it.[17] Therefore it is necessary when men or women want to leave the world that they accept their need for each other in a monastery.

However much the founders of the New Monastery (later called Cîteaux) were aware of this tradition, they yearned to live like the Desert Fathers. They sought out what they called, in a Biblical phrase, "a place of terror and great solitude" (*locus horroris et vastae solitudinis*, Deut 32:10) far from the madding crowd, deep in the countryside, and requiring the hard work of the monks to make what they called a desert bloom.[18] In recent years historians have pointed out that most of the time, the monks actually came to areas already settled by peasants and so were misrepresenting the facts in claiming to tame a frontier.[19] But the desert myth in fact provided an important incentive to Cistercian life, and it is necessary to distinguish between the way the monks visualised their new settlements and the actual social geography of these places. For the monks who came to Esrum in the North of Zealand, for example, they were colonising a wilderness, and they probably kept the Danish name of the place in their Latin charters because it reminded them of the Old Testament name Esron, which the church father Jerome had called *juxta eremum*, "next to the hermitage".[20] Thus by an accident of language Esrum pointed to the desert myth for its origins.

In order to settle what they considered to be a wilderness, monks had to work hard and forget their social origins in the lower aristocracy. Until the end of the twelfth century, the first generations of Cistercians learned by doing. They drained marshes, cut down trees and planted fields. One of the popular stories to emerge from this period concerns how Mary and two other female saints came down from the hills above Clairvaux at harvest time, when the brothers were sweating in the August heat.[21] The holy women went from brother to brother and dried the sweat off their foreheads. This is a gesture of compassion, but also of recognition that the Cistercians worked hard and needed comfort and even consolation. Here is a spiritual sensuality of a type that characterises early Cîteaux and its many daughters quickly spreading throughout Europe.

The early Cistercians believed that the spread of the Order to the far corners of Europe and the monks' cultivation of the land (with the help of lay brothers) were manifestations of God's blessing on the new monasticism, which claimed to follow the Rule of Saint Benedict more faithfully than previous monastic movements had done. The Cistercians created, as I have shown elsewhere, "a valley of fruitfulness".[22] Here they saw the equivalent to what the Massachusetts pilgrims in the seventeenth century created as a 'city on the hill'.

The desert bloomed, both spiritually and materially, and the monks sent out new foundations to the very ends of the known world. In their own terms, based on

Psalm 71:8, *a mari usque ad mare*, or in the song sung today by patriotic Canadians and Americans, "from sea to shining sea". In this development the sensual world was essential, for the monks calculated their success on the basis of the number of daughter houses and the acquisition of new lands to cultivate. At the same time, however, the monks recognised that their primary goal was a spiritual one: the monastery existed in order to praise the Lord through prayer and song in choir, and it was essential to keep a strict discipline, which included getting up in the middle of the night for vigils. Unlike their Cluniac brethren, the Cistercians did not allow themselves to go back to bed after this office: they forced themselves to remain awake, to pray and meditate, something that their modern successors in the Cistercian Trappists do to this very day (and which is not easy!).

In so doing, the Cistercians were once again following the lead of the Desert Fathers. A section in "The Sayings of the Desert Fathers" is entitled, "That one ought to pray without ceasing and soberly".[23] One of the most memorable anecdotes here concerns abbot Macarius, who was asked how to pray. His answer was simple: "There is no need of much speaking in prayer, but often stretch out your hands and say, 'Lord, as you will and as you know, have mercy upon me.' But if there is war in your soul, add, 'Help me.' And because he knows what we need, he shows us his mercy".[24]

The Cistercians, as monks before them, made use of the words of the Psalms of David, in praying and singing them through the monastic week. But they always began at the start of vigils with the simple prayer, repeated three times: "*Domine, aperi labia mea:* Lord open my lips". The thought was that the first time the prayer was said, the monk was distracted and sleepy. The second time he was beginning to concentrate but still not quite together. Hopefully the third time the prayer was said, he began to hear the words and to open his lips, both spiritually and physically. Prayer was regarded as a physical act, the making use of the body's functions in order to speak and sing and thereby to get into touch with the self and to put both body and soul into the wonderful presence of God. Far from despising their bodies, monks were taught to make the best use of them in order to let their song rise forth and fill their churches.[25]

Bernard and the Transformation of the Self

The young Bernard of Clairvaux (1090-1153) would have been aware of the desert tradition and its incitement to limit the claims of sensuality in order to enrich the spiritual life. He followed in the steps of the Fathers in seeking to pray at all times.

In the words of his friend William of Saint Thierry, "His whole self became absorbed in the spirit, his whole hope steered towards God, his whole memory engaged in one great spiritual meditation or gaze".[26]

William was careful, however, to insist that Bernard took proper care of himself. He says that Bernard cared for his body in so far it was necessary for "its serving of the spirit".[27] The Latin passage is difficult and has confused editors, but the meaning seems to be that Bernard did not try to destroy his body. In the very next chapter, however, William described how Bernard considered sleep to be a waste of time: "To this day, he keeps vigil beyond the humanly possible and is ever complaining that no time is more wasted than when he sleeps". William mentioned how Bernard would get irritated at brothers who "snore too loudly" or lie in bed "untidily": "He rebukes such sleeping as carnal and worldly".[28]

William did not spare any details in describing Bernard's digestion. Because of his many fasts and vigils, "his ruined stomach promptly throws up, undigested, whatever he forces down his throat".[29] Bernard experienced "the gravest torment" in letting food pass through his system: "Whatever residue still lingers to nourish the body, serves less to sustain him in life than merely to postpone his dying". William admitted, however, that Bernard's habit of denying himself food had become so natural to him "that even if he wished to indulge further at some meal, he scarcely could".[30]

Bernard's anorexia, if that is the correct term for his refusal or inability to take or keep food in his system, caused the local bishop so much concern that he appealed to the General Chapter at Cîteaux and arranged for Bernard to be moved to a hut outside the monastic precinct, where he could be looked after by a servant who was to make sure that Bernard ate properly.[31] According to William, Bernard was not pleased with this arrangement and had the greatest contempt for his caretaker. At one point in his stay Bernard was served raw blood instead of butter but he apparently did not know the difference.[32] This anecdote made such an impression on his followers that it was included in the summary of Bernard's life, which is found in the popular *Golden Legend*, stories of the saints compiled at the end of the thirteenth century by the Dominican preacher Jacobus de Voragine.[33] After a year or so he returned to his community, and for the rest of his life he was plagued by ill health, probably a result of the way he had treated himself as a young monk.

Saints in medieval culture are often described in terms of their ascetic excesses and attempts to kill the impulses of the body. Bernard belongs to this group, but he is exceptional because he himself tells us about the price he paid for his zeal. In one of his Sermons on the Song of Songs, delivered to the monks at Clairvaux in the 1130s, he used his own self as an example to encourage the brothers: "I am not ashamed to admit that very often I myself, especially in the early days of my conversion, experienced coldness and hardness of heart, while deep in my being I sought for him whom I longed to love". Bernard explained that he felt completely alienated from any sense of the presence and love of God, "my soul melted away for sorrow, even to the verge of despair".[34]

The condition that Bernard here described is known in monastic literature as *acedia*, sometimes translated as 'sloth' but really a form of depression, in which the individual finds himself or herself unable to feel anything for the beliefs that are supposed to sustain her life. The Desert Fathers recognised *acedia* as a genuine problem, sometimes a result of the devil's intervention, but more often a symptom of loss of meaning in vocation and daily life.[35] Bernard's solution was to remind himself of other people, "the sight of a good and holy man" or even the memory of a dead or absent friend. Then he could get into contact with his feelings: "My tears were my food day and night" (Ps 41:4).[36]

Bernard admitted being mortified by the fact that instead of being lifted up by the thought of God, he was more affected by the awareness of another human being: "I feel ashamed that the remembrance of human goodness should affect me more powerfully than the thought of God". He spoke and wrote of his own limitations and frustrations, of course, in order to encourage the monks whom he addressed, "Many of you too, I feel, have had similar experiences, and have them even still".[37]

This conclusion reveals a great deal about the sense world in which Bernard functioned. He was looking for ways to deal with the dreaded *acedia*: "One and the same food is medicine for the sick and nourishment for the convalescent; it gives strength to the weak and pleasure to the strong. One and the same food cures sickness, preserves health, builds up the body, titillates the palate".[38]

Bernard was speaking here of spiritual food, the nourishment that comes through human contact and example. He was making a statement of faith in the value of human community, especially as found in the monastic way of life. He believed that, in being aware of each other, monks would grow in humility, "brotherly love…and good desires".[39]

This point of view is remarkable in view of the Desert Father tradition. There the individual is encouraged to maintain a safe distance from other people. This caution is not primarily the result of a fear of sexual attraction. Certainly the Desert Fathers were aware that when people share an everyday life, they could begin to fantasise about sharing each other's bodies. But the main concern was that, in getting involved in the needs of others, the desert dweller would forget the primary reason for leaving human company in the city: to live in the presence of God, to turn every act and word into prayer, to forget one's self and one's own needs, including those leading to social bonding.[40]

For Bernard, once he had gotten through his rigorous ascetic program and near- **101** ly wrecked his health, it became apparent that he needed others. He thus seems to have chosen to ignore the desert tradition and to contribute to a new appreciation of friendship in the monastic life, one of the leading traits of twelfth century culture. In insisting that his friend William of Saint Thierry remain with him at Clairvaux, Bernard indicated the value he placed on friendship.[41] William apparently wanted to return to the monastery where he was abbot, but Bernard would not hear of it. His strength of will is indicated by the fact that after refusing to obey Bernard, William became ill and so had no choice but to remain at Clairvaux in accord with Bernard's will.[42] Here we see one more indication of Bernard's command of the senses. William became physically ill, an experience of the physical senses, seemingly because Bernard wanted his friend to remain sensually close to him. Bernard insisted on the physical, sensual presence of his friend.

In my view Bernard could not live without his friends and so refused to part with them. By insisting on affectionate bonds, he was putting aside the monastic emphasis on asceticism and *apatheia*. Bernard considered human bonding to be a natural part of monastic life and did not apologise for expressing his need for others. In recognising his feelings for others, he found his way out of depression, even though he would have preferred to do so by thinking about the love of God. But for Bernard there could be no conflict between loving God and loving one's friends.[43]

Asceticism versus Sensuality:
Two Medieval Cultures?

If we read further in Bernard's Sermons on the Song of Songs, we will find a profound sensuality. By allegorising the sensual language of the Song, Bernard was able to express his own inner needs and yearnings: "Let us return to the words of the bride and listen attentively to what she says, that we may learn to relish what she relishes".[44] The bride can be the individual soul or the Church, but she is most of all a sensual being who yearns for fulfillment in the groom, who is Christ or God.

At times Bernard's lyrical praise of the groom ends in a prayer to God, as when he speaks to Wisdom, "sweetly powerful and powerfully sweet, with what skill of healing in wine and oil do you restore my soul's health. Powerfully for me and sweet to me."[45] This evocation of God's healing power speaks of the soul, but Bernard makes use of material objects, wine and oil, to visualise the function of God's wisdom.

We thus come to the great paradox of Bernard and of the monastic culture to which he contributed. On the one hand there is a quest for purifying soul and body, in diminishing bodily functions and concentrating on spiritual life. On the other hand there is a spiritual sensuality, the enjoyment of companionship with other people in the monastic life, the keen appreciation of good conversation, uplifting stories, and upright examples. For Aelred of Rievaulx (1110-67), whose writings on the spiritual life Bernard encouraged, this sensuality could go so far as to allow touching and holding hands in the monastery.[46] Today, however today we might look upon such forms of physical contact and ask whether they had a sexual element. There was no problem with the practice in the twelfth century though: Aelred believed that the monastery had become a kind of heaven, *paradisus claustralis*, where monks were each other's friends and could advance in their lives with each other's help.

There could be problems in a monastery if the abbot favored a few friends. Bernard does not deal with the potential problem though, and it is important to remember that his primary friends were his biological brothers, who entered Cîteaux with him and looked after his needs. The brothers made sure that Bernard did not go too far in his self-denial, and they were also critical when it came to the miracles that, from an early point, were seen as his doing.[47]

For Bernard there was no conflict between sensuality and asceticism, since he attained what we might call a spiritual sensuality that checked him from the extreme behavior that had characterised his youth. The impulse to asceticism could be balanced with a sense of joy in words that lifted Bernard and his audience to a perception of God's presence in the world. I do not mean to idealise this way of life, only to point out that for Bernard and his generation, a balance was apparently achieved. Bernard began with the extreme asceticism of the Desert Fathers and succeeded in a short while in more or less destroying his digestive system. He also, as abbot, at first demanded endless sacrifices of his monks, even telling them that in entering the monastery they had to leave their bodies behind. But his regime became milder, as he saw that the affective bonds of monastic life did not require such asceticism. Instead of the destruction of the body, there could be a celebration of life in building monasteries in beautiful places and giving them names that celebrated the light that permeated them. Bernard became a model for his brothers: attentive, aware, and uniting a spiritual dimension with renewed attention to the needs of the body.

As in almost all golden ages in history, the great moment soon passed, and coming Cistercian generations looked back with awe and veneration at Bernard and his times.[48] But the balance between body and soul, asceticism and sensuality, materiality and spirituality: this sense of combining opposites quickly disappeared, though the memory of Bernard, his words and actions, remained.

Bernard's Afterlife:
New Forms of Sensuality as Holiness

The sources we have for Bernard's life, especially the *Vita Prima*, so central in getting him canonised in 1174, provide us with many ways in which to see how he made use of his senses in order to attain the holiness that was his goal. I have hardly touched on the response to Bernard outside the Cistercian world, but it is sufficient here to point out how his physical presence had great importance for large numbers of people, who flocked to him with their illnesses and other troubles.[49] The saint as miracle-maker makes use of the sensual world in order to transform it through spiritual power. Here Bernard resembles other medieval saints by performing miracles both in life and after death. The dead Bernard's miracles were such a problem for the monks of Clairvaux that the abbot of Cîteaux – when he came to pray at Bernard's funeral – told him to stop performing healings for lay people.[50] Only in this way could the monks of Clairvaux have the peace and quiet they needed in order to live their monastic lives of prayer and work.

In this case, Bernard had become too physical. His dead body contained a power that was sought out by all sorts of people. But Bernard after death continued to manifest himself in new ways that combined the sensual with the spiritual worlds. In the *Exordium magnum cisterciense*, we thus find a great collection of stories from about 1200 concerning the Order's first century. This was a narrative of how a monk at Clairvaux once saw Bernard at prayer in front of the crucifix. At one point the figure of Jesus on the cross bent down and embraced the abbot.[51] This vision seems to have had a powerful effect on Cistercian spirituality and its content was spread far and wide in medieval Europe, as can be seen in images made of Bernard [ill. 12].[52]

The *amplexus* or embrace, as it is called, became one of the favored ways of showing Bernard's saintliness. It even came to Denmark and was used in the 1490s on a new altar commissioned at Esrum Abbey by the abbot Peder Andersen.[53] Here, at the

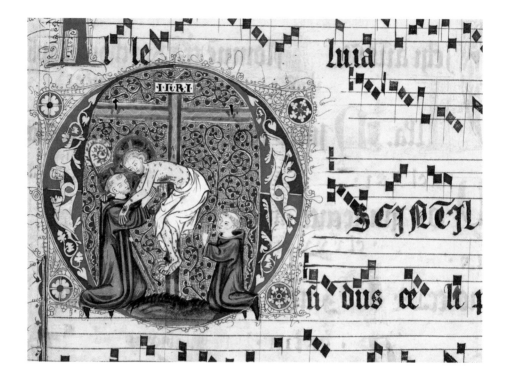

[**III. 12**] Bernard being embraced by Christ bending down from the cross, known as the *Amplexus*. The story appears in Cistercian literature by about 1200 but is not seen in art before the first half of the fourteenth century, as shown here in a Gradual from the Cistercian women's house of Wonnental in Breisgau, Baden (c. 1345). Badische Landesbibliothek Karlsruhe. BLB, Cod. UH 1, fol. 195r.

end of the Middle Ages, Jesus was seen as a man with a substantial, physical body. His embrace is not what I would call passionate, but it is certainly intimate.

Even more radical in expressing the sensuality of Bernard's spirituality is the story found in a panel from an altar on Majorca soon after 1300, but also evident in an Icelandic Mary-saga from the thirteenth century [ill. 13].[54]

We see or hear of how Mary showed her gratefulness to Bernard for his teachings about her by giving him milk from one of her breasts. Mary's milk is considered to be a form of wisdom that Bernard imbibed, so by praising Mary he came to increase his own insights into sacred mysteries. There can hardly be a more sensual, if not sexual, image, with the celibate monk chastely sucking from the breast of God's mother. This image used to be shown as a stained glass window in the Trappist-

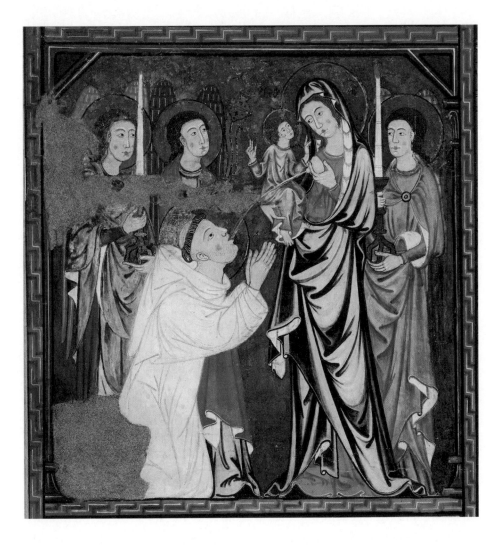

[**III. 13**] The *Lactatio:* Mary squeezes her breast to provide milk for Bernard, an image that first appears here in the retable of the Knights Templar's church in Palma de Majorca, from about 1290. The story of the lactation does not appear in literature until a few years later. Museo de Mallorca, Palma.

Cistercian abbey of Gethsemani in Kentucky. According to one of its monks, Bible-Belt Protestant visitors would catch sight of it and almost cry in disbelief, "What's that?" Contemporary Protestant Americans could have great difficulty in accepting such a physical expression of Cistercian spirituality.

Bernard was remembered as a great lover of Mary. More than a century after his death this memory formed itself into the story of the *lactation*, the giving of milk from the Virgin's breast. For the Cistercians there was no difficulty in reconciling this form of sensual experience with the spiritual life of Bernard and his place in the Order. Since the sixteenth century, Catholic and Protestant forms of Puritanism have driven us far from medieval perceptions of reality. In Bernard's writings, his hagiography and *Nachleben*, however there are attempts to reconcile the physical, sensual world with the spiritual.

A final manifestation of Bernard's presence in the spiritual-sensual dimension is found in his relics. It was not by accident that, Bernard's remains were removed from his tomb and dispersed during the French Revolution.[55] For the denizens of the Revolution, Bernard was much too physically present to be allowed to remain where he was. His relics were therefore mixed up with those of other saints. So, from the 1790s it became impossible to speak of Bernard's own remains. For centuries prior to this moment, however, the tomb of Bernard at Clairvaux had been a place of pilgrimage for members of the Cistercian Order. They felt that in approaching the physical remains of the saint, they could come close to his spiritual power and presence in their lives.

Relics were portable and could be brought almost anywhere, and so they became almost an industry, especially in the late Middle Ages. Already in the twelfth century, however, we are told of a relic of Bernard that had made its way to Denmark. The hair and beard of Bernard, as well as his tooth, brought there by Archbishop Eskil of Lund, had been taken to a Cistercian monastery, probably Esrum Abbey in Northern Zealand. Here the devil was furious at losing a sure catch, a Count Niels Grevsun, who had entered the monastery and hence secured his salvation. In revenge the devil attacked another brother and caused what appears to have been an epileptic fit. When Bernard's relics were applied to the man's chest, he cried out in German, presumably his native language, "Take it away, take it away, remove Bernard... Alas how heavy you have become, Bernard, how weighty, how unbearable you are for me".[56] Bernard was present in a spiritual manner through the physical fact of his body part.

A Difficult yet Sensible Saint
in a Single Medieval Culture

If we return to Bernard in his lifetime there are innumerable miracle stories which are often ignored in modern literature, because they are considered to reflect medieval superstition. But Bernard made it possible for lay people to seek him out for the sake of physical help and cures, as in a story of how a deaf boy was brought to him in 1148, at the Cistercian General Chapter in Cîteaux. Bernard prayed for the boy and then put his hands on him and asked if he now could hear. He shouted, "I can hear, Sir, I can hear!" In gratefulness the youth "hugged Bernard so tightly that the others could scarcely tug him loose".[57] The boy is said to have reacted physically to the fact that he could hear: his embrace of the abbot breaks all the usual strictures that Cistercian monks we are not to have physical contact with other men or with women.

Sometimes Bernard himself was rumored to go too far in his physicality. At least one of his enemies, Walter Map, narrated how Bernard once lay upon a youth in order to bring him back to life, but the boy failed to get up. Walter Map's response was "I have heard before now of a monk throwing himself upon a boy, but always, when the monk got up, the boy promptly got up too".[58] The language here implies that the monk was supposed to give the boy an erection, and in this way Bernard and his Cistercians were being accused of what we today might call sexual abuse.

There is a thin line between the deaf boy's tight embrace and the charge that Bernard abused boys. But Walter Map's slander shows us that medieval people were not ignorant about the boundaries between spiritual sensuality and overt sexuality. Bernard was remembered as a man who could drink the milk of the Virgin, embrace the figure of Jesus on the cross, and be hugged by a boy, while at the same time he lived the ascetic life and failed to distinguish blood from butter. In so doing he was a saint, one blessed by God, and so the Cistercians looked to him for spiritual power and insight. It is not by accident that Dante chose Bernard as the final guide in Paradise to the glory of God.

Bernard grew in the later Middle Age, in the sense that he was seen in new and different ways in uplifting stories (*exempla*) and in religious art. A recent study of Bernard's representation in art has shown that the fourteenth and fifteenth centuries took Bernard out of the cloister and showed him as laypeople perceived him.[59] Also, the contents of edifying stories changed: while in the *Vita Prima* he gave knights beer in order to convince them to stay at Clairvaux and become monks, in the *Golden*

Legend more than a century later, the knights have become students, who are given wine instead of beer.[60] But the point is the same: Bernard made use of the physical world in order to enhance the spiritual universe that he built up in and around his monastery.

I have no desire to make Bernard (or any other medieval saint, for that matter) more appealing than he actually was. For some of his opponents, such as poor Abelard, he was a monster. For Pope Eugenius III, who had been Bernard's monk at Clairvaux, the abbot of Clairvaux made demands that could not be met. But for many people who came to Bernard in search of healings or other miracles, he was more than human. We turn to such figures according to our own needs and construct them according to our own worldview. But the primary sources tell us that Bernard did not destroy his body: he restricted it and in youth probably went too far in doing so.

Thanks to the criticism of his monks, however, Bernard found a balance between asceticism and sensuality that enabled him to live to the relatively old age of 63. He did not hate his body, even though he disliked giving it the time it required for sleeping. He learned to accept the material life that made its demands and to transform it through his participation in divine power. In Bernard, reason and affectivity, *ratio et affectus*, joined in a powerful and convincing way. He may be a difficult saint for us to comprehend, but to those who sought to touch him in order to gain cures for their illnesses, matters were quite straightforward. Bernard was a man of God.

The abbot of Clairvaux needs to be seen in terms of his miracles, for these made him available, not only to other monks, but to the common people as well. In one story, Bernard's brothers tried to stop him from performing these acts, apparently because they attracted unwanted attention to the monastery. For Bernard it could be hard to accept this criticism, "they frequently taunted and abused [him] even to tears".[61] Here we can see a link between the world of the senses and its medial conveyance: Bernard's miracles made his ascetic life available for virtually everyone in medieval society, or at least those who could get physically close to him. Once he was dead, the miracles could be mediated into the far corners of the medieval world, for the saint in heaven was available to all those who sought him out.

In Bernard I see one medieval culture, not two, the product of the union of body and soul. The Cistercians avoided any temptation to dualism and sought to unite body and soul in the monastery. In the first decades of the twelfth century they created their new Order and transformed monastic life. Bernard in his battered body contributed to this union. It is this body to which the crucified Christ was seen to bend down and embrace. Here we meet spirituality and sensuality at one and the same time, mediated through wonderful stories that conveyed hope and meaning to all kinds of people.

Notes

1 Webster 1994, p. 644, "holy"; p. 1187, "sanctity".

2 Cicero *In Verrem* II, 5,19: "vir in publicis religionibus foederum sanctus et diligens."

3 Attwater 1980, pp. 7-8.

4 Vauchez 1997, pp. 13-14.

5 Sulpicius Severus, *Life of Martin of Tours*, III.

6 William of Saint Thierry, *Vita Prima Bernardi* I, 20; PL vol. CLXXXV, col. 238; trans. Cawley 2000, p. 20.

7 See Henning Laugerud's chapter on *Memory*, cognition and sensation in this volume.

8 Brown 1982, pp. 10-15.

9 Waddell 1966, 6, xiii, p. 85.

10 Waddell 1966, 11, v, p. 108.

11 Brown 1971, pp. 80-101.

12 Waddell 1966, 11, xv, p. 109.

13 McGuire 2010, pp. 13-15.

14 Waddell 1966, 11, xiv, pp. 108-109.

15 Waddell 1966, 11, xxviii, p. 110.

16 Ward 1976, pp. 185-187.

17 *Benedikts Regel*, trans. Jensen, 1.

18 See *Exordium Cistercii* I, in Waddell 1999, p. 179.

19 McGuire 1991, pp. 282-288.

20 Haastrup 1985, p. 100.

21 Legendre 2005, p. 289.

22 McGuire 1991, pp. 282-286.

23 Waddell 1966, 12, p. 111.

24 Waddell 1966, 12, x, p. 113.

25 McGuire 2011, preface.

26 William, *Vita Prima* I, 20; trans. Cawley 2000, p. 20.

27 William I, 20; trans. Cawley 2000, p. 21.

28 William I, 21; trans. Cawley 2000, p. 21.

29 William I, 22; trans. Cawley 2000, p. 22.

30 William I, 22; trans. Cawley 2000, p. 22.

31 William I, 32; trans. Cawley 2000, p. 32.

32 William I, 33; trans. Cawley 2000, p. 33, who comments "Dark red blood, in any form, could not be confused with yellow dairy butter", so he suggests "a spread, or dip…like British Marmite".

33 Jacobus 1969, p. 468. For a more general and comprehensive account of practices of consumption in the Middle Ages, see Jette Linaa's chapter on medieval consumption in this volume.

34 Bernard, *Sermones in Cantica* XIV, 6; trans. Walsh 1977, p. 102.

35 As according to abba Poemen, nr. 150; trans. Ward 1976, p. 158. Also Syncletica, nr. 27; trans. Ward, p. 197.

36 Bernard, *Sermones in Cantica* XIV, 6; trans. Walsh 1977, p. 102.

37   *Sermones in Cantica* XIV, 6; trans. Walsh 1977, p. 103.

38   *Sermones in Cantica* XIV, 6; trans. Walsh 1977, p. 103.

39   *Sermones in Cantica* XIV, 6; trans. Walsh 1977, p. 103.

40   McGuire 2010, pp. 33-34.

41   *Vita Prima* I, 33; trans. Cawley 2000, pp. 32-33.

42   *Vita Prima* I, 60; trans. Cawley 2000, pp. 53-54.

43   McGuire 2009, pp. 248-249.

44   *Sermones in Cantica* XIV, 7; trans. Walsh 1977, p. 103.

45   *Sermones in Cantica* XVI, 15; trans. Walsh 1977, p. 124.

46   Walter Daniel, *Life of Ailred*, trans. Powicke 1978, p. 40.

47   *Vita Prima* I, 45; trans. Cawley 2000, p. 43.

48   *Vita Prima* I, 35; trans. Cawley 2000, p. 35; William of Saint Thierry's reflections on the golden age at Clairvaux.

49   *Vita Prima* I, 64-68; trans. Cawley 2000, pp. 60-62.

50   *Exordium magnum* II, 20; ed. Griesser 1961, p. 117.

51   *Exordium magnum* II, 7; ed. Griesser 1961, p. 103. Translated in Ward & Savage 2012, pp. 136-137.

52   France 2007, pp. 179-204.

53   France 2007, pp. 195-196; McGuire 1991, pp. 227-249.

54   France 2007, pp. 205-238; McGuire 1991, pp. 189-225.

55   Vacandard 1902, vol. II, p. 555.

56   McGuire 1991, pp. 125-126.

57   *Vita Prima* IV, 40; trans. Cawley 2000, p. 97.

58   Map, *De nugis curialium*, ed. James 1983, p. 81.

59   France 2007, pp. 339-354.

60   *Vita Prima* I, 55; trans. Cawley 2000, p. 49. Jacobus 1969, p. 476.

61   *Vita Prima* I, 44; trans. Cawley 2000, p. 59.

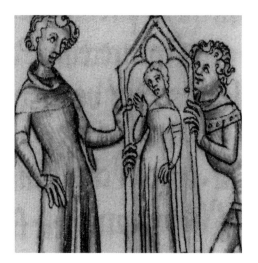

112

[**REPRESENTATION**] How do we describe our beloved? This chapter investigates the question of sensory representation in the medium of non-religious, medieval, narrative literature. Taking a post-medieval idea of medium and representation as point of departure, I suggest understanding representation as the production of reality (in contrast to representation as a correspondence with reality). This concept of representation makes the relation between reality and literature opaque. A short introduction to the article establishes a rough overview of this problematic relation and then turns to the main focus: a particularly complicated, but also illuminating sample text, namely passages from Chrétien de Troyes' *Cligès*. The passages exemplify the representation of the beloved in the medium of courteous literature. As the analysis will demonstrate, representation becomes less an image of the woman and more a self-portrait of both the narrator and perhaps also of Chrétien himself. Furthermore the example seems to show that describing (and thus sensing and understanding) the woman is as difficult as approaching and experiencing 'presence' in itself.

REPRESENTATION

Courtly Love as a Problem of Literary Sense-Representation

113

[Jørgen Bruhn]

Manufactured Representations

In this chapter I will focus upon the question of literary representation in non-religious, narrative, medieval literature. Starting from an understanding of representation as creation of meaning – rather than representation as a correspondence with an outer world – I offer a rough taxonomy of representation in medieval literature. After that I will show how the production of meaning necessarily involves sensorial aspects. Chrétien de Troyes' chivalric romance *Cligès* from the second half of the twelfth century provides a salient example of this phenomenon.

As compared to the majority of contributions in this book I emphasise texts that could, at least from the viewpoint of post-medieval thinking, be termed 'literary texts'. These are relatively detached from the all-important religious, 'hagiosensorial' dimensions of medieval thinking.[1] I roughly sketch problems of representation in medieval literature, and hope to demonstrate that – even in non-religious texts – considerations and representations of the senses are inherent to what may at first sight be considered a solely verbal representation. In other words: reading medieval literary representation in the light of twentieth century theory will enable me to understand that literary representation is never 'only' verbal language being processed as symbolical signs. Consequently, medieval literary representation exemplifies the more universal fact that representation per definition involves non-literary and even non-aesthetic aspects, namely the senses.

For a literary scholar, for instance Georg Lukàcs in his influential historico-philosophical study *Die Theorie des Romans*, which was written during World War I, medieval mentality and artistic creation is understood in contradistinction to the

REPRESENTATION

problems of modernity in the Renaissance and Baroque. Lukàcs based his historical framework on the idea that Antiquity and the Middle Ages are characterised by an un-mediating and philosophically unproblematic homogeneity that has been lost from the Renaissance and onwards. Rewriting the Hegelian philosophy of history in the guise of literary forms, Lukàcs distinguishes the Greek and medieval epics from the novel. Indeed, by radicalising Lukàcs' position a bit, his ideas may be summarised in the following manner. Literature from pre-Renaissance epochs was understood in terms of consolidating ideological and philosophical systems, first in Greek thinking, and later on in Christian thought. This produced what was considered adequate artistic forms. According to Lukàcs, antique and medieval authors experienced no problems in establishing artistic relations between man and world. Using the terminology of Grusin and Bolter in *Remediation: Understanding New Media*, we might say that Lukàcs considers pre-modern culture a culture of *immediacy*.[2] More precisely: before modernity, *representation* in its current meaning did not exist. That this was *not* the case has been shown abundantly in contemporary research into medieval literature and culture, which has tirelessly described and discussed the intricacies of representation in the Middle Ages.

Being closely related to but not identical with equally complex terms like *mimesis* or *realism*, even 'medium/media' and 'mediation', the term *representation* has a long and complicated history. I choose to work with a non-medieval concept of representation and mediation, i.e. an idea of *media* as an opaque device directed towards something in distinction to the concept of *medium* in the medieval sense of the term, where medium produces presence. Translating Hans Henrik Lohfert Jørgensen's distinctions between medieval and modern understandings of 'media' and 'medium' into my special interest here, I would say that the modern concept of representation is based on an understanding of *media* of communication and signification, whereas medieval representation is based on an understanding of *medium* as a channel or vessel for transferring an *efficacious message* (e.g. prayer, blessing, consecration, oath, or legal announcement), *quality* (e.g. healing power, divine grace, holiness), or *substance* (e.g. the sacrament, spiritual or bodily presence, the Word of God incarnate in some shape of mediator or mediatrix).[3] The contemporary understanding of media is conditioned by distance and difference, whereas the medieval notion of medium, in the form suggested here, is a tool reducing distance and even producing presence.[4]

In a seminal study of post-medieval representation, Christopher Prendergast's *The Triangle of Representation* uses a distinction that relates to the division between representation as a sign *replacing* something, i.e. a symbol representing reality, versus someone *representing someone else*, for instance a representative in a parliament.[5] When this double meaning of representation is taken into consideration, the political aspects of representation comes to the fore: to represent is per definition an instance of choice, of letting one possibility be representative instead of another. Representation and power is thus – as W.J.T. Mitchell demonstrates in his conclusion to *Picture Theory* – intimately related: representation without power is unimaginable – and power devoid of any representational dimension is self-contradictory.[6]

Stuart Hall, in his essay in *Representation: Cultural Representations and Signifying Practices* suggests a productive distinction between theories of representation focused on either the *object of representation* (reflective theories) or the *representing subject* (constructivist theories).[7] Whereas reflective theories ask to what extent a sign represents reality faithfully, the constructivist approach sees representation as a subjective act, which partly produces reality. Reflective theories of representation focused on the object refer to a theory of correspondence where truth may be established by finding the corresponding relation between a sign and its referent. I pursue a theory of representation, indebted to contemporary constructivist thinking, which is focused on showing how subjects, in intense interrelations with the surrounding world and the available signifying systems, *produce* versions of the world via the process of representation. In other words, emphasis is less on the object of representation and more on the representing subject. I am interested in discussing ways in which narrative literature enables readers and writers to encounter versions of reality as these are represented via, for instance, incorporated points of view in fictive persons. Understood in this manner, fictive representations, such as narrative literature, do not offer versions of the world; instead they give us versions of manufactured subjectivities, and these subjectivities may in turn offer versions of the world. In this optic, one way of defining the medium of narrative literature may be to describe it as manufacturing representations of the world. The question is what happens when I transfer this admittedly non-medieval idea of representation to medieval literature?

In order to answer this question I wish to begin with a few examples of literary representation from the high and late Middle Ages, and afterwards I shall analyse a fragment of a larger text (a chivalric romance written by Chrétien de Troyes around 1175) in greater depth. In conclusion I rephrase the question of representation into terms of the relation of literary representation and the senses.

Problems of Literary Representation
in the Middle Ages

Problems of representation, which are not difficult to find in medieval literature, may be divided into three categories: a) some texts are stressing problems with sensing the world 'correctly'; b) a group of texts where the problematic nature of representation seems to be agreed upon by both the writer and the (informed) reader; and c) a group of examples stressing a (double) indescribability.

a) One example of the cognitive problems of grasping the world in a way that seems appropriate, would be the opening of Chrétien de Troyes' chivalric romance *Perceval* from c. 1180. Here, Chrétien creates an opening scene, where the young Perceval is unable to frame the impressions of seeing and hearing the spectacle of the approaching human beings as what they are; namely threatening knights. This lack of comprehension creates a comical effect when Perceval insists on seeing and approaching them as if they were angels.

The function of such cognitive mistakes is that they can be effectively cleared away inside the fiction, such that the protagonist understands the supposedly true nature of reality. For the reader of the fiction reality has been known from the beginning. In Dante's *Divine Comedy*, scenes that follow this structure abound: several of the mistakes of 'Dante the pilgrim' who directly experiences "Inferno", "Purgatorio", and "Paradiso" are set against the extended knowledge of 'Dante the writer', i.e. the fictive narrator who later *describes* the terrible and the exalting experiences of 'Dante the pilgrim'. The result of this clash is the *Divine Comedy* itself. In these cases, Dante and Chrétien show that the sensual impression may be overwhelming for the protagonist, with false images that he is only later able to 'see through' in order to access the real world. Chrétien and Dante create representations of fictive individuals whose access to reality suffers from a deficit. In her contribution to this volume, Kristin Aavitsland discusses this fundamental deficit by analysing other cultural artefacts. She argues, convincingly, that after the Fall of Man, human senses are "corrupted and have lost their potential to experience the glory of God".[8] This deficit, which is founded in theological dogma, is nevertheless fundamental for all medieval representational practices, even a so-called 'secular' writer like Chrétien.

b) A host of other problematic representations concern the less direct examples of medieval authors who debate problems of interpretation and representation in their texts. Marie de France's elegant, but also disturbing, adaptation of the Tristan-myth, "Chevrefoil", ca. 1180, may function as an example here. In order for the myth to fit her favoured literary genre (the rhymed short story-like "lais"), she deftly cuts out everything but the most necessary material concerning the star struck lovers and condensates the many different versions of the Tristan-material into a brief narrative. Marie de France construes her own surprising climax to the story when Iseut is forced to recognise a sign from Tristan while travelling through the woods; but as if this was not enough, Iseut must even decode a message inscribed on a wooden stick. *How* Iseut manages to decode the message, and *what* that message actually consists of is difficult, if not impossible, to actually deduce from the text, which remains secretive. Perhaps Isolde is meant to read a "T" for Tristan on the stick ("When he had prepared this staff/He autographed it with his knife")[9] and draw her own conclusion. This seems reasonable from a realistic point of view: how can much writing fit onto a hazel twig anyway? Or perhaps she is meant to read a much longer message on the stick (here rendered in the English translation by Judith P. Shoaf):

117

> This is the gist of what he wrote,
> The message he sent her, as he spoke:
> That he'd stayed there for quite a while,
> Waiting, lingering in exile,
> Spying, trying to learn or hear
> How he could find a way to see her,
> For without her he cannot live.
> For those two, it's just like with
> The sweet honeysuckle vine
> That on the hazel tree will twine:
> When it fastens, slips itself right
> Around the trunk, ties itself tight,
> Then the two survive together.
> But should anyone try to sever
> Them, the hazel dies right away,
> And the honeysuckle, the same day.
> 'Dear love, that's our story, too:
> Never you without me, me without you!'[10]

As has been noted, such examples almost inevitably create a meta-fictional effect, raising questions about the possibilities and problems of literary representation, here focused on *what* is being said, or *written*, and what role the inscribed message may have in the larger narrative structure.[11]

The functions and effects of literary representation, as compared to my Perceval example above, are distinguished by creating a *balance* between the author and the readers. There is a balance between the abilities of the sophisticated writer and the competent reader; together they create a harmonious relation between representation and the world around the perceiving subject inside the text. In this category, the complexity and difficulties of representation are not diminished, but it does not create any problem.

c) Another aspect of Dante's *Comedy* can exemplify a different question of representation in medieval literature, namely the indescribability-topos, so cherished by Dante. Danish scholar Hanne Roer shows how Dante theorises this in his work *Convivio* from the beginning of the fourteenth century by describing the indescribability-topos as the impossibility for the human intellect to *cognitively grasp* divine creation on the one hand and the impossibility to *artistically represent* this divine creation on the other.[12] This enables Dante to verify the truthfulness of his own literary fiction by claiming that what he is about to describe may seem too fantastic to be true, here from a classic English translation of Paradiso: "O how all speech is feeble and falls short/Of my conceit, and this to what I saw/Is such, 't is enough to call it little".[13]

However, even in the marvellous thief-scene in *Hell*, Song XXV, Dante (both as a pilgrim in the plot and as the writer creating the text) is eager to show how the representational apparatus – literature – is *weaker* than the intentions of the writer-figure that Dante creates. Things seem so fantastic that Dante the writer both challenges and defies classical authors, Lucan and Ovid,[14] but at the same time he needs to excuse himself for his seemingly unbelievable descriptions.[15] Or to continue my comparison with Kristin Aavitsland's argumentation of medieval religious representation: the indescribability-topos is the result of the fact that not only are Man's senses corrupted – even the object of our representations is, in religious terms, only the "recognition of God."[16] I will try to show below that this religious representational paradigm is also a condition for non-religious literature, for instance Chrétien.

Representation and the Senses

In the following I would like to rephrase the problem of medieval literary representation in terms of the relationship between sense and representation in the examples. The three types of examples above border on the question of the senses, because creating literary versions of the world is necessarily related to the senses. Indeed, the three types of text referred to above may be described not merely as literary problems of representation, but also as questions of the senses and perception. The first case of Perceval's misunderstanding may be reformulated in terms of Perceval making 'false' mental images related to his mother's descriptions of angels. In Marie de France's Tristan-version the discussion concerned the possibility of, practically, physically, writing a long verbal message on a piece of wood (or not), as well as being able to actually *see* the stick in the wood and identify it as a message from Tristan. The case of Dante's indescribability topos deals more with the fact that Dante, via his two alter egos (the 'pilgrim' and the 'writer'), represents other worlds to which we may have mental access (for non-believers amounting to fantasy, for believer's being truthful), but no actual sensual experiences. Consequently, readers may find it hard to understand and/or believe. In other words: literary representation in the Middle Ages is related to the senses.

In order to focus on this question of representation and the senses, I will discuss the 'indescribability' topos in an extended example from what is often considered a very typical aspect of medieval secular culture: the representation of love in chivalric literature. I have chosen a fragment of one of Chrétien de Troyes' romances, *Cligès*, which will illustrate the degree to which the indescribability-topos proves an interesting testing ground for considering the relation between the senses, representation, and literature. The analysis of the specific fragment is meant, therefore, to disclose more general problems related to the question of representation and the senses.

Chrétien's *Cligès* is, like Marie de France's text discussed above, a version of one of the classical stories of medieval and even post-medieval fictional mythology, the Tristan-motif. For Anthime Fourrier, Chrétien's *Cligès* is clearly a reply to *Tristan:* it has been called both an 'Anti-Tristan' and a 'Super-Tristan', but Fourrier prefers the snappier "Neo-Tristan."[17] I have analysed the text's two basic problems in another context. For the male protagonist: how to be a knight without being violent. For the female protagonist: how to make love while staying a virgin.[18] Here, however, I want to discuss the text from another angle, questioning instead the problem of the senses as related to the question of representation or perhaps rather, un-representability.

The fragment I wish to analyse is among the much-debated parts of Chrétien's oeuvre because of its masterful, but also complicated rhetorical construction. It is basically a monologue conducted by the main character of the book, the young knight Alexander, who is anxiously trying to describe his beloved Soredamors. The monologue is a detailed discussion of the nature and effects of love, of watching the beloved. As part of the monologue, the basic question of how to represent the beloved object becomes a crucial theme, too. I will show that the secular text offers parallels to the theological problem of both perceiving and representing God.

Alexander's extended monologue occupies about two hundred and fifty lines (624-870) out of a total of ca. 6800 lines of *Cligès*. The monologue begins with the topos of 'love as illness', continues by discussing 'love as a hard master' followed by a description of love's arrows: the final section in the first part concerns his two eyes and his heart that have turned out to be his worst enemies (because they inflict the pain of love on him). The second half of the monologue functions as Alexander's return to the arrow-metaphor in order to describe Soredamors. To begin with, the 'love as pain'-metaphor leading to the 'love as master'-metaphor are textbook examples of a troubadour-vocabulary and it seems topical, not to say banal. Re-told in this manner, the text seems clear enough. When analysed in greater detail things get more complicated and interesting however. In the following I will make my way through this fragment, hopefully stressing the overall theme of this chapter: the relation between medieval literary representation and the senses.

How can it be, Alexander wonders at the opening of the monologue, that arrows can penetrate his body without leaving any visible wounds? Alexander's own answer is: because the arrows enter through the eyes. But the eyes are not hurt either, and the reason, according to Alexander, is that the eye is simply a receptacle whereas the real forces and vulnerability lie in the heart. That is why the arrows may pass the eyes into the heart without damaging anything.[19] This question is the core of the section, and it is almost literally repeated a few lines later.[20] Probably mimicking the scholastic rhetoric, Alexander tries to explain this puzzling fact, but the answer, which is supposed to be a rational and non-metaphorical explanation, is filled with new images in need of interpretation. In prose-translation the lines go as follows: "For is the heart in one's breast not like the flaming candle within a lantern? If you remove the candle, no light will shine forth; but as long as the candle burns the lantern is not dark, and the flame shining within does not harm or destroy it."[21] This mock-physiological discussion moves on to the next metaphoric cluster, regarding the relation between the eyes and the heart.[22] Alexander constructs yet another metaphor with the window as the main metaphor: "It is the same with a pane of glass: no matter how thick or solid, the sun's rays pass through without breaking it".[23]

It is probably a church's stained glass window that is being referred to here, and the idea is that it is penetrable by light without being broken. This image was a common medieval metaphor for the Virgin Mary, in particular in religious descriptions of church windows. Chrétien, I will argue, wants his alert reader or listener to catch both the religious and the sexual undertones (penetration) of Alexander's pseudo-scholastic reflections. As we shall see below, the question of penetration will return in other forms in the fragment.

Alexander continues the series of metaphors by implicating some rather obscure comments on the eyes as mirrors in the direct continuation of the lines quoted above:

Yet no matter how bright the glass, it will not help you to see unless some brighter light strikes its surface. Know that the eyes are like the glass and the lantern, for through the eyes comes the light by which the heart sees itself and the outside world, whatever it may be. It sees many different objects.[24]

The metaphors do not offer any clarification, and the two opposing theories of visual perception (see my description below), extramission and intromission, mix in a way that generates questions rather than answers. This technique seems to be intentional on the part of Chrétien, not only in this passage, but also in the following part of the fragment.

Alexander, in this section, has tried to represent his feelings and sensations in four different registers, according to Peter Haidu: a medical, a courtly, a scholastic, and a soldierly register, all included in a monologue.[25] Finishing this, he moves from his own inner feelings to a representation – a portrait – of Soredamors.

The Portrait

Now I shall tell you how the arrow that has been entrusted to my care is made and shaped. But I am afraid I might fail, and the arrow's shape is so splendid that it would be no surprise if I did. Yet I shall direct all my efforts to describing how it appears to me. The nock and feathers are so close together, if one looks carefully, that they are divided only by the thinnest line; and the nock is so smooth and straight that there can be no question of any imperfection.[26]

It takes a while before the reader or the listener is capable of relating the description of the precious arrow with the thing it allegorically represents, namely Soredamors. Parts of the arrow are compared to what the reader slowly recognises as Soredamors' lovely hair, the extremely straight parting of her hair and her eyes.[27] The arrow *is*, in other words, Soredamors. After having established this, Alexander leaves the arrow-allegory for a while in order to produce a more traditional portrait. However, as Colby notes, "The hair, parting, forehead, and eyes of Soredamors were very beautiful; but they were nevertheless describable", which is not the case when it comes to the nose, the cheek, and the mouth. Consequently, the indescribability-topos comes into play, but in a special way: the features are described in the form of questions, as if the descriptions are imprecise and unsatisfactory but necessary all the same. The questions seem to accept the double indescribability condition discussed above: an indescribable and only barely understandable phenomenon (God – or the woman) and an insufficient representational tool (the human sense apparatus combined with language or with an image, see ill. 14).

The description of the cheek with the help of the rose and the lily are examples of this negative description: "And whose tongue is skilled enough to describe the symmetry of her shapely nose and shining face, wherein the rose suffuses the lily and slightly softens its glow to enhance her face?"[28]

A rose is compared to a lily, and the lily to its own disappearance and illumination, thus in one sense disappearing and in another being likened to the lamp, which was part of the earlier metaphor of the heart. Alexander moves farther down the body of his beloved, and he seems to get more and more excited as he describes the whiteness of the throat. As he, i.e. his eyes and his description, travels downwards he must admit being submitted to the condition of a double indescribability because of his lacking linguistic abilities, but also because he has quite simply not seen her body below her naked throat. As the threatening erotic sensuality of her body inevitably approaches, Alexander breaks off. We may speculate that in order to control his sexual arousal, while at the same time describing the object of it, he is forced to use a strange metaphor: not only the symbol of Amor's Arrows, but the metaphor of the physical form of the arrow itself. Therefore, sexual (and comic) connotations haunt the description. Indeed, it is hard to overlook the sexual allusions hidden in the phallus-like arrow penetrating its quiver, and the only part of the arrow he can actually see is the notch which may visually be connected to the form of the female sex. Eyes, quivers, and – earlier on – church glass, are part of a larger system of different versions of penetration, but not in any simple or unidirectional way. While being

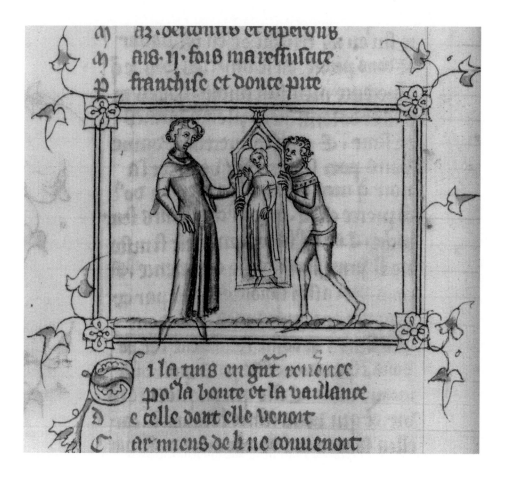

[**III. 14**] The representation of love – the love of representation: The communication between lover and beloved is mediated by a portrait of the fine lady, allowing the lover to envision and approach the otherwise unapproachable object of his amorous desire. Via the near-lifesize image, the lover is admitted a glimpse of the beloved, which at the same time (re)presents her picturesque beauty to him and prevents him from encountering her face to face. Frontispiece miniature from Guillaume de Machaut's *Le Livre du Voir-Dit,* Paris, c. 1370-1377. Paris, Bibliothèque Nationale, MS fr. 1584, fol. 235v.

penetrated by the arrows of love, symbolised, and allegorically represented by Soreda-mors, Alexander at the same time tries to penetrate Soredamors with his verbal description.

Due to the monologue's complexity, it has been widely discussed in the literature. Colby described the portrait in the tradition of twelfth century literature and rhetorical treaties, with two crucial aspects: the functional (or narrative) dimension and the ornamental (or aesthetic) dimension. Peter Haidu has underlined that the monologue is a portrait of Alexander, or, as I would put it, a representation of Alexander representing. Ruth H. Cline argues that the leading principle behind the reflections on the vision and the arrows of love, as well as on the relation between the eyes and the heart, are to be found in Chrétien's reading of Averroës: "A reading of Averroes will show that the method by which the eye operated was still a hotly debated topic in Chrétien's time, and that his metaphors are completely in line with at least one theory".[29] The theory referred to by Cline is the Platonic theory of 'extramission', stating that visual perception is a result of light rays sent out from the eyes, which stands in opposition to the theory of 'intromission' where visual perception is created by way of the object.

Dana Stewart, on the contrary, argues that it is highly unlikely that Chrétien might have read Averroës who was translated only after 1200.[30] Also, she claims that Chrétien is not arguing for a Platonic idea of vision ('extramission'), as Averroës does, but on the contrary expresses a distinctly Aristotelian theory of vision ('intromission'). Dana Stewart's interpretation is probably the most convincing concerning the sources of optical theory, but she cannot explain the conspicuous metaphoric levels related to other conceptions of the senses and representation. This may be because her reading only concentrates on the idea of optics as a source, not as part of a larger metaphoric and representational system.[31]

However valuable as the cited articles and books are, in particular from the viewpoint of establishing a historical and philosophical context round the question of senses and representation, my own interpretation will approach Alexander's monologue in another way, namely by seeing the portrait as an ekphrasis. This will result in understanding how the portrait is producing (virtual) senses instead of mirroring sensual impressions.

The Portrait as Ekphrasis

The portrait of Soredamors should be related to a description in Chrétien's preceding romance *Erec et Enide*, namely the description of the two thrones given to the eponymous newly-wed couple. Both descriptions are verbal (literary) representations of non-linguistic entities. Also, the descriptions use a number of traditional poetic and rhetorical methods concerning difficult representations, the abovementioned negative descriptions, the topos of inexpressibility (Curtius), and indescribability (Colby). The shared elements suggest that the portrait of Soredamors could be considered as an 'ekphrasis'. While modern definitions of ekphrasis often define it as a "verbal representation of a visual representation",[32] antique and medieval definitions of ekphrasis focused on the notion of 'enargaia', i.e. a creative act of vivifying an object for the reader.[33] Ekphrasis is an important sub-category of literary representation. W.J.T. Mitchell's work on ekphrasis, notably in his essay "Ekphrasis and the Other", allows us to search for another thematic opposition in Alexander's portrait of Soredamors, namely between what is visible and what is expressible.[34] In extension, questions of power, language, and love must be addressed in relation to the role of the senses.

I interpret Alexander's repeated and often ambiguous allusions to vision and the eye as signs of this struggle. Using Mitchell's terms regarding the power aspects of ekphrasis, it becomes clear that Alexander meets his other, the beloved Soredamors, by turning the mystical presence of a living woman into an object. His verbal monologue is, in other words, a failed attempt at mastering the non-verbal. Outside himself he finds what we could call the visual, the corporeal – or the Real in Lacanian terms. That is, the 'it' outside the symbolic order of language and representation in modern ideas of representational media. Briefly returning to the medieval understanding of 'medium', we could call it the lack of establishing a convincing or satisfying presence.

Following an older idea of ekphrasis, embedded in the idea of enargaia, the representational problems sketched above may show that Alexander, and probably also Chrétien, is *produces* a feeling of presence for the beloved phenomenon while describing it, thus creating an effect of enargaia, which is beyond narrative control. From such a constructivist point of view, as formulated by Hans Henrik Lohfert Jørgensen, "a construction of the medieval sensorium, [...] produced not only distinctive sensual experiences but also distinctive ways of organising sensation and setting up the senses."[35]

So, even though Alexander's description is hyperbolically positive, it also shows his immense difficulties of employing language for representation, i.e. transforming a non-linguistic sensual presence (Soredamors) into a linguistic artefact. Because of the inherent problems in this descriptive process, the portrait also turns into a self-portrait of Alexander; we learn quite a lot about Alexander by following his description of his beloved.

Literature:
in-between Medium and Media

Other contributors to this book show how a 'hagiosensorium' structures medieval conceptions of representation and mediation. An invisible, godly presence produces a complicated sensuous system of mediating practices in medieval society. I argue that a hagiocentric structure does not inform the highly systematised practice of courtly love, but the representational problem of relating medium and sensorium persists. In my main example, Chrétien, via the fictive figure Alexander, struggles to express a relation between the sensible and the sayable in words: the sensible facts in the monologue – if we follow a 'bureaucratic' division of the senses, belong to the vision and a kind of inner feeling of Alexander which is supposed to be transformed into a verbal image of the bodily features of Soredamors – based on the feeling of love. Both visual impressions, and the inner feeling of love, are characterised by being highly difficult to represent in a verbal, literary form. As I have tried to show above, however, the problem is also that the presence as well as the sensual features of the beloved are not only re-presented, but in fact produced. This is the reason, I argue, why Chrétien has been forced to use an almost scholastic system of argumentation on the one hand, while deconstructing the same argumentative form in his complicated and partly contradictory metaphorical system in the text on the other. He is, in other words, a victim of the double indescribability mentioned above in more than one instance; Alexander's inadequate tools of representation meet the un-expressible beauty of Soredamors. Alexander tries to overcome this complex problem by establishing what he believes to be a rock-steady ground, namely the senses. Unfortunately, the senses – *seeing* the beloved, *feeling* love in one's heart – turn out to be highly complicated factors in themselves. Even if Chrétien employs both optical theory, typical and almost banal courtly metaphors, and frames it in a mock-argumentative framework – almost copying scholastic thought – he does not succeed. Being in love does not make sense even if the senses are a crucial part of love.

The attempt to stabilise the feeling of love by way of the senses is, Chrétien's *Cligès* seems to say, doomed to fail.

The senses thus occupy an ambiguous position in the fragment I have discussed, and perhaps in the wider field of medieval secular literature. The senses may be referred to – and here I return to my sketch in the beginning of this chapter – as faulty. They may be discussed as parts of a plot, or they may partake actively in the problem of indescribability by not being described, but constructively produced during the description, as was the case in the Soredamors-portrait. So, even if indescribability may at first seem a liminal phenomenon of literary representation, it may be the topos that most convincingly exemplifies the question of the senses and its relation to representation. A medieval author like Chrétien obviously struggles to construct the senses as the relatively stable foundation that makes his abstract perceptions and ideas comprehensible. But problems arise at the very moment he tries to found his ideas on the senses; amorous feelings enter the body via the eyes, the eyes are related to the heart, the heart is supposed to decide for the body, in the same way that the light relates to the darkness of an unlit lamp, or the light penetrating windows. These processes – as well as their subtle emerging interrelations and internal hierarchical structure – are supposed to be represented by way of language. This results in paradoxical constructions, like the "vision of the heart" and the "feeling of the eyes": synesthetic sense-mixtures that contradict the bureaucratic compartmentalisation of the senses. Literature – exemplified by a spectacularly complex passage in Chrétien's *Cligès* – turns out to occupy a place between 'medium' (producing presence) and 'media' (standing in for non-present objects); literature aims at a simultaneous production of presence, while attempting to represent absent phenomena.

127

Notes

1   See Hans Henrik Lohfert Jørgensen's chapter on the *Sensorium* in this volume.

2   Bolter & Grusin 1999.

3   See Hans Henrik Lohfert Jørgensen's primer *Into the Saturated Sensorium* introducing this volume.

4   See Hans Ulrich Gumbrecht 2004, where he argues for a renewed focus on the aspects of what I here refer to as the medieval functions of 'medium'.

5   See Prendergast 2000, pp. 5-6.

6   Mitchell 1994.

7   Hall 1997, p. 15.

8   See Kristin Bliksrud Aavitsland's chapter on *Incarnation* in this volume.

9   Shoaf 1991-1996.

10   Shoaf, 1991-1996.

11   For instance in Krueger 2003.

12   See Roer 2004.

13   Dante 1871 translation, v. 120-122.

14   *Inferno* XXV, l. v. 93-97.

15   *Inferno* XXV, l. v. 140-144.

16   Aavitsland this volume.

17   Fourrier 1960, p. 123. When I quote from or refer to *Cligès* in the following I place William W. Kibler's English translation (1991) in the main text with the Old French original in the footnotes, referring to the verse-numbers of Poirion's Chrétien-edition (1994).

18   See Bruhn 2010.

19   Poirion 1994, 701-702; Kibler 1991, p. 131.

20   Poirion 1994, 712-713; Kibler 1991, p. 131.

21   "Donc est li cuers el vantre mis,/Ausi com la chandoile esprise/Est dedanz la lenterne mise."; Poirion 1994, 714-716; Kibler 1991, pp. 131-132.

22   For an investigation into the question of the representation as well as the function of the heart in medieval (both religious and non-religious) literature, see Webb 2010.

23   "Autresi est de la verrine:/Ja n'iert si forz ne anterine/Que li rais del soloil n'i past,/Sanz ce que de rien ne la quast"; Poirion 1994, 723-726; Kibler 1991, p. 132.

24   "Ne ja li voirres si clers n'iert,/Se autre clartez ne s'i fiert,/Que par le suel voie l'an mialz./Ce meïsmes sachiez des ialz,/Con del voirre et de la lanterne:/Car es ialz se fiert la luiserne/Ou li cuers se remire, et voit/L'uevre de fors, quex qu'ele soit;/Si voit maintes oevres diverses"; Poirion 1994, 728-735; Kibler 1991, p. 132.

25   See Haidu 1969, p. 71.

26   "Or vos reparlerai del dart/Qui m'est comanderez et bailliez,/Comant il est fez et tailliez./Mes je dot molt que ge n'I faille:/Car tant en est riche la taille,/N'est mervoille, se je I fail,/Et si metrai tot mon travail/A dire ce que moi an sanble./La coche et li pennon ansanble/Sont sip res, que bien les ravise,/Que il n'a c'une devise/Ausi con d'une greve estroite,/Mes ele est si polie et droite/Qu'an la coche sanz demander/N'a rien qui face a amender."; Poirion 1994, 768-782; Kibler 1991, p. 132.

128

27 Alexander is thus making a description beginning at the top of the body, from hair towards the body, as was the standard descriptive practice according to Colby 1965, p. 154.

28 "Et qui a boche se deliver,/Qui la façon seüst descrivre,/Del nes bien fet et del cler vis,/Com la rose oscure le lis,/Einsi come le lis esface,/Por bien anluminer la face"; Poirion 1994, 813-817; Kibler 1991, p. 133.

29 See Cline 1971, p. 264.

30 In Stewart 2003.

31 Spearing 1993, (referring to Cline) shows that the idea being expressed here is of antique origin but in Chrétien's time the question of vision and love was not yet settled, even if the connection between love and visuality was a commonplace. This might be an explanation of the divergent tendencies in Chrétien's use of metaphors of love at first sight.

32 This is one among many definitions that are critically discussed and evaluated in Scholz 2007.

33 See Wandhof 2003, in which the thrones in *Erec* occupy an important place.

34 In Mitchell 1994, pp. 151-181.

35 See Hans Henrik Lohfert Jørgensen's chapter on the medieval *Sensorium* in this volume.

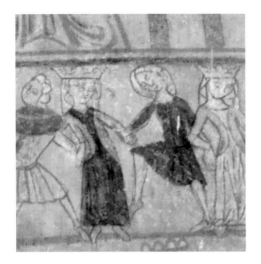

[REMEDIATION] This chapter focuses on medieval media and on the change that occurs in their relations to each other. Originally, media were separate parts of a certain social and geographical environment, the media reality of the epoch being defined by public subgroups that were localised around functionally separate centres of communication. In the late Middle Ages these subgroups were mixed and the media boundaries of segregated subcultures suspended. Media phenomena such as intermediality and remediation therefore become relevant, and the notion of remediation is introduced at the beginning of the chapter by presenting the work of Bolter & Grusin. As one example of this transformation, the relations between the medieval popular ballad in Denmark and Sweden and church paintings are described. The ballad is an intermedial art form that is remediated into paintings on the church walls together with other art forms such as theatre, legends, and proverbs. At the end of the Middle Ages some Scandinavian workshops even take up motives from satirical texts and jocular ballads that are remediated into *Mahnbilder,* and thereby take on a new function for the churchgoer. This is part of a process where the whole space of the church is remediated as a backdrop for the cult and the worship of mediated cult objects.

REMEDIATION

Remediating Medieval Popular Ballads in Scandinavian Church Paintings

131

[Sigurd Kværndrup]

The World of Media Remediated:
The Sensorium of Man Transformed

The notion of remediation has changed its meaning over the past decade; or rather it has taken on a new dimension. Earlier remediation would be defined as the act of providing a remedy. The new dimension of the notion was produced by Jay D. Bolter and Richard Grusin however in *Remediation: Understanding New Media* (1999). Here they define the notion as incorporation or representation of one medium within another medium. Underlying this important work was the process of media digitalisation. This was so all-embracing that, over a very short time, almost all technical media changed from analogue to digital communication:

> In this last decade of the twentieth century, we are in an unusual position to appreciate remediation, because of the rapid development of new digital media and the nearly as rapid response by traditional media. Older electronic and print media are seeking to reaffirm their status within our culture as digital media challenge that status.[1]

The authors use 'remediation' in order to argue that the new visual media achieved cultural significance by refashioning and paying homage to earlier forms of media such as painting, photography, film, and television. Additionally, they note that earlier media incorporated and refashioned their predecessors: photography remediated painting, film remediated theatre and photography, and television remediated film

REMEDIATION

and radio. These twentieth century media changes had great implications, not only politically – as Bolter and Grusin discuss later with Walter Benjamin's famous essay from 1936 "The Work of Art in the Age of Mechanical Reproduction" as a backdrop – but also in the way art and media are experienced, thereby influencing man's very sensorium.[2] Indeed, when the world of media is remediated, man's sensorium is transformed – an idea that underlies major works on media and the senses by Marshall McLuhan and Walter Ong.[3] The purpose of this chapter is therefore to show how Bolter & Grusin present us with useful tools to understand certain aspects of artistic or qualified media in the Middle Ages and their special way of appealing to the senses.[4]

The Double Logic of Remediation

First, let us take a closer look at *Remediation*. Bolter & Grusin begin by analysing a futuristic film, *Strange Days*, in which a technological wonder called "the wire" makes it possible for a user to experience the most perfect virtual reality, and they add: "If the ultimate purpose of media is indeed to transfer sense experiences from one person to another, the wire threatens to make all media obsolete."[5] The authors stress that the film demonstrates the double logic of remediation: "our culture wants both to multiply its media and to erase all traces of mediation: ideally, it wants to erase its media in the very act of multiplying them."[6] This 'double logic' is the interplay between *immediacy* and *hypermediacy*. With hypermediacy, mediation is highlighted, which is typical for the earlier twentieth century: "The Medium Is the Message" as McLuhan maintained in *Understanding Media*.[7] With immediacy and transparency as the goal, the medium is erased like in virtual reality or in flat screen-television. These technical media seek to place a viewer in the same space as the objects viewed. On the way, the authors add interesting historical perspectives to their post-modern thesis: European culture has shown an insatiable desire for immediacy since the renaissance. For Bolter & Grusin this is a standard notion – even if they are also aware that the invention of linear perspective in paintings was contested by other pictorial systems without the same pretensions to transparency.[8] However, one could also stress that it represents a 'pictorial turn' from a multisensory and oral to a primarily visual way of thinking. The present publication, among other things, aims to problematise this standard notion – also named "the great divide" by Mark Smith[9] – and to show that the Middle Ages, using other media tools while appealing to other senses, also shared the goal of placing an observer in immediate connection with a (holy) object. Bolter & Grusin, on the other hand, give a few but fine examples from the Middle Ages when they explain the notion of *hypermediacy*. The medieval fascination with and exploration of the material medium itself is shown in the case of the manuscript medium where elaborately decorated initial capitals integrate text and image. The cathedrals are seen as an amalgam of hypermediated works of art, inscriptions, stained glass, relief statuary, and richly decorated altarpieces, combined in an enormous celestial space. In the important chapter "Networks of Remediation", they go deeper into explaining the two terms:

> We have so far used the term immediacy in two senses: one epistemological, the other psychological. In the epistemological sense, immediacy is transparency: the absence of mediation and representation. It is the notion that a medium could erase itself and leave the viewer in the presence of the objects represented, so that he could know the objects directly. In its psychological sense, immediacy names the viewer's feeling that the medium has disappeared and the objects are present to him, a feeling that his experience is therefore authentic.[10]

It is easy to see how important *immediacy* has been for the relationship between medieval objects of art and an observer, not least when the object of representation is the Divine. This feeling of deep identification is essential for the knowledge that you are being heard by God.

> Hypermediacy also has two corresponding senses. In its epistemological sense, hypermediacy is opacity – the fact that knowledge of the world comes to us through media. The viewer acknowledges that she is in the presence of a medium and learns through acts of mediation or indeed learns about mediation itself. The psychological sense of hypermedia is the experience that she has in and of the presence of media; it is the insistence that the experience of the medium is itself an experience of the real. The appeal to authenticity of experience is what brings the logics of immediacy and hypermediacy together.[11]

If you look at the non-realistic, figurative language of the Middle Ages, very code- and media-conscious as it is, Bolter & Grusin may be right in this analysis. Pictures, but also relics and other holy objects, were not transparent as immediacy, but rather gave access to the holy by means of and with the medium – thus a sort of mediated immediacy or indirect spontaneity. If you realise that immediacy is defined differently in the Middle Ages – more like a perceptible contact with the holy, than like a transparent representation of the holy – then this somewhat categorical historiography is transformed. In fact, the medieval situation has a certain similarity with our contemporary media paradox as described by Bolter & Grusin: a hypermediacy that produces immediacy exactly through the articulation of the media and their strong multisensory presence.[12] Now, let us take a look at the development of medieval media from the point of view of a media historian.

Media and the Medieval Public

Historical research into the media of the Middle Ages is a fairly new chapter in medieval studies. Based on a number of separate studies, Werner Faulstich published *Medien und Öffentlichkeiten im Mittelalter 800-1400* in 1996 – a work focusing so much on "human media and written media" (*Menschmedien und Schreibmedien*) that perhaps these concepts ought to have been included as a subtitle. Faulstich convincingly argues "Teilöffentlichkeiten" (public subgroups), localised around functionally separate centres of communication defined the media reality of the epoch. Faulstich mentions "Hof/Burg" (court/castle), separate from "Land/Dorf" (countryside/village), separate from "Kloster/Universität" (monastery/university), separate from "Stadt" (city). On its own, but capable of integrating with all the other public subgroups we find the "Kirchenraum" (the space of the church). Faulstich lists 15 distinctive media, which are divided between the human and written, noting that in fact the number is more or less the same as today. Clearly absent from Faulstich's theory, though, are images and building-media.

In his work, media means technical media – including 'the human', using body and voice for recitation, speech and song. The term is not used to describe what Elleström defines as a "qualified medium", i.e. an art form like the ballad or the ecclesiastical fresco.[13] This medium is summarily categorised, alongside pictorial media like glass mosaics, as the media Wall, obviously meaning church-wall, whereas the trappings of the private residence, tapestries, and paintings, are not touched upon. Faulstich explains this glaring absence with the lack of media scientific research on the subject!

He points out two waves of remediation in the Middle Ages (naturally without using the term itself). *First* the obvious gradual remediation of "man the medium" into "writing the medium", however, in such a way that this communicative "improvement" was "solely based on the media of the ruling class belonging to a minority"[14], while it had little impact on the majority of the people. Yet, he concludes that the traditional human media, like the court jester, the singer, narrator, preacher, and academic suffer a loss of function in matters of education, fostering of children, and world knowledge in the late Middle Ages. This is due to the increasing importance of the printed types of communication becoming more and more organised as an independent market through the book, the letter, and the chronicle, causing the decline of an oral culture, which is based on tradition and mnemonic skills.

The *second* remediation occurs at the end of the late Middle Ages in the relations between public subgroups. The course of events constituting this second remediation, runs from the Black Death, which caused the European economy and communication infrastructure to collapse, through a significant popularisation of culture to a renewed population growth in the second half of the fifteenth century, centred around cities whose citizens increased their powerbase, economy, and influence. Thus, the aristocratic and feudal societies of the Early and High Middle Ages were transformed into the estates of the realm, creating stronger nations and states. Also, the traditional boundaries between public subgroups were broken down by the inter-systemic media of the age acting as the main force of change: "This was in part the case with the letter as a medium of battle, likewise so for the beggar monks and especially concerning the travellers. Thus a decline in traditional systemic media started – they became common and therefore dysfunctional"[15]. The fool was no longer a courtly speciality, countryside plays and peasant games were influenced and replaced by ecclesiastical plays and by the games of city culture. The travelling university scholars were no longer hired as priests or ecclesiastical teachers, instead they sought their livelihood in worldly trades.

In the following chapter I shall give some Swedish and Danish examples of Faulstich's thesis, showing how an oral medium, the popular ballad, is transformed and remediated into images on church walls – most of them in the latter part of the Middle Ages.

Remediation of Ballads in Medieval Scandinavian Churches

The medieval popular ballad was born as an intermedial art form with a rich combination of modalities and means of expression: the Scandinavian ballad, like the Anglo-Saxon, is constituted through a media-integration of text and song, carried out with one or two singers, answered by a 'chorus' like in the antiphon, implying perhaps that the church was also present at "the birth of the ballad".[16] A well-known couplet Christmas carol from the Middle Ages has the same four beats as the ballad and the same rhyming system and burdens:

Puer natus est in Bethlehem (solo, four beats)
Halleluja, Halleluja (burden with four beats)
Unde gaudet Jerusalem (solo, four beats)
Halleluja, Halleluja (burden with four beats).

It is possible that we are at the root of the strophic ballad here, though it was moved from the church to other performance arenas by singers and lay people: to the churchyard, to the boat, the meadow and the market, each new arena leaving semiotic marks and situated speech acts on the textual world of the ballads.[17]

It is further discussed in ballad research whether chain dancing was also originally an *integrated* part of this qualified medium, or whether ballads were merely sometimes performed as dances in a looser *combination* with the song. In my opinion, the strophic medieval ballad is best interpreted as a ring-dance that may also be performed as a song.[18] The dance-genre, named *choros*, has roots back to the church of antiquity with its background in Greek and Jewish festive traditions, as shown by Backmann 1952.[19] According to Backmann, *Chorea* was disseminated as a joyful medium by the church.[20]

Cathedrals were open, not only to prayer and preaching, but also to the performance of various art forms. One of these, of course, was the singing of hymns, where the very church room served as an early medium and *performance arena* for a diversity of *artes*.[21] Among the gestural art forms that – according to Backmann – might be performed with churches as an arena, was the *choros*, French *carole*. It combined ring-dance and poetry with interaction between solo- and choir singing. The story is complicated by the fact that during the development of *chorea*, the Roman Church time and again banned carolling in churches and in its surroundings. Nonetheless, churchyard dancing continued, as if this *performance arena* close to the realm of the departed was essential to the art form.[22] On the other hand, there *are* very few records of ballads and ballad performances from the Middle Ages. This has raised the question: Is the ballad a medieval art form at all? Dante Alighieri gives an important key to understanding why this may be so in his *De vulgari eloquentia*: He compares *balata* with *canzone*, and says that the *canzone* is a finer art form than the *balata*; it is therefore recorded by "friends of the book", whereas the *balata* is not: The *canzone* has a text, which may stand alone, where the *balata* needs *plausores* (dancers and clappers) to be performed. Thus, the ballad cannot be reduced to the modern category of literature, but transgresses it by also involving music and performance media. It is a so-called intermodal and multisensory art form, appealing to all the senses in animate, intermedia performances. The dance is very often shown and, in a way, re-mediated *within* the Danish ballads, as for instance in the famous dance about King Valdemar the Great and his mistress Tovelil, who is baked to death by the jealous queen (referring to events in the 1160s, but probably younger):

> The Danish king would not be denied,
> And sent his horse to be at her side
> *In truth, King Valdemar loves them both.*
>
> And there they dance in the court of the queen,
> And many fair maidens there are seen.
>
> They dance four or five in a ring,
> While proud Tovelil sang for them.[23]
>
> The dance is trod by eight by nine
> While Tovelil then sang a rhyme.
> *In truth, King Valdemar loves them both.*[24]

The Ballad as Visual Art

In an earlier study, *The East-Nordic Ballad* (2006), I have shown that medieval ballads (like the quoted) may remediate other media like dancing and singing, including intermediality in several ways. In the very combination of dancing, singing and dramatic story telling, it is an *overt* intermedial art form. It is an important part of my hypothesis, however, that the East-Nordic ballad functions in *covert* interaction with a fourth art form: *images*. Many of the initial, formulaic ballad scenes (e.g. 'mother and daughter sewing' or 'knight and virgin gambling with cards') are also found in medieval pictures, such as woven tapestry, embroidery and painting.[25] An example from the new translation of Danish ballads:

In her bower sits Hillelil
None knows my sorrow save God –
She sews her seem so ill.
There is none living to whom I may tell my woe.

She sewed with silken thread her seam,
When she should sew with gold a-gleam

She sewed with silken thread her seam,
When she should sew with silk the seam.

And then unto the queen they go:
None knows my sorrow save God –
'So badly Hillelil does sew.'
There is none living to whom I may tell my woe.[26]

Pictorial scenes like these are remediated into stories that may function as a visual point-of-departure for the ballad maker, with possible feedback to the painter/artist. Normally being illiterate, the maker is also more apt to imagine ballad scenes as pictures than remembering them in the form of poetry. The scenic storytelling in ballads is similar to the tableau method of storytelling, well known from church paintings. In the ballad story, the silent figures are given voice, and through the force of music, the story often develops in a few scenes from this pictorial daily-life into gruesome tragedies and panicked situations, which the chain dancing evokes and attempts to expel. The dialectic between images and ballad texts may go both ways, and the adaptation and remediation of ballads is part of the change in style and purpose of the church room in the late Middle Ages. One of the best-known examples of this is from Sweden.

In 2009, the 500th anniversary of the great Swedish painter Albertus Pictor's death was celebrated and his collected works from more than 20 churches were published.[27] He represented three or four ballads in the central fields of the vault's fourth bay in Floda church (Södermanland, c. 1480). We see Ogier the Dane slaying the giant Burman, and here Albertus even quotes the ballad on an inscription band: "Hollager dans han wan siger af Burman" (Ogier the Dane won victory over Burman).[28] Furthermore, we see Sven Fötlink fighting a troll[29] and Didrik of Bern in single combat against Wideke Welandsson.[30] Finally, Albertus painted the struggle

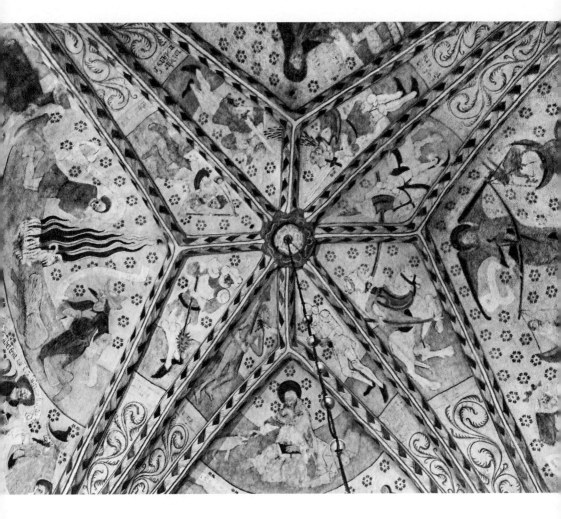

[**III. 15**] Four ballad-heroes in single combat. Wall-painting by Albertus Pictor in the church vault of Floda (the Mälar-area, Sweden, c. 1480). Photo: Tommy Olofsson.

between David and Goliath.[31] Thus, Albertus has juxtaposed a legendary ballad of a biblical motive with three popular, heroic ballads, which all show a 'Christian' fighting a 'heathen' [ill. 15].

Here we see the case of a medium that belongs to the oral culture of the late Middle Ages remediated as frescoes on a Swedish church vault. The key to interpreting these illustrations of single combat between ballad-giants is a nearby picture of the duel between Cain and Abel; thus, the pictures should be seen and interpreted as a *psykomaki* – a spiritual battle between the pure of heart and the poison of envy. Formally, the structure of the decoration follows the need of 'filling the spaces' that arise from the elaborate architecture in this large village church with its many vaults. Generally, meaningful coherence in the church decorations is established either through epic sequence, as in the many stories about Mary and the birth of Christ, or through metonymic echo-spaces around a Biblical or cultic motive, like in Floda.

The latter method is especially common in the late gothic period, often creating strongly *hyper-mediated* church walls in a rich interplay of pictorial reference, architectural detail, and decorative effect. Here, finally, one may see ludic, theatrical paintings, especially *drolleries* and grotesques, where the iconographic meaning is difficult to decode, but where many of the pictures seem to have parallels in jocular and satirical ballads that are not well known today.[32]

Other Examples from Denmark

Arising from a newfound collection of medieval ballads in the Swedish town of Växjö, a project at the Linneaus University demonstrated that the pictorial world of ballads is also mirrored in a number of Danish church paintings from 1300 onwards.[33] In the church of Ørslev (South Zealand), we have an early example of incorporating and remediating the ballad as a medium, where the typical subject matter of knightly ballads is depicted together with a demonstration of the ballad dance. It is probably no coincidence that the church is situated contiguously with Bråde, one of Denmark's greatest medieval manors (now Holsteinborg), then belonging to the bishopric of Roskilde [ill. 16].[34]

The image on the eastern wall of the south chapel is from approximately 1320. Its motive is a chain-dance beneath a painting of the holy wedding of Christ and Mary, symbolising the intimate union between God and his congregation.[35] The chain consists of three beautiful, crowned virgins, and six men. Some seem to be nobles, whereas the first and the last carrying the sun and the moon look more like comedians. The dancers demonstrate the different types of steps that belong to the ballad dance, thus endowing the painting with a visual sense of rhythm that correlates to the movements of the dance. The trumpet-playing hare is probably a symbol of a secular musician. This perhaps implies that his profession was suspicious, since the hare acts as a symbol for the Devil in some of the ballads.

The image is part of a larger composition: In the opposite corner of the holy wedding, you see a knight offering the church to John the Baptist to whom the church and a nearby holy well were consecrated. Below, a devil is putting faeces in a barrel

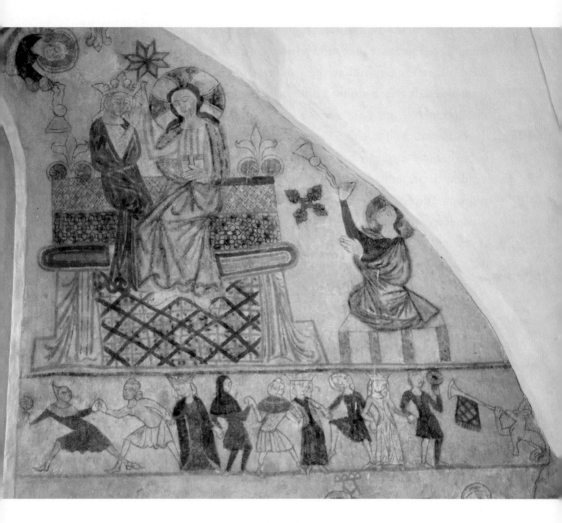

[**III. 16**] The ballad dance under the holy wedding (the south chapel in the church of Ørslev; South-Zealand, Denmark, c. 1320). Photo: Sigurd Kværndrup.

of wine, which is then ready to be consumed by a holy man with a halo. Beneath this, Christ is beaten and crucified, and Mary laments at the cross. Beneath the chain dance, four priests hold or raise the holy chalice, which is ready to be worshipped. Above the chain, the holy wedding takes place in Heaven, and the logic may be that just as chain-dancing at weddings was usual on earth, so it is in Heaven.[36] Two bands above and beneath the chain imply that the ballad dance takes place in a liminal zone between earth and Heaven. The totality of the chapel's decoration is hard to inter-pret. There is a clear appeal to all five senses, and it even seems logical that it invites a meditative viewer to raise her eyes and her heart from earth to Heaven, and through the sublime medium of the ballad dance understand that the joy on earth is nothing compared to the blessedness you shall have in heaven. At the same time, one may experience a discreet warning against believing too much in the vainglory of drinking and dancing.

In the south chapel, there are two more paintings with motives from the formulaic world of the courtly ballads. To the left you see a wooing scene, followed by the wedding to the right. Above them are painted scenes from the life of the Virgin Mary and from the birth of Jesus to the family's refuge into Egypt. The whole decoration in the chapel seems to be devoted to Mary, whom you also see mourning at the cross on the east wall. The third wall in the chapel has been decorated too, but it has not been possible to decipher it [ill. 17].

In this particular image, chalices are also raised, but here we observe a typical scene from a knightly wedding ballad where virgins with golden goblets on their white hands are courteously welcoming noblemen as their guests. The scene is found in many ballads; here from the translated, Danish ballad "Torben's Daughter and her Father's Slayer":

> And then they rode to Sir Torben's farm
> *Under the swale –*
> There stood his daughter so full of charm.
> *Comes the dawn and the dew drifts over the dale.*
>
> There stood his daughter so fair and grand,
> *Under the swale –*
> With a golden goblet in each hand.
> *Comes the dawn and the dew drifts over the dale.*
>
> She filled the goblets up to the brim,
> *Under the swale –*
> Her father's slayer, she toasted him.
> *Comes the dawn and the dew drifts over the dale.*[37]

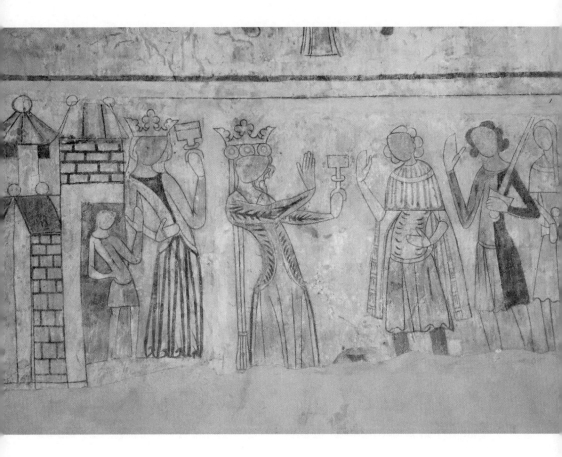

[Ill. 17] The virgin "standing outside" (the gate) "with a golden goblet in each hand", welcoming virtuous suitors (the south chapel in the church of Ørslev; South-Zealand, Denmark, c. 1320). Photo: Sigurd Kværndrup.

On the south wall's right side, you see the wedding between the noble virgin and her wooing knight. Two beautiful horses are ready to carry the newly wedded couple to the knight's farm. As in many ballads, a musician plays the fiddle at the wedding, and the singer assures us that "no gold was spared for musicians and mountebanks" [ill. 18].

This is far from the only ballad painting in the churches, though many are legendary ballads whose heroes are also saints. Why are such motives painted on church walls? Why are the music, the dance and the tales of ballads remediated in the space of cultic and liturgical media with their own forms of singing, performing, and storytelling? The explanation may be that the popular ballad is regarded as a liminal

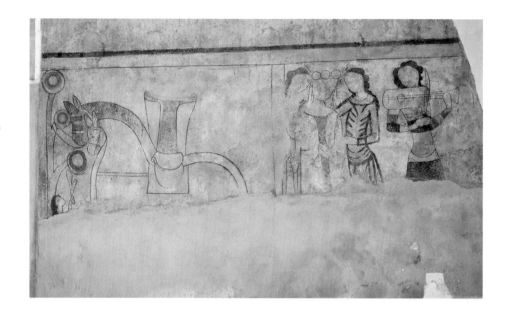

[**III. 18**] The jester plays at the virgin's wedding (the south chapel in the church of Ørslev; South-Zealand, Denmark, c. 1320). Photo: Sigurd Kværndrup.

medium that is able to establish and mediate communication between the sensual and the holy world: between the spaces of popular entertainment and amusement and the spaces of cult and liturgy. The following example is from the waning of the Middle Ages where the painters often hit more sombre notes (Nørre Alslev, Falster 1500).

The Dance of Death

The Dance of Death, on the western arch leading to the tower-room of the church in Nørre Alslev, is not exactly a remediation of a ballad, but of a literary genre. This is in turn a further development of a kind of penitent sermon, the *Memento Mori*. However, contrary to the norm for death dances – as in nearby Lübeck – the Dance of Death in Nørre Alslev is shaped as a choir dance (*choros*): the dancers hold each other's hands as in a ballad chain, and they move from right to left, like in the ballad, but with a heavy stride. Comparing the two dance-frescoes, one immediately notices that it is only the half-rotten dead who jump and dance merrily like all the dancers in the church of Ørslev. The other participants, from the peasant with his shovel to the nobleman, the bishop, and the king, wade mechanically and stiffly onwards like

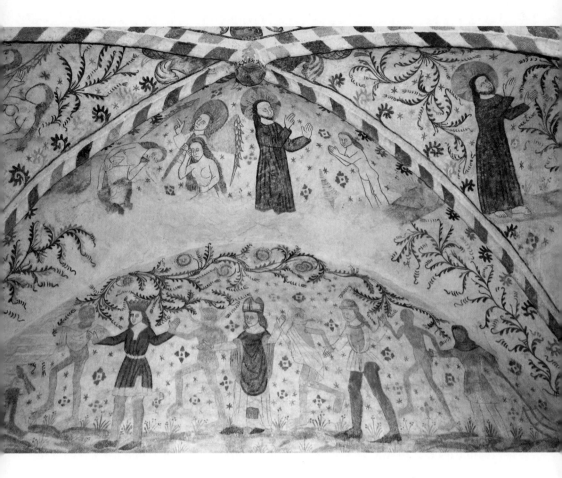

[Ill. 19] The dance of death (the west wall of the church in Nørre Alslev, Falster, Denmark, c. 1500). Photo: Sigurd Kværndrup.

people who do not really want to join in, even if they are forced to do so. The Dance of Death visualises an egalitarian principle possibly hailing from the mendicant orders.[38] Farthest to the left, where the maw of Hell could also have been located, we notice a fragment of a musician and his instrument, which is probably the drone on a bagpipe [ill. 19].

The painting is clearly one of the many *Mahnbilder* from the late Middle Ages, showing the transitory nature of earthly life and perdition's terrifying consequences at the hour of death. Nevertheless, the frieze also encompasses a radiant and sensual multitude of voices in the ornamentation, which encircles, indeed permeates, the scene. Below, Creation is seen in the form of fertile soil, herbs, and flowers trickling forth. Above, a vine from the tree of life is visible, pointing beyond death as a symbol of salvation; it springs from the left hand corner of the painting and could possibly be seen as an encouraging alternative to the dance of death. Between these two poles, flowers rise from earth towards Heaven, like the prayers of man, and stars fall from Heaven like the grace of God. Below the mural was the font, above it the creation and fall of Adam and Eve. Its style is typical for the important Elmelunde work-shop,[39] and the Danish art historian Søren Kaspersen sees the combination of warn-ing and hope for the children of Adam as typical for decorations executed near the centre for the worship of the holy Birgitta in Maribo on the island of Lolland, in the proximity of Nørre Alslev.[40]

Satirical Drama and Jocular Ballads, Remediated

The church paintings from the late fifteenth century Scandinavia also contain a number of decorations with strong satirical elements. This is given in a style so free and daring that it can astonish even a spectator of our time. The best-researched part of this tendency is the remediation of Danish medieval theatre, in studies by Haas-trup and Kaspersen.[41] The church of Linderöd in Scania has another fine example from 1498 of medial sectors being mixed together, thus portraying an outspoken boundary breakdown between the public subgroups that Faulstich has shown. On the northern wall of the nave, a mural depicts a young man holding one of his clogs in his left hand, while waving his right hand. It would seem that he is signalling a sad goodbye to Christ in the church's choir. What is going on? The painting stems from a range of jocular ballads that describe the loss of a young man or woman's sexual innocence, using the popular image of the lost shoe or slipper. To whom the man with the clog has lost his innocence is shown in the painting with astounding open-ness: right under the man a woman's anatomy is seen from below. Another picture shows a man trying in vain to shoe a cat, a task, which according to ballads and proverbs is as impossible as recreating virginity after it is lost. Above this ballad, we see Adam and Eve falling out of Eden while they mourn the conditions of mankind on earth. In the mural's remediation of both Biblical narrative and ballad motif, it creates a new visual exegesis of what it is that man really falls into [ill. 20].[42]

[**Ill. 20**] The young man with a lost clog (the north wall in the church of Linderöd, Scania, Sweden, 1498). Photo: Tommy Olofsson.

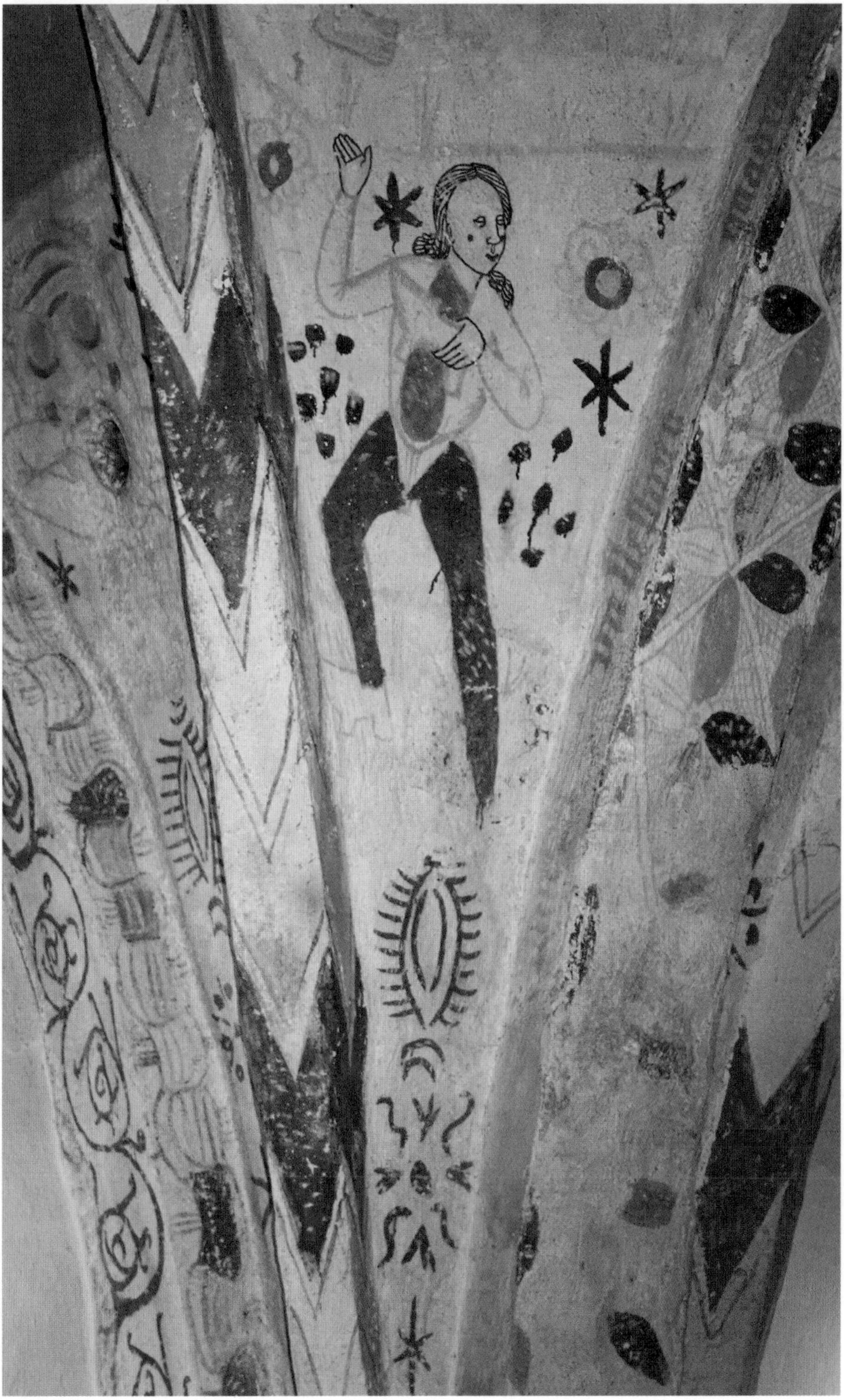

Orality in Images:
A Multisensory Remediation

Towards the end of the Middle Ages, the decoration of many churches seemingly changed and also attracted profane means of expression, leading to a multisensory remediation of many different art forms into images on the church walls. One explanation for this is that new classes and the mendicant orders had a strong influence on the decoration of the churches, where it had formerly been the prerogative of the aristocracy and the clergy.[43] Thus, parts of the oral cultures were now remediated into images on the church walls, even before they were recorded in printed media. Another explanation is that the very space of the church was transformed and the function of its walls changed. In the earlier Middle Ages, church paintings might have had a ceremonial and hieratic function; in the later Middle Ages they also acquired a moral and edifying function. The church walls would tell moral stories for the churchgoers or show the glory of God's creation, even in images from real life. Not least, suggestive *Mahnbilder* would highlight the dangers that arise from sin and the fall of mankind [ill. 19 and 20]. In this way, the church room itself became the most important mass medium of its time, addressing literally *everybody* and presenting *all aspects* of the culture – remediating all media, including visual and performative, oral and literary, liturgical and theatrical media.

Notes

1   Bolter & Grusin 1999, p. 5.

2   Bolter & Grusin 1999, p. 73.

3   See McLuhan 1965, esp. part II, pp. 77-105; Ong 1982.

4   See Elleström (ed.) 2010.

5   Bolter & Grusin 1999, p. 3.

6   Bolter & Grusin 1999, p. 3.

7   This is the title of chapter 1 in McLuhan 1965, pp. 7-21.

8   Bolter & Grusin 1999, p. 24, discusses this with Panofsky's *Perspective as Symbolic Form* (1927).

9   Smith 2007, p. 8 ff.

10   Bolter & Grusin 1999, p. 70.

11   Bolter & Grusin 1999, pp. 70-71.

12   In "The Modalities of Media" Elleström discusses Bolter & Grusin 1999: "It is a very inspiring book, full of interesting observations relevant for intermedial studies, but the authors' notions of media and remediation are conspicuously vague. In their view, a 'medium' seems to be all kinds of modalities [...] and all kinds of media as (not) defined by McLuhan." Elleström 2010, p. 47.

13   See Elleström 2010, pp. 12-17, where he distinguishes between technical media (such as a book, a TV-set, a stage), basic media (like word, song, dance, picture,) and qualified media (meaning art forms with a specific history).

14   Faulstich 1996, p. 269: "bezogen nur auf die Herrschaftsmedien einer kleinen Schicht."

15   Faulstich 1996, p. 270: "Partiell den Brief als Kampfmedium, sodann die Bettelmönche und vor allem die Fahrenden. Damit ging ein Verfall der traditionellen systemischen Medien als solcher einher – sie wurden ubiquitär und infolgedessen dysfunktional."

16   An important point in Pound 1921, and Kværndrup 2010. Colbert 1989 proves that the Scandinavian ballad is of medieval origin in *The Birth of the Ballad*.

17   An allegorical legend takes place at Christmas in the German village of Kölbigk in 1021, recorded in four countries: Twelve dancers abducted the vicars' daughter and carolled with her in the very churchyard during mass time, singing a typical couplet ballad stanza with one burden: "Equitabat Bouo per silvam frondosam, ducebat sibi Mersuinden formosam/ Quid stamus? Cur non imus?" (Bovo rode through the leafy woods, taking with him the beautiful Merswind. Why are we halting? Why don't we move on?). The special reason for the recording being that the dancers were punished by the Lord with constant dancing; after a year this was, however, reduced to shivering, explaining perhaps the reason for getting the illness of Saint Veits dance.

18   In accordance with Gummere 1907, and others.

19   Backman 1952.

20   A document from the hand of the East Roman Emperor shows Nordic dancers as early as 950 at the court of the Emperor Constantine VII Porphyrogennetos in Constantinople, where "axmen" from heathen Scandinavia entertain him at Christmas with ring-dances (*chorea*). This could also be understood as an example to the effect that chain dancing may also have local and even heathen roots.

21 See Dreyer 1997, and Kværndrup 2010. The concept of *Performance arena* is from Foley 1995. The concept points to the actual scenes wherein some oral performance was conducted, and to the expectations that are inherent in the reception of a qualified oral medium.

22 See Sachs 1937. Bourcier 1978 gives several examples of ecclesiastical prohibitions against caroling in churches; thus Pope Zacharias as early as 774 decreed a ban against "les chants et caroles des femmes à l'église", p. 52. And Bourcier adds that the persistence of the bans proves the persistence of the dance.

23 This stanza, together with the next, represents a fine example of the so called *incremental repetition* (with Gummere 1907), a stylistic device typical for partly improvised oral poetry; this is seen in all the quoted ballads.

24 Translation by Broadbridge 2011, p. 64. The ballad is number 121A out of 535 types with several thousand variants in DgF (The Ancient Ballads of Denmark). The collection of ballads began as early as 1550 in Denmark where many hundreds were written down.

25 A fine collection has been preserved from the destructions of war, in photos by Kurth 1926.

26 Broadbridge 2011, p. 61. "Hillelil's sorrow" is DgF number 83.

27 Albertus Pictor lived from approximately 1440 to 1509.

28 The ballad "Holger Dansk och Burman" (SMB 216; DgF 30); SMB means *The Medieval Ballads of Sweden*. Jansson 2009 argues to the effect that Albertus had probably heard these ballads, part of the oral culture as they were.

29 The ballad "Sven Fötling och trollet" (SMB 210; DgF 31).

30 The source could be a ballad. The plot is known in the West-Nordic *Didriks saga af Bern*.

31 This may also refer to the ballad "David och Goliat" (SMB 200, only known in Sweden).

32 An example of this is given at the end of the chapter.

33 The project was carried out by the Linneaus University docent and poet Tommy Olofsson, together with the author of this chapter. It has resulted in more than a thousand photos of church paintings. The work, *The Middle Ages in Word and Image*, was published in Sweden 2013. The photos in this chapter are by Tommy Olofsson, except for those from Ørslev Church, which are by the author.

34 The church is described in Hermansen & Nørlund (ed.) 1938; the decorations in Haastrup (ed.) 1989, pp. 895-913. The decoration was restored by Jakob Kornerup in 1886. The National Museum of Denmark has lately discovered new paintings in Ørslev. Ulla Haastrup writes about the paintings in the south chapel, that they are parallel to worldly decorations, and that dancing- and wedding-scenes among others are known from a private house in Bern, Switzerland from the early fourteenth century. See also Haupt 1995.

35 Or, as the crowned woman has no halo around her head, the painting may show the Danish queen Ingeborg who – at the time of the painting – ended her days as a nun, thus being 'the bride of Christ'.

36 See Kaspersen 1979.

37 Broadbridge 2011, pp. 51-52. The ballad is printed in DgF as number 288. The ballad is not a typical knightly wedding-ballad, as the virgin is abducted by her wooer who has killed her father.

38 See Rosenfeld 1956 and Kaiser 1983 with German dance macabre-texts.

39 See Hammer 1990. About the dance of death in Nørre Alslev: Hammer 1990, pp. 79 ff., 139 f.

40 See Kaspersen 2013, forthcoming.

41 See Haastrup 1980, pp. 135-156: "The wall paintings in the parish church of Bellinge (dated 1496), explained by parallels in contemporary European theatre", and Kaspersen 1988.

151

42 The painting is analysed by Tommy Olofsson in Kværndrup & Olofsson 2013, pp. 12-21.

43 An important point in the many works of the late Axel Bolvig; see Bolvig 2002.

152

[**DEVOTION**] The body, the senses, and the five perceptual organs were activated and incorporated in late medieval devotion.
The present chapter addresses visual illustrations and textual descriptions of devotional *practice,* understood as the actual bodily
movements, the use of objects, the uttering of words, the mental
exercises, and the application of the senses involved in devotional actions. Through the performance of sometimes very intricate clusters of mental and physical actions, the material body
and the spiritual soul were locked in a reciprocal relationship, influencing each other and joining forces in a mutual attempt to
reach God. A central focus of the chapter is to shed light on how
practice strategically served to establish this reciprocal relationship and in particular how the senses were made to play an instrumental role in the process. It does not study sensory perception of specific devotional *objects,* but instead concentrates on
the corradiation of perceptive impressions that meet and merge
in and through practice, i.e. the structural role of the senses in
devotion as such. It is argued that compound and synaesthetic
forms of sensory perception were integral to late medieval devotional practice.

DEVOTION

Perception as Practice and Body as Devotion in Late Medieval Piety

[Laura Katrine Skinnebach]

The Practice of Devotion

Devotio or devotion was one of the main preoccupations of late medieval life. It was continuously dealt with in visual material and a large body of various writings. Devotion was not merely to *believe* something to be true – the existence of God – but to integrate this belief into one's entire life, so that it influenced and determined views, actions, attitudes, and relations.[1] In the widely reproduced and popular devotional text *De Imitatione Christi*, Thomas a Kempis (1380-1471) wrote: "At the Day of Judgement, we shall not be asked what we have read, but what we have done; not how eloquently we have spoken, but how holily we have lived."[2] In order to be a true devoted Christian one had to *live* a life in constant awareness of the significance of all actions. *Devotio* was the heartfelt and active expression and declaration of faith, and was the core element of both *vita activa* and *vita contemplativa*. At the same time devotion was an extremely comprehensive term covering an extensive range of actions that were continuously reproduced but at the same time constantly subject to alterations and debates, which resulted in new variants side by side with old ones. What these actions had in common was that they attempted to interact with God and had the immanent element of *something done*.

This active aspect of devotion may fruitfully be studied as *practice*. Ludwig Wittgenstein once stated that the practice of language comprises not only the words themselves and their meanings, but also the "actions into which it is woven [...]".[3] When attempting to understand the meaning of language one must, according to Wittgenstein, approach how it is effectuated in specific situations instead of looking at single words and their grammatical relations to other words. It then becomes a study not of language as something definitive, but of how language is given meaning and becomes meaningful through its use, that is, through how it is practiced. When regarding devotion in parallel terms, as *practice*, the investigation of it becomes a study of the *actions* of devotion. It is a study that is interested in the composition of devotion, how the different elements of devotional practice, the combination of movements, gestures, objects, words, and locations are activated during the process and how they relate to one another as each of these elements are in turn activated in the devotional process. It is ultimately a study of meaning-production itself and how specific aspects of devotional practice – in this case actions that involve perception – are given meaning in a specific context.

The practice of devotion can be studied in a large variety of material traces. Donations, testaments, pilgrimage, altarpieces, murals, book-illuminations, devotional guides, books of hours, theological treatises, disputations, music, liturgical books, and architecture informed, aided, and instructed the devout on *how* to live and, thus, represent expressions of medieval devotional life and the practise of it. For the purpose of the present investigation, I focus on a few of these expressions, limiting the scope to a selection of prayers from four, Danish, late-medieval devotional books originally used and produced in the late fifteenth and early sixteenth centuries.[4] In these books – which belonged to Marine Issdatter, Johanne Nielsdatter Munk, Anna Brade, and one unknown owner – most devotions are explained in introductory *rubrics* (Lat. *ruber* = red, because they were written in red ink). Sometimes these rubrics describe punctilious and intricate patterns of movement, gestures, words, locations, and objects; other times they are simple, mentioning only the name of a specific saint and a short prayer. These rubrics recount how devotion is performed and composed and, thus, have a focal position in the argument.

As a supplement – but also as a point in itself – I have included two central devotional instructions, The *Itinerarium mentis in Deum* written by the Franciscan friar Bonaventure (1221-1274) and *The Nine Ways of Prayer of St. Dominic*, also known as *De modi orandi* compiled about 1280 by an anonymous Dominican friar. These two books have many things in common with the Danish material and demonstrate that devotional books produced in the thirteenth century had been widely absorbed by mendicant, monastic, and lay practitioners in the fifteenth and sixteenth centuries, so that it followed some of the same strategies and logic regarding the use of body, senses, and perceptual processes as means for religious experience and progress. It has often been argued that medieval cultural interaction exceeded the dichotomies historians tend to draw between accepted and unaccepted, learned and lay, between orthodoxy and the 'popular', and the present investigation illustrates that this was indeed the case.[5] Although the Danish primers, to which I refer in the present chapter, originally belonged to monastic women or women of the nobility, they include material that would have had a wide appeal and may have circulated beyond these limited groups.

The theological guides and writings – and Bonaventure's book in particular – contain extremely thorough descriptions of the *technical* aspects of ascending, that is, *how* man who is bound to a material body is able to experience the immaterial God. This question of man's access to the experiences of God was completely fundamental in medieval theology of devotion with Dionysius the Areopagite (late fifth to early sixth century) and John of Damascus (c. 655-750) as central figures. Later it was treated by the Dominican Thomas Aquinas (1225-1274), in his writing on the senses (most notably in his commentary on Aristotle), which is also referred to in the present study. Whereas Bonaventure describes, in great detail, how the process of human perception may be engaged and used in the service of divine experience, Thomas Aquinas argues – in continuation of Bonaventure and inspired by Aristotle – that the senses mediate between the soul and the material world. Although these two prominent theologians belonged to different orders, their ideas on devotional perception share many similarities and seem to have been implemented into more ordinary forms of devotion. Their ideas concerning the body and the senses permeate – as will be shown – the structure of devotional practice as illustrated by the Danish examples.

Exceeding the Body-Soul Distinction

Questions concerning the devotional significance of the body were tremendously important in the late Middle Ages. The debate and ambivalence concerning how God could be manifested through matter, and how matter could be incorporated in the practice of devotion, frequently surfaced in theological disputes, treatises and devotional guides. Questions concerning how to *deal* with the body lay at the very core of these reflections, because of the paradoxical nature of the relation between the human body and the divine spiritual soul. The result was not a complete rejection of the flesh, as much as it was an attempt to embrace it.[6]

There are numerous examples that indicate how the body was in*corporated* in the practice of devotion. In female monastic devotion fasting was used as a means to intensify the devotional experience, and not merely as means to discipline a disobedient, material body.[7] And although severe, self-inflicted pain and castigation – common as it was in mendicant circles in particular – could be seen as an attempt to suppress the body, it was also a way in which the close bond between body and soul became effectively and physically manifest to the self, while at the same time adding to the devoutness of the soul. As Caroline Walker Bynum, who has devoted much of her research to topics that relate to questions concerning the importance of body and matter in medieval faith and spirituality, has stated: "Control, discipline, and torture of the flesh is, in medieval devotion, not so much the rejection of physicality as the elevation of it – a horrible yet delicious elevation – into means of access to the divine."[8] The most significant example of this is perhaps the intense interest in the blood of Christ exhibited by medieval theologians and devotional practitioners. The holy blood was regarded as the ultimate sign of God's humanity and, thus, as a means to access God precisely because it represented physical bodily life – and also death – itself. As Bynum has stated, "[…] given fifteenth century physiological assumptions, blood was the stuff of – and life of – the body, yet its spilling was violation and dying; blood came forth in both death and progeny; it leaped onto those it saved and those it accused; it was continuity and rupture, presence and absence."[9] Blood represented the link between man and God because it was the ultimate sign of likeness and Incarnation.

Incorporation of body and perception in devotional practice became one of the main strategies, aiming at constituting one devout entity, body and soul in corporation.[10] The ways in which this incorporation could be brought about were numerous and can be found in the very organisation of devotional practice. In the prologue to *The Nine Ways of Prayer of St. Dominic*, the writer explicates the purpose of his text by making the following observation about the connection between body and soul:

> However, what we must say something about here is the way of praying in which the soul uses the members of the body in order to rise more devoutly to God, so that the soul, as it causes the body to move, is in turn moved by the body, until sometimes it comes to be in ecstasy like Paul, sometimes in agony like our Saviour, and sometimes in rupture like the prophet David.[11]

Through the physical body, the soul, which makes the body move according to its will, is able to express its devotional experience. The body may also, if used in the correct way, intensify the devotional state of the soul. What the author of *The Nine*

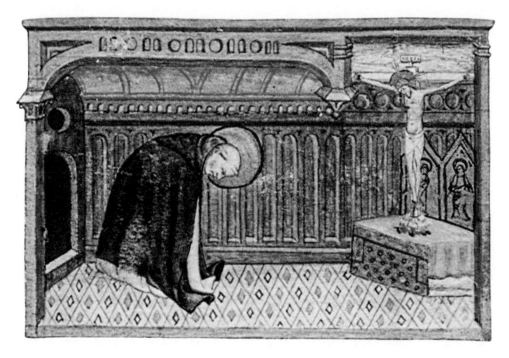

[**III. 21**] St. Dominic bowing head and heart before the alter with the bleeding crucifix as the ultimate sign of the impact of his prayer. Illustration from Cod. Rossianus 3
dating from c. 1330. The Vatican Library.

Ways underlines here is that there exists a reciprocal relationship (Lat. *reciprocus* =
interdependent, mutual) between body and soul. The soul ultimately moves the
body to act, and may in fact move it in a way so that it is put to devotional use: when
the soul moves the body, the soul is in turn moved by the body.

The main theme of the booklet is, then, to provide inspiration and guidance in
the *practice of body-soul reciprocity.* The first practice described is based on the
assumption that the prayer of a man who humbles himself 'pierces the clouds'. The
practice is performed by "bowing humbly before the altar as if Christ, whom the
alter signifies, were really and personally present and not just symbolically."[12] The
writer describes in detail how St. Dominic supposedly did it:

> So the holy father, standing with his body erect, would bow his head and his heart
> humbly before Christ his Head, considering his own servile condition and the out-
> standing nobility of Christ, and giving himself up entirely to venerating Him.[13]

Dominic gives "himself up entirely" with body and soul by bowing head and heart together, a parallel physical and mental bow. By putting the bodily limbs in the service of the soul, the two aspects of human nature conform to each other and become one entirely devoted person. To the writer, St. Dominic represents the perfect example of how body and soul can become one in the devotional veneration of Christ, how the whole human being is absorbed in the performance of humility.

The devotional effect of the practice and how it fulfils its devotional *end* is illustrated by the small accompanying image [ill. 21].[14] It shows Dominic before an altar with a crucifix. But the crucifix is no longer merely a statue. Christ is "really and personally present, not just symbolically", literally soaking the altar-cloth with the blood streaming from His feet. Through St. Dominic's simultaneous performance of inner and outer humility, Christ may now be perceived with mind and bodily alike. In fact eight out of the nine images in the booklet depict Dominic before a crucifix that, as the result of his devotion, bleeds extensively from hands, feet, and sidewound. A crucifix is mentioned explicitly as a devotional aid in one of the practice descriptions (no. 4), which underlines the continuity of meaning in texts and images in this version of the *modi orandi*. Both provide examples to follow and imitate, indeed the images make it even more imploring by foregrounding the outcome. The bleeding crucifix vividly illustrates that the prayer performed by St. Dominic has actually been received and exchanged for an experience of the presence of Christ. [ill. 22].

The attempt to establish a reciprocal relation between body and soul was not particular to the booklet or something exclusively Dominican or monastic for that matter. Similar strategies permeate other devotional guides, including Danish, medieval, devotional books. A Danish medieval prayer book from the fifteenth century, which originally belonged to Marine Issdatter from the Bridgettine monastery in Maribo, contains the following short practice:

> Notice [*Mærk*] what is written in the following
> The first with genuflection for the annunciation / the second curtsying with hands folded across the knees for his sweat / the third kneeling with hands lifted upwards / the fourth lying prostrate also to his sweat / the fifth standing with hands crossed over the chest to his laceration / the sixth kneeling and between each time kissing the ground to his coronation and carrying of the cross / the seventh standing cross-wise to his crucifixion / the eighth sitting down with hands crossed over the lap to his descent from the cross / the ninth Ad Veniam for his burial / the tenth with genuflection for his resurrection and ascension and for the assumption of Virgin Mary.[15]

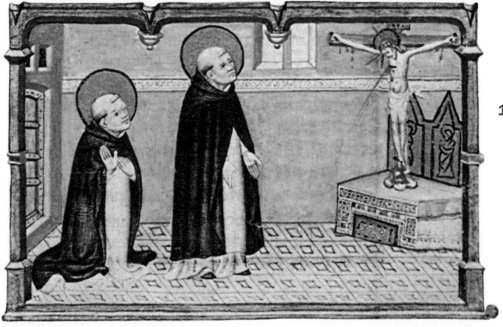

[**III. 22**] The fourth way of praying according to *De modi orandi* of St. Dominic. The image accompanies a text describing how Dominic would sometimes stand before the altar and "fix his gaze on the crucifix, looking intently at the cross and kneeling down over and over again, a hundred times perhaps [...]". The writer states that after a while he would look as if he had managed to penetrate heaven in his mind. The resulting practice has a visible impact on the crucifix, bleeding as it is from hands, feet, and sidewound. Illustration in Cod. Rossianus 3 from c. 1330. The Vatican Library.

The practice differs from other practices because it does not include a prayer text. It is simply composed of different bodily movements, each of them performed in commemoration of different events in the life and Passion of Christ and Virgin Mary. The events are ordered chronologically in the same way as the stations of the cross, and the movements are most often chosen for their associative function; kneeling and kissing the ground accompanies the carrying of the cross, which commemorates how Christ stumbled under the weight of the heavy cross; the crucifixion is accompanied by a bodily position similar to a cross; Christ's burial is commemorated *ad Veniam*, i.e. by lying face down on the ground.[16] Physical movements and mental practices are performed simultaneously so that body and soul are reciprocally integrated. Furthermore, the bodily positions and their mimicry of Christ during the Passion create at close connection between the body of the devout and the body of Christ. It is as if body and mind enacts the Passion together and thus establishes a mental as well as physical imprint of it.

The distinction between body and mind, between Christ and devotee, is blurred, which is underlined and nurtured by the introductory words of the rubric "Mærk væl thette". The Danish verb "mærk" means both to take *notice* of and to *feel* as well as it means *mark*. "Mærk" is, then, a word that refers both to a physical and a mental practice as well as how that practice makes its *mark* on the practitioner. Body and soul are mutually influencing each other, pursuing the same goal: to be fully imbued and imprinted with the life and Passion of Christ. Although physical images are not explicitly mentioned this does, however, not exclude the possibility that the bodily movements could have been performed before a series of physical images showing the different stations of the Passion of Christ, underlining to the practitioner the similarities between the body of the devotee and the suffering body of the incarnated God in the visual depiction. In any case the mental experience of the Passion – marked by the text or aided by a physical image or inner images stored in memory – merged and reciprocated with the actions performed by the devoutly obedient and productive body.

A very different practice that further exemplifies the integration and mutual involvement of body and soul can be found in a Book of Hours from around 1480. It originally belonged to the niece of Jens Iversen Lange, bishop in Aarhus, Denmark 1449-1482, Johanne Nielsdatter Munk, a lady of the nobility who was married to the head of the Imperial Court (*Rigsråd*) Oluf Mortensen Gyrstinge. The practice consists of a short rubric and ten fairly long prayers devoted to the Virgin Mary. The rubric states that a person who devoutly (*meth gudælighet*) reads the prayers before the image of the Virgin for thirty days with one burning candle will, without a doubt, be heard regardless of whatever sorrow that person is in.[17] Between each of the ten prayers the practitioner is instructed to stand up while reading ten *ave maria*, suggesting that the prayers are performed kneeling. The prayers follow the chronology of the life of the Virgin beginning with the Annunciation and gradually, one by one, the long readings unfold the mystery of the Virgin birth. Simultaneously the body is activated and moves in accordance with the structural alternation between the two kinds of prayer; the contemplative readings and the repetitive recitation of the *ava marias*. The ten long contemplative prayers demanded inner reflections on the miraculous Incarnation and were thus accompanied by a humble physical position while the *ave marias*, most likely 'read' from memory, saluted and reached out towards the graceful Virgin who would, as a result of the practice, provide protection and aid (as the rubric stated). At the same time the candle, which would have been purchased or produced and lit in advance before the image of the Virgin, illuminated the visually rendered features of the Virgin in accordance with the prayer's progressive enlightenment of the soul to the amazing nature of the Incarnation.

The three examples above are taken from very different devotional contexts, thus underlining that the reciprocal relation between body and soul was not only a matter of interest in specific devotional circles. It was not merely a monastic concern either; it characterised devotional professionalism and lay devotion alike. Practice of devotion generally strived towards transcending the paradoxical relation between body and soul by transforming the relation into a mutual dependence. The constant attempt to establish a devout character – a virtuous *habitus* – involved the practice of reciprocity where body and soul followed each other closely, firmly integrated, making common cause in contemplating God. In late medieval devotional practice the body was not reduced to a mouthpiece for the expressions of the soul, but was a devotional agent in its own right. Devoutness was impregnated onto the soul as the body was formed into a *figura* of devoutness. Through the practice of devotion the threshold between body and soul was effectively pierced and exceeded, leaving the whole organism saturated with devotion.

The Process of Devotional Perception

The reciprocity between body and soul aided and enforced the pious experience. The establishment of a reciprocal connection relied very much on the *practice of perception*, which carried a distinct meaning in the medieval context. The practices described in *The Nine Ways of Prayer of St. Dominic*, as well as Marine Issdatter's and Johanne Nielsdatter's devotional books involved a whole variety of perceptual actions that covered almost the entire physical sensorium. As the examples have shown, the practice of perception was not confined to the use of devotional objects such as images, prayer books, prints, or other kinds of *devotionalia*.[18] It also comprised other perceptual aspects that could be experienced with the physical and mental senses in combination. Touching the cold floor with one's – occasionally bare – knees, while kneeling in prayer; smelling the odour of incense in the church room, shifting between standing and kneeling, tasting the sweet words of prayer, lighting a candle, or listening to one's own voice uttering the different virtues of the Virgin are all examples of sensory practices and impressions that made up the devotional performance. Muscular movements and actions that involved perception were – just as devotional objects – able to establish a cognitive link between the sensible world, *sensibilia*, and the internal intelligence, *intelligibilia*. As Henning Laugerud has argued perception could ultimately mediate divine presence by referring the perceiving agent to that which the sensible world signified.[19] Beholding an image of Christ, for example, would refer the beholder to Christ. In a similar manner other forms of perception would do the same; by letting the senses smell, hear, see, feel, and taste holy sensibles, the mind would be referred to what the sensibles signified. The smell of incense, the sound of prayers or words from Scripture, the feeling of the floor or the body formed as a cross etc. were sensory actions that carried a well-established devotional meaning and signified God.

Sensory perception of material circumstances should thus be understood on the background of this reciprocal and permeable relationship between body and soul. The body was a perceiving organ that incorporated the material world through the senses. At the beginning of the fifth century St. Augustine wrote in his *De Trinitate* that:

> [...] although an inanimate body does not sense anything, yet it is through a bodily instrument [*instrumentum*] that the conscious soul is mixed with the body senses, and it is this instrument that is called sense.[20]

The instrumental sensorium mediated the surrounding physical world to the mind and the inner senses. In a devotional context this *liminal* function of the senses was treated with a certain ambivalence: the senses were regarded as faculties without a will of their own, and thus no ability to filter good from evil. Sensory incorporation of the outer world, of sensibles, could, then, potentially have both positive and negative effects on body and soul, and the consequences could be grave as an English writer stated around 1440 in the text called *Jacob's Well*:

> Keep your sight from lecherous sights and your ears from lecherous hearing and your mouth from lecherous speech and your nose from dishonest smelling and your limbs, hands and mouth and your other members from lecherous touching. These are the five wits and gates through which the enemies enter the heart.[21]

The senses were regarded as passages between the human soul and the world outside and these passages had to be carefully attended to in order to prevent them from indulging in sinful perception. Or else the soul would fall to the enemy. In other words, the senses had to be guided and guarded by a virtuous *habitus*, as Thomas Aquinas argued, that is, dispositions to act in a certain – good – way located in each individual soul as a result of previous practice.[22] This was a recurring theme in medieval theology, but it was equally predominant in devotional guides and prayer books. A prayer to the Virgin Mary from the anonymous AM 418,12° concludes with the following typical petition: "help me to true peace in body and mind […] and guard my five senses".[23] In this specific case a rubric promises that the one who performs the prayer with a humble heart and in commemoration of the Virgin, will be granted 100 days of indulgence and "see" the Virgin at the hour of death.[24] Guarding the sensorium was, then, also a practice of purification of the passage between inner and outer, resulting in an ability to sense more clearly, in this case to be able to actually *see* the Virgin when passing from this life to the next.

In spite of the grave prospects, it was an undeniable fact that the bodily senses could also – if applied and used correctly and reciprocally – mediate God. Many medieval descriptions of the process leading to contemplation in fact began with sensory perception. Aquinas stated in *Summa Theologica* that: "it is natural to man to attain to intellectual truths through sensible objects, because all our knowledge originates from the senses."[25] From the preliminary considerations of the sensual world, the process gradually ascends towards a divine level, the perfection of contemplation. One of the most comprehensive descriptions of this process is the *Itinerarium mentis in Deum* written in 1259 by the Franciscan St. Bonaventure. He divided the way to contemplation into six stages corresponding with the six powers of the soul: the senses, the imagination, the reason, the intellect, intelligence, and the sparkle of the ground of the soul (*sensus, imaginatio, ratio, intellectus, intelligentia* et *apex mentis seu synderesis scintilla*).[26] Concerning the first step towards contemplation Bonaventure writes:

> Whoever, therefore, is not enlightened by such splendour of created things is blind; whoever is not awakened by such outcries is deaf; whoever does not praise God because of all these effects is dumb; whoever does not discover the First Principle from such clear signs is a fool. Therefore open your eyes, alert the ears of your spirit, open your lips and apply your heart so that in all creatures you may see, hear, praise and worship, glorify and honour your God lest the whole world rise against you.[27]

This first step is the basic sensory experience of the world, that is, experiencing God *through* the world. God has left certain signs or vestiges (*vestigia*) in the world: "In order to contemplate the First Principle, who is most spiritual, eternal and above us, we must pass through his vestiges, which are material, temporal and outside of us."[28] So the way to God is in its nature a kind of *passing through* the sensory *instrumentum*.

The second step is the understanding of God *in* the world. The world, macro cosmos, reaches the soul, micro cosmos, through the five senses. Here sensory phenomena, not in the form of substances, but in the form of likenesses, *similitudines*, are absorbed by perception, guided by lust and judgment. *Similitudines* are created in a *medium* between sensible substance or *sensibilia*, and the senses. Sight perceives colours, Bonaventure states, as well as heavenly and luminous bodies; touch perceives solid and earthly bodies; taste, hearing, and smell perceives everything in between, that is, liquids enter through taste, phenomena of the air enter through the ears and all that has the form of steam enters through the sense of smell. Colours, light, textures, liquids, steam etc. are media or certain forms that the similitudes can take, and these media transport the similitudes to the outer senses in the form of sense-impressions.[29]

From here, on the third step, the outer senses are transferred to the inner senses where the cognitive faculty *ratio*, perceives it. Both Bonaventure and Aquinas maintained that the soul possessed four internal sensory faculties that processed the outer sensory objects mediated by the body's perceptual *instrumentum:* common sense, phantasy/imagination, estimation, and memory.[30] The inner senses were not construed as equivalent to the five outer senses, but described as apprehensive abilities that processed the sensory perceptions passing from the outside world, into the mind, through the bodily senses. The disparate sensory perceptions mediated through the proper senses were brought together in the common sense (which I will return to below). The sense data gathered by the common sense were then retained and preserved by phantasy/imagination in the form of *phantasms* or internal images. The estimative power received the intention of things (this was beyond the ability of the perceptive organs, because it had spiritual character) and memory stored them for later use. These internal senses form the basis of human perception and cognition.

The fourth step is the door to Christ (or Christ as the door). Only by grace is man able to overstep this boundary and 'regain' the senses of the soul in order to 'sense' Christ internally.[31] On the fifth level man beholds – with the restored inner perception – the invisible reality of God. Using the inner eye is to learn to see again, as Bonaventure explains. Finally, on this sixth level, man is able to sense internally, with his new restored senses, everything the human thought is unable to comprehend. The spirit has exceeded the world of sensibles and itself, and is illuminated by God, while at the same time it recognises itself in the sparkle of the ground of soul, as the image of God.[32]

According to Bonaventure's description the way to contemplation must begin by passing through the corporeal, temporal *vestiges* of the material world until it can be led to the inner truth of God. But this was a practice that required involvement of the soul. The senses had to be able to grasp the divine through a gradual formation of a devout soul. The virtuous sensorium was, then, a sensorium configured to sense the holy, a *hagiosensorium*.[33] The hagiosensorium was established through the practice of reciprocity; when body and mind together engaged in pious perception, it could potentially reinforce the intensity of the discernment. However, this placed a great responsibility on the devotional circumstances, or quite simply what the senses were turned towards. In order for the senses to transport sensory perceptions of material *sensibilia* to the inner sensory faculties in a positive and virtuous way, they had to engage in devout perception.

Immutation of the Senses

The process of sensing – perceiving the world through the sensory *instrumentum* – was described by Bonaventure as sense-impressions passing though the sensory apparatus in the form of similitudes mediated by colours, light, textures, liquids, steam etc. In his *Sententia libri De anima* Thomas Aquinas described this particular part of the process in a similar but much more detailed fashion as a *change* in the senses (*immutatio*).[34] The human senses are, according to his view, immutated by what they sense, so that they somehow become *like* the objects: "[…] it follows that, whilst at the start of the process of being acted upon the faculty is not like its object, at the term of the process it has its likeness."[35] This does not mean that the senses are composed of *sensibilia* but that they are affected and changed by them since the sensory capacity is a potentiality.[36] As Aquinas states in *Summa Theologica*, "[…] the perception of sensible forms comes by an immutation caused by the sensibles […]."[37] Later in the commentary he adds further that "if they [the senses] were intrinsically made up of the objects they perceive, their perceptions would not presuppose any exterior sensible objects."[38]

There are, according to Aquinas, two kinds of immutation that can be applied to the proper senses: natural (material) and spiritual (immaterial).[39] The sense of sight perceives only in the latter immaterial and spiritual way, whereas the other senses do both. Beholding something red does not transform the eye materially so that it changes into the colour red, but the eye perceives the configurational state of the colour.[40] In this respect the sense of touch is different. When the skin touches an object that is cold or hot, the material quality of the object is transferred to the skin. At the same time, however, the spiritual aspect of the *sensibilia* is mediated to the sense of touch. The ability in materiality to represent the invisible, divine and immaterial was not in spite of their material character but closely connected to it. The function of the sensitive soul was to receive sense data transmitted from a sensory object (proper or common) through a medium that immutated the senses and then change them into phantasms, a sort of pre-cognitive state of form. Whereas phantasms were related to the sense data in the sense that it retained information about its material form, the intellect grasped instead the quiddity (Lat.: *quidditas* = essence or what-ness) of the material objects. The senses apprehend things as they *are* whereas imagination may apprehend something extra-material. This also means that sense objects – what we put before our eyes, ears, skin, tongue or nostrils – may potentially have a focal impact on the soul, since the senses are the gates to the soul. It follows, as has been stated above, that the senses can be affected in both harmful and positive ways.[41] The positive influence on perception changes one's disposition by actualising its potentiality, not by destroying anything, but by adding to it. An image of the Virgin and Child would, for example, affect the senses and the soul in a positive direction, whereas a 'lecherous' sight would have the contrary effect. The use of devotional poses (kneeling, standing erect, lying *ad veniam*) and movements (shifting between kneeling and standing), speaking (and thus tasting) and reading or listening to devout words, attempting to cry or touching specific objects (given that it was performed with a true heart) should be understood in this light: bodily actions and sensory activation stimulated and immutated the senses in a similar fashion.

Sensory perception and the use of *sensibilia* were, thus, acknowledged to hold a central position in the practice of devotion. As a result the practitioner would – ideally – be conformed to inner devoutness, which would in turn affect the body in a reciprocal manner. An example taken from a Danish devotional book produced between 1400 and 1500 for an anonymous owner is particularly illuminating. The practice consists of an extended rubric that describes in detail a rather elaborate devotion to the Virgin Mary followed by a fairly short prayer text.[42] The rubric informs that the practice is supposed to begin at the day of the Virgin Mary during Lent (the feast day for the celebration of the Annunciation to the Virgin Mary is 25th of March) with the reading of sixty *ave marias*, while the petitioner kneels in honour of the Virgin and the joy she felt when she heard the words from Gabriel's mouth. On the same day, the practitioner should make a string, read one *ave* while kneeling, and tie a knot on the string. On the next day the practitioner simply ads one knot and reads two *ave marias* and this continues one year around until the next Annunciation day; every day one knot and one *ave* is added to the procedure. It is also required that a candle should be kindled in the honour of the Virgin as long as the daily practice is performed (in the beginning just for a very short while, and towards the end considerably longer). On the last day of recitation the full amount of *ave marias* are performed before the image of the Annunciation with a candle – this time the size of the candle is up to the practitioner – and it should be left burning when the recitation has ended. But the devotional practice is not yet complete. On Saturday the practitioner has to produce a wax candle the size of the distance between the mouth of Gabriel and the mouth of Virgin Mary (supposedly as measured on the image), and while the candle burns, continuously recite as many *ave marias* as possible. This should be observed for nine days, every day ending with a prayer:

> O Virgin Mary I offer you these numerous ave marias and this candle in praise, adoration and honour for the great happiness you received in your heart from the mouth of the angel Gabriel when he announced the birth of the son of God, that he should become man in your holy body. Amen.[43]

In the first half of the practice the fingers aid the mind by keeping track of the *ave marias* corresponding to the amount of knots on the string. The focus of the mind is aided by the tactile count of knots and articulated through the mouth, the organ of taste and speech. Simultaneously the body is arranged in a kneeling position. If each *ave* took approximately fifteen seconds to recite, the practitioner would on the last day of the devotion have to endure one and a half hours of kneeling, counting, and reciting, and the body would most likely be severely agonised and *sensed*. After one and a half hours of praying – either mumbling or speaking aloud – the mouth would already for quite some times have been feeling dry, affecting the sense of *gustus*. Sight would sense the image and the burning candle, smell would sense the odour of warm wax, and hearing would register the monotonous repetition of the same words over and over again.

This particular devotion involved the senses in an all-encompassing fashion; every sensory faculty is preoccupied with devotional perception, all of them immutated and changed in a manner that would refer the mind to the devout undertaking and transformation. Furthermore, the monotonous performance of the same movements and perceptual exercises would gradually implement a close link between specific sense-impressions and what they signified (humbleness and devoutness towards the Virgin). A devout habitus would be solidly formed and imprinted in body and mind.

In the second part of the practice, the amount of recitations are no longer regulated by the knots on the string, but instead by the length of the candle whose size is given by the distance between the mouth of the virgin and the mouth of Gabriel on the visual depiction. The whole practice that has gone before is now condensed in the measurement of the candle and the offering of it before the image. The image becomes momentous, because it adds yet another dimension to the practice, that further strengthens the focus on the Annunciation. The preparatory actions of measuring the distance turn the mind towards Gabriel's words of announcement, words that are also the foundation of the prayer *ave maria*: "Hail Mary, full of grace, the Lord is with Thee; blessed art Thou among women and blessed is the fruit of Thy womb, Jesus. Holy Mary, Mother of God pray for us sinners now, and at the hour of our death." Likewise, the mind would be reminded of Mary's response to Gabriel's words: *Fiat mihi secundum verbum tuum* ("Be it done to me according to Thy word"), which would be the right answer by any pious Christian to anything happening to him or her. In this way the physical act of taking the measure of the candle, the topic of the image, the mental focus, and the words of the prayer, all coincide in a practice that unifies mental and bodily actions in one mutual concentration on the mysteries of the Annunciation to the Virgin and the miraculous Incarnation. Body and soul, material objects and perception, intentionally cooperate and aim towards the same objective, the same *end*, and their interplay seems to intensify the practice. This example shows how the practice of mental and physical actions is engaged in order to immutate the senses and ultimately facilitate devout perception. The practice culminates with the converging of all the senses on the contemplation of the words of Annunciation, which can be seen, tasted, heard, touched, and smelled with inner and outer senses, body and mind concurrently. The sacred words may now be integrated and contemplated with the entire sensorium. Perception is pivotal in the practice mentioned above. It builds up slowly, gradually increasing the requirements of time, mental concentration, and physical stamina until it reaches a climax when the perceptive body and the perceptive soul have accomplished unification towards the end. The performance of preparations beforehand, the combination of movements, and reading, the engagement of inner and outer senses in pious perception, makes up a devotional structure that requires full concentration in all its parts. The *sensorium* is open to material and immaterial impressions that corradiate and merge as a result of practice and is left marked by the enterprise. The active application of the bodily *instrumentum* in the practice of devotion – kneeling, praying, standing, speaking devout words, beholding, and touching objects etc. – should be regarded as an attempt to affect and immutate the senses, and impel the process of perception in a positive direction. As such, the materiality of devotion and the establishment of reciprocity between body and senses lie at the very core of practice, but only because of the amalgamation of body and soul that follows as a consequence of the operation. The physical change occurring in the sensory instrument as a result of the practice of sensing itself, could potentially lead to a change of the inner sensorium. Furthermore, the virtuous sentiments of the soul would pervade the actions of sense. In the practice of devotion, *homo exterior* and *homo interior* were no longer separate natures, but conformed and concerted according to the same aim; to address God with the whole organism. It was, however, not only body and mind that amalgamated during devotional practice. The whole process of practice was imbued with a sense of convolution where all the single parts entered into a complex relationship with the others. This was particularly evident with the devotional incorporation of senses and, as we shall see below, an intentional application of so-called compound sensory phenomena. Through the practice of devotion the senses were coiled together and merged into a pious instrument, a *saturated sensorium*.

Composite Sensorium

At the second step of the *Itinerarium mentis in deum* Bonaventure takes much interest in the description of the senses and their individual perceptive abilities as mentioned above, but Bonaventure was also aware that some phenomena could not be perceived with the singular senses. These are the so-called compound phenomena that are experienced with more than one sense at the time:

> Through these doors [the five particular senses], then, enter both simple bodies and composite bodies made of a mixture of these. We perceive with our senses not only these particular sense objects, which are light, sound, odour, taste and the four primary qualities which touch apprehends; but also the common sense objects, which are number, size, shape, rest and motion.[44]

The five senses have different specialities, and their particular elements, bodies, and phenomena enter the soul through their respective media, whereas the "common sense objects" are perceived collaboratively. The different devotional examples mentioned above indicate an extended use of such composite sensory phenomena. The practitioner sometimes had to *move* geographically in order to get to a particular image or place mentioned in the rubrics, or make preparations beforehand such as purchasing a candle and perhaps measuring it to fit a specific chosen devotional prescription (e.g. *size* or *shape*). Motion was also an issue in cases where devotion made use of different bodily positions, such as kneeling and standing alternately while reading specific prayers. The specific poses – often combined with inner contemplative exercises – would be moments of *rest*, although only to some extent, since some poses – like standing erect with arms to the side such as to figuratively look like a cross or crucified person – most likely took a lot of effort. *Numbers* were frequently used, especially when it came to repetitive recitations of *pater noster* and *ave maria*, where aids in the form of a rosary, a string with knots or a specific amount of candles were needed in order for the practice to be efficient. But the practice of counting was also applied in cases where devotions stretched over many days, even months or years. Finally, the common sense object's *shape* and *size* where constantly in play; not only were they activated whenever a devotional practice made use of objects with specific shapes and sizes that could only be perceived with a combination of the proper senses (such as an image or tactile object, or even the experience of size and shape of a specific place), but they were also applied to the devout organism that *shaped* itself in devout forms and, as shown above, significant poses and sentiments that adjusted ones physical and mental size according to the devotional situation (to kneel humbly or to stand with arms stretched out towards God as in the prayer from Johanne Nielsdatter's book mentioned above).

In symmetry with this mixed nature of the common sensibles, the mind was also able to experience sensory perception *as* mixed. Aquinas, being inspired by Aristotle, described *sensus communis* or common sense as the ability of human perception to integrate physical sense perception.[45] *Sensus communis* was not regarded as five individual inner senses, or as a sixth sense, but simply the sense of the conjunction between the five senses. In the common sensory principle, the bodily sense-impressions are gathered and merged into one interior sensation.

The composite potentiality of perception was to a very large extent present in the performance of devotional practice. By preoccupying as many receptive organs as. possible as well as actively pushing their perceptual limits beyond the performance of

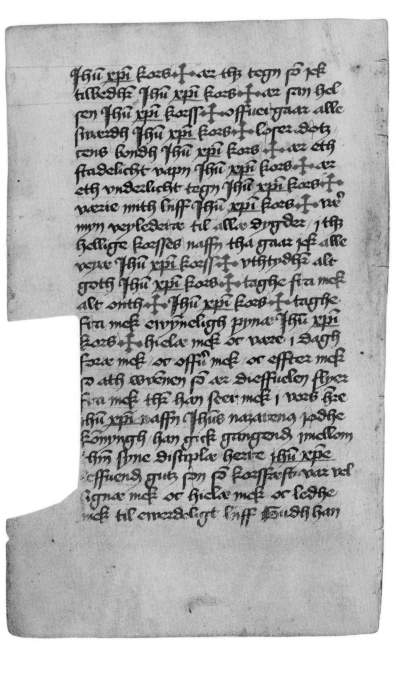

[III. 23] The Cross prayer from Anna Brade's prayer book dated 1497. The combination of words and the ultimate sign of Christ, the Cross, stimulate an amalgamation of body and mind. Every single prayer in Anne Brade's book is equipped with a small image in the margin. In this particular case, however, the image has been cut out. Thott 553, 4°, fol. 9v. The Royal Library in Copenhagen.

'proper sensation' the full perceptive capacity of the human mind was simultaneously and reciprocally activated. Such practices strategically strived towards a sensory configuration that was both composite as well as composed (in the *sensus communis*). Thus endowed with a saturated sensorium, the devotee was apt to transgress other thresholds as well and the distinction between inner and outer was permeated in the process. This form of sensory practice is clearly present in descriptions of devotion from the late medieval period. One example is a cross prayer from Anna Brade's primer from 1497 [ill. 23].[46]

This specific version of the cross prayer makes extensive use of the *sign* of the cross.[47] It is inserted every time the word *"kors"* (cross) is mentioned in the text, and the rubric prescribes that the practitioner makes the sign of the cross with her right hand every time she encounters the word/sign while reading it (fourteen times all in all).[48] The practice would earn the practitioner an indulgence of 1000 days.

The practice involves an intricate combination of sensory perceptual actions combining primary and common sensibles: the practitioner sees the words and cross-signs, touches the book and makes the sign if the cross in front of the body, tastes and hears the sound of the words that invoke the cross' protective powers, moves, rests, repeats and shapes. But what makes this practice even more intersensory in character is the fact that it could, as the rubric states, be 'read' in no less than four different ways: by reading it, hearing it, carrying it, or by merely seeing it (*"hwo som bær henne pa sigh screwen/ eller hører henne læse/ eller selff læss eller seer for sigh"*) [see ill. 24].[49] The prayer covered and converged almost all sensory aspects; it guaranteed that, no matter *how* it was performed, no matter what perceptual composition was used, it would provide protection and indulgence. The simple fact that it was written in a prayer book guaranteed that every time the owner brought it with her, she would be under the prayer's protection. Alternatively she could copy the prayer and crosses onto a piece of parchment, seal it in a small container and carry it around her neck, or sew it into her clothes, as many others did in this period, and still be guarded by its beneficial effect.[50]

The cross-prayer illustrates that texts and signs could be operative even if they were not perceived in ways we today would regard as the conventional sensory channels: through eyes, ears or mouth. Words and cross-signs against the body, the shape and size of the object (book or consealed parchment) felt as the body moved, perceived and absorbed by the sense of touch; it all served to generate a devout awareness of the presence of the crucified Christ. Composite sensibilia – motion, rest, shape, size, and number – and the common sense *sensus communis* were integrated

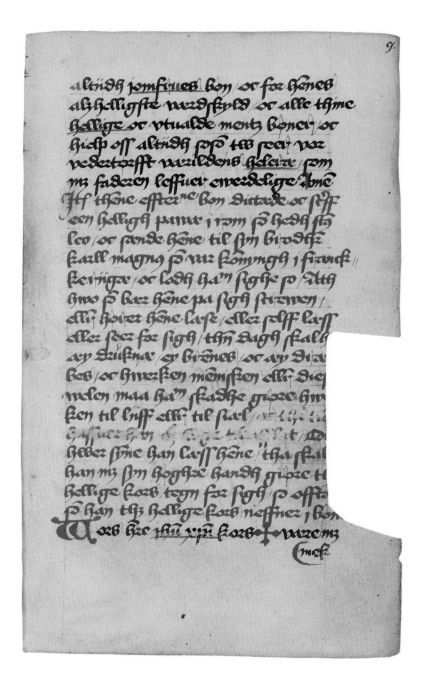

[**III. 24**] The rubric introducing the cross prayer in Anna Brade's prayer book. A post-Reformation owner of the book erased the sentence promising indulgence: "oc ther til haffuer han M dage til afflat". The rubric is written on the *recto* of the prayer text (previous illustration), leaving also this page with a lacuna where the image should originally have been. Thott 553, 4°, fol. 9r. The Royal Library in Copenhagen.

into the practice of devotion as a supplement to the incorporation of the primary senses. The result was an almost full coverage of the entire human sensorium, a complex interplay between inner and outer senses. Devotional practice could then be performed in ways that consumed the whole perceptive capacity of man and required its absolute attention. The functionality of practice would rely entirely on this awareness, intensified as it was through the coalescence of the senses.

174

Synaesthesia

Prayer books, devotional guides, images, and other devotional material shed light on late medieval devotional practice and in particular the position of the body and the senses. Different physical and mental actions and exercises were ordered in a way so that body and soul became mutually constitutive in the devotional process, establishing one conformed and united organism reaching towards God. One of the most important ways in which this was done, was through the use of the bodily senses. Devotional objects played an important role in this respect, but the practice of devotional perception itself was of even greater significance. Perception was regarded as the most basic step on the way to contemplation and in the practice of more ordinary forms of devotion this shines through as well. Devotional practice was often structured so that the use of the outer senses reciprocally influenced the use of the inner senses. When the outer senses sensed something of devotional significance (the cold church floor, the names of the Virgin, the eternal light, the face of a suffering saint) these vestiges immutated the senses and were transferred to the inner senses where they were processed into intellectual reflections, phantasms and sometimes even divine extra-material experiences.

Medieval devotional practice expresses a complex understanding of sensory perception that does not confine each individual sense into dealing with a limited area of perception. The type of sensory reception demanded by the examples mentioned above could be characterised as *synaesthetic*. Synaesthesia is a term currently used to describe the ability in some humans to have cross-referential sensations, like if someone is able to experience a tone as blue. A synaesthetic experience is when one sensory experience automatically is connected with a sensory experience in another sensate modality although this second modality has not been affected by any sense-impression. In traditional psychology and neuroscience the ability to have co-sensing has been regarded as a malfunction of the sensory apparatus. Modern reseach in neuro-psychology is beginning to understand it as a much more common phenomenon[51] and in this respect is shares many similarities with Aristotle's definition of the term *Sunaistanesthai* as simply meaning co-sensing or with-sensing. He used the term to describe a feeling shared by many, a communal sense-experience.[52] In the beginning of the Christian era the meaning shifted so that it became more related to *sensus communis*, designating the kind of sensation that occurs when multiple physiological affections meet *one* person simultaneously. When these affections meet, they are experienced as completely joined so that their derivation cannot be decided.[53] There is no sensory orientation or specific 'place' of origin.

Medieval devotion nurtured a sensibility for *synaesthetic* experiences, to establish joined sensations in which the sensations of the singular proper senses could not be separated, but were completely merged into one all-encompassing experience of venerating God. Devotional perception was performed by an undivided external/internal sensorium where each sense was no longer confined to absorbing only their primary sensory objects but fused into one cognisant organ. The human sensorium was saturated in devout perception. In this way the practice of perception established a state of loss of sensory direction and by insisting on mixed perception of material *sensibilia* the mind seems to have been pushed towards extra-material contemplation and apprehension.

Notes

1   von Achen 2007, p. 24.

2   What Thomas touches upon here is a question of the insignificance of knowledge in the spiritual and devotional life. It was indeed a recurring theme in spiritual and theological writings, for instance also in *The Cloud of Unknowing* and the writings of Jean Gerson. English translation from Thomas a Kempis 2005, p. 6.

3   Wittgenstein 2007, §7.

4   For a more thorough treatment of the subject, see my Ph.d. dissertation: Skinnebach 2013 (unpublished dissertation).

5   Bynum 1986 & 1992 as well as Ryan 2006 & Hamburger 1998.

6   See Bynum 2011 & Kristin B. Aavitsland's chapter on *Incarnation* in this volume.

7   Bynum 1987.

8   Bynum 1989, p. 182.

9   Bynum 2007, p. 257.

10 Boitani & Torti 1998; Hamm 2007 & Skinnebach 2013 (unpublished dissertation).

11 Tugwell 1982, p. 5. According to Tugwell the text circulated widely in Dominican milieus and beyond up to the fifteenth century. Cod. Rossianus 3 on which Tugwell's small booklet is based, was produced c. 1330 in the south of France and belonged to the Cartheusians of Porta Coeli in Valencia, now in the Vatican Library.

12 Tugwell 1982, p. 6.

13 Tugwell 1982, p. 6.

14 In Cod. Rossianus 3 each of the nine practices are supplied with an illustration. Some of the frescoes in the Convent of San Marco, Florence, dating from the mid fifteenth century, painted by Fra Angelico and his assistants, clearly derive from the Dominican practice of prayer as described in the *modi orandi*. See Bartz 2007, p. 68.

15 Gks 1614, in MDB IV, no. 962. The original Danish text reads: "Mærk væl thette som her effther screffuit stander / Thet førstæ meth knæfald for bebodelsen / Thet annet stande neghende oc lægge hændernæ pa kors ower knæenæ til hans swedh / Thet tridie standhe pa knæ meth opløffte hænder / Thet fiærde liggæ korswiis oc til hans swedh / Thet fæmte standendæ oc hændernæ lagde korswiis pa brystet til hans flængelse / Thet siætte pa knæ oc mellom hwert tiw kyssæ iorden til hans tornkronelsæ oc korsbærelse / Thet siwende stande korswiis til hans korsfæstelsæ / Thet otende sidde nedher oc lægge hændernæ korswiis pa skødet til hans nedertagelse aff korssit / Thet nyendæ Ad veniam for begraffuelsen / Thet tiændhæ meth knæfall til hans opstandelse oc opfarelsæ / oc iomfru maria optagelse". The Danish text is quoted from *Middelalderens Danske Bønnebøger*, a publication of a selection of Danish medieval devotional books (prayer books and Books of Hours) by Nielsen 1946-1982 (in the following referred to as MDB). All English translations by philologist David Folkmann Drost and the author.

16 Although the owner of the book belonged to a Bridgettine monastery, this practice is very different from the specific Bridgitine way of the cross described in Gotfred of Ghemens print called *De femten steder, Vorherre tålte sin pine på*, which list fifteen stations as opposed to the usual fourteen stations. See Dahlerup 2010, p. 329 f.

17   "Huo som thisse æffter skreffne bøner læsær i xxx dage meth gudælighet for iomfru maria billet oc meth ieth brinendæ lyus, tha vordær then menniske hørdh, e huat drøffwilse then menniskæ pa kallær iomfru maria, vden alle thyffwel, och thet hauer mange menniske prøuet meth thisse bøner oc hauer fonghet hielp aff iomfru maria, oc ther skulle læses x aue maria standindæ opp i melle huer bøn oc sa bønen." Cod. Holm. A 42, MDB I, no. 28.

18   See especially Camille 1994, 1996 and 1998; Hamburger 1998; Marks 2005.

19   Laugerud 2005.

20   The full quotation reads: "Sensus autem oculorum non ab aluid sensus corporis dicitur nisi quia et ipsi oculi membra sunt corporis, et quamuis non sentiat corpus exanime, anima tamen commixta corpori per instrumentum sentit corporeum et idem intrumentum sensus uocatur." Augustine: *De trinitate*, *On the Trinity*, 11, 2, 2. English translation from Hill 2012 has been slighty altered by the author. Hill has translated Augustine's "corpus examine" to "unconscious or lifeless body", which I have changed into "inanimate" because this term indicates more clearly that Augustine perceived the relation between body and soul as complementary.

21   "Kepe ii sy3te fro leccherous sytes & iin erys from leccherous heryng and ii mowth fro leccherous speche and ii nose fro dyshonest smellyng and ii lymes handys & mowth & iin oiere membrys fro leccherous towchyng. iese ar ii v wyttes & 3atys through whiche ie feendys entryth ie herte." From Jacob's Well. Salisbury Cathedral MS 103, fol. 122. I quote from Woolgar 2006, p. 12.

22   Thomas Aquinas' treatment of human acts and *habitus* in *Summa Theologica*, *ST* II, Q. 49-89. For a further treatment of my understanding and use of the term see Skinnebach 2010 & 2013 (unpublished dissertation).

23   "[…] hielp mek til san fredh bodhe til liif ochs iæl Hielp mek sancta maria til eet stadelight hoob · kerlighe troo · ydmygheet och raadh · at wernæ myne fæm synnæ · At fuldkomme the vii miskundelighe gerningher […]". AM 418,12˚, MDB II, no. 344.

24   "Innocensius pawe i rom han gaff alle the som thenne bøn ydmygelighe læs meth fuldkommeligh hugh oc hierthe iomffru maria till loff oc hedher C daghe till afflat aff syne synder Oc skal thet menniske vidhe o snarlighe see iomffru maria · naer hans døtz timæ kommer […]". As n. 23 above.

25   "Est autem naturale homini ut per sensibilia ad intelligibilia veniat, quia omnis nostra cognitio a sensu initium habet." *ST* I, Q. 1, art. 9, Latin quotes refer to Busa 1980, vol II, and English translations to *Summa Theologica*, 1920.

26   Bonaventure: *Itinerarium mentis in Deum*; *The Journey of the Mind to God*, I:6. In the following all Latin quotes refer to Peltier 1864 whereas English quotes refer to Cousins 1978.

27   "Qui igitur tantis rerum creatarum splendoribus non illustratur, cæcus est: qui tantis clamoribus non evigilat, surdus est: qui ex omnibus his effectibus Deum non lauded, mutus est: qui ex tantis indiciis primum Principium non advertit, stiltus est. Aperi ergo oculos, aures spiritualis admove, labia tua solve, et cor tuum appone, ut in omnibus creaturis Deum tuum videas, audias, laudes, diligas et colas, magnifices et honores, ne forte contra te universus orbis terrarum consurgat." *Itinerarium* I:15.

28   "[…] quaedam sint vestigium, quaedam imago, quaedam corporalia, quaedam spiritualia,

quaedam temporalia, quaedam aeviterna, ac per hoc quaedam extra nos, quaedam intra nos: ad hoc, quod perveniamus ad primum principium considerandum, quod est spiritualissimum et aeternum et supra nos, oportet, nos transire per vestigium, quod est corporale et temporale et extra nos, et hoc est deduci in via Dei; oportet, nos intrare ad mentem nostram, quae est imago Dei aeviterna, spiritualis et intra nos, et hoc est ingredi in veritate Dei". *Itinerarium* I:1.

29 *Itinerarium* II:4.

30 *ST* I Q 78 art 4.

31 *Itinerarium* IV:3.

32 *Itinerarium* VII:1.

33 See Hans Henrik Lohfert Jørgensen's chapter on *Sensorium* in this volume.

34 The Latin word *immutatio* (from the verb *immuto*) means *changed* and should not be confused with *immutabilis* which means *unchangeable*.

35 "Et propter hoc sequitur, quod secundum quod patitur a principio, non est similis sensus sentienti; sed secundum quod iam est passum, est assimilatum sensibili, est tale quale est illud." II:7, Latin text: Thomas Aquinas: *Sententia libri De anima* in Busa 1980, vol. 4. English translation by Foster and Humphries 1951 in *Commentary on Aristotle's de Anima*. See also Pasnau 1999.

36 *Commentary* II:7.

37 "[…] perceptio formarum sensibilium sit ex immutatione sensibilis […]", *ST* I Q 78 art. 4.

38 *Commentary* III:1.

39 *Commentary* II:20.

40 Stump 2003, p. 251 f.

41 *Commentary* II:11.

42 The full rubric in Danish reads as follows: "Her effther scriffues nogher lesning till iomfrw maria oc skall begynnes wor frw dag i fasthe; fførsth skall mand lesse paa sine knee iij synne xx aue maria iomfrw maria till loff for then store glede hwn fick. Wor frw dag i fasthe skal mand begynne en lesning aff iomfrw maria, Skall mand giøre en snoor oc skall man falle paa syne knee, saa skal ma lesse første dag en aue maria oc knytte en knwde paa snoren, annen dagen ii atther paa syne knee, Saa skal man lesse fremdelis hwer dah ieth aar om kring till wor frw dag i fasthe kommer igen, Oc skal man hwer dag [øghe] en knwdhe oc en aue maria til oc skal man lesse them offuer alle sammen hwer tidh hand øgher till, Skall man hwer dag lesse them paa syne knee meth eth lywss medhen bønerne ware, skal man offre them gud oc iomfrw maria till loff hedher oc ere ffor then store glede hwn fick i syt hierte aff gabriell engels ord ther han bebode hynne at føde gudz søn oc gudz søn skulle worde man i hynnes iomfrwelige legomme, Saa skall man bedhe iomfrw maria om thet ath hwn wille for see thet meniske oc hwn wille werdis till at bede for thet menniske til gwd at hand wille forsee thet menniske effther syn willie. Første at aars daghen haffuer eth endhe saa skall hand lesse them alle offer, saa skal mand taghe then samme snoor oc gøre eth lywss offuer hynne hwor stort hand will, saa skall man setthet for iomfrw maria beledhe som gabriel engel bebode hynne oc icki slycket medhen ladet wdh brendhe." AM 784,4°, MDB IV, no. 1134.

43 "O iomfrw maria ieg offrer teg thesse wthalighe aue maria till loff hedher oc ere oc thette lywss till loff hedher oc ere for then store gledhe ther tw fick i thit hierte aff gabriell engels mwndh ther

hand bebode teg at fødhe gutz søn at hand word mand i thit legomlige legome. Amen."
AM 784,4°, MDB IV, no. 1134.

44 "Intrant igitur per has portas tam corpora simplicia quam composita, ex his mixta. Quia vero sensu percipimus non solum haec sensibilia particularia, quae sunt lux, sonus, odor, sapor et quatuor primariae qulitates, quas apprehendit tactus; verum etiam sensibilia communia, quae sunt numerus, magnitudo, figura, quies et motus," *Itinerarium* I:3. See also Hans Henrik Lohfert Jørgensen's reference to Bonaventure's *Itinerarium* in his chapter on *Sensorium* in this volume.

179

45 *STI* Q 78 art 4.

46 Thott 553, MDB II, no. 170. The dating of the text is written on the last page of the book: "Thenne bogh lodh syster Anna bradis atter scriffue/ Aar effter gudz byrdh Mcdxcseptimo". Anna Brade was abbess in Maribo.

47 An almost identical but slightly shorter version of the practice can be found in Johanne Niels-datter's Book of Hours, Stockholm A 42, MDB I, no. 69.

48 "Wors herre ihesu christi kors † være meth mek Ihesu christi kors † ær thet tegn som iek tilbed-her Ihesu christi kors † ær san helsen Ihesu christi korss † offuergaar alle swærdh Ihesu christi kors † løser døtzcens bondh Ihesu christi kors † ær eth stadelicht vapn Ihesu christi kors † ær eth vnderlicht tegn Ihesu christi kors † værie mith liiff Ihesu christi kors † være myn veyloderæ til allæ dygder/ i thet hellige korsses naffn tha gaar iek alle veyæ Ihesu christi korss † vthtydher alt goth Ihesu christi kors † taghe fra mek alt onth † Ihesu christi kors † taghe fra mek ewynneligh pynæ Ihesu christi kors † hielæ mek oc være i dagh foræ mek/ oc offuer mek/ oc effter mek so ath wvennen som ær dieffuelen flyer fra mek ther han seer mek i vors herre ihesu christi naffn Ihesus nazarenus iødhe konnyngh/ han gick gangendis imellom them syne disciplæ/ herre ihesu christe leffuendis gutz søn som korsfæst var velsignæ mek oc hielæ mek/ oc ledhe mek til ewerdeligt liiff Gudh han skywlæ mek ihesus han værne mek christus værie mek/ gudh vænde fra mek alt onth/ I naffn gudh faders oc søns oc then hellige andz Amen pater Aue". See n. 46 above.

49 The entire rubric reads: "Item thenne efterscreffne bøn dictæde oc screff een hellig pawæ i rom som hedh sanctus leo oc sæde henne til syn brother karll magnus om var konnyngh i franckkeri-igæ/ oc lodh hannum sighe so/ Ath hwo som bær henne pa sigh screwen/ eller hører henne læse/ eller selff læss eller seer for sigh/ then dagh skaln h[an] æy druknæ/ ey brennes/ oc æy dræbes/ oc hwerken mennisken eller dief[f]welen maa hanum skadhe giøre hw[er]ken til liiff eller til siæl/ oc ther til haffuer han M dage til afflat/ o[c] hwer synne han læss henne/ tha skal han meth syn høghre handh giøre thet hellige kors tegn for sigh/ so offtæ som han thet hellige kors neffner i bøn[en]." See n. 46.

50 Numerous examples have been studied by Skemer 2006.

51 Some recent scholars have seriously challenged this understanding of synaesthesia, arguing that "synaesthesia might provide a more productive model for conceptualizing perceptual processes than the conventional sense-by-sense approach [...]". See Howes 2009A, p. 226.

52 Heller-Roazen 2007, p. 81; Chrétien 2004, p. 123.

53 A Greek writer, Priscian of Lydia, who was active in Persia in the sixth century, defined it as the sensation that occurs when sense-impressions are joined so that they can no longer be divided.

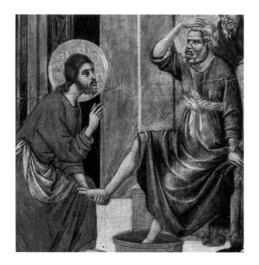

180

[**RITUAL**]   This chapter discusses the combined uses of several media in medieval church rituals. Assessing the application of a (modern) notion of ritual to medieval liturgical ceremonies, it points out how these 'rituals' worked through a sensory combination of words, music, architectural setting, and movement within that setting. Also visual artefacts and in some cases, the 'sacramental' use of material objects were involved. In a particular ceremony, carried out since Antiquity on the basis of John 13:1-17, the narrative of Jesus washing the feet of the disciples, the singing of chants was combined with the actual washing of the feet of either monks or poor people. The combination of words and melodies with elaborate *melismas,* and the further sensorial staging and setting of the ceremony produced a 'polyphony' of media, which can be analysed by way of early medieval notions of sacrament. The chapter also demonstrates how this sacramental 'polyphony' of media remained important for medieval ceremonies, even when the notion of sacrament was theologically narrowed during the twelfth and the following centuries.

RITUAL

Medieval Liturgy and the Senses: The Case of the Mandatum

181

[Nils Holger Petersen]

Medieval Liturgy and Intersensorial Liturgical Performance

Medieval liturgy constitutes an important, complex, yet ill-defined area to which the modern term 'ritual' has frequently been applied in modern scholarship. I shall take my point of departure in the notion of liturgy in order to return to a discussion of 'ritual' in that context. The term 'liturgy' was not used in the Middle Ages, and there does not even seem to be a single unifying term in use during the Middle Ages for the contemporary concept of 'liturgy'.[1] As John Caldwell points out, however, this does not refute 'liturgy' as a relevant term in modern scholarship. Indeed, it would probably be impossible to avoid it, considering its pervasive use in scholarship of the last hundred years. However, it is important to realise that as used nowadays, for instance defined as, "the ritualised public celebration of the faith of the Church,"[2] it is part of a modern abstract understanding of the character of public worship, which seems anachronistic for the variety of public devotion in the Middle Ages.

Indeed, attempts to characterise what properly belonged within 'the liturgy' and what did not, have in recent scholarship been seen as an untimely backwards projection of views based on much later Catholic sensibilities from the sixteenth century.[3] Terms like para-liturgical and extra-liturgical, not found in the Middle Ages, have sometimes been used in previous scholarship (also in the twentieth century) to characterise certain ceremonies, types of ceremonies, or even special types of chant, found in liturgical manuscripts, as not 'really' liturgical. Such ideas are connected to the notion of an 'official' medieval liturgy; again a notion for which there is no actual evidence, although certain liturgical elements were obviously more generally acknowledged than others and, indeed, omnipresent in manuscripts.[4]

RITUAL

In spite of this terminological problem, I shall continue to use the notion of 'medieval liturgy', acknowledging that there is no well-defined medieval phenomenon that completely corresponds to the term, recognising also, however, a modern scholarly need to approach medieval public worship in a general way as this in recent times has been defined more or less in analogy with the definition above for 'medieval liturgy'. However, I shall assume that whatever is found in a medieval manuscript for church ceremonies does indeed belong to the 'medieval liturgy', as I use the notion, at the place and time in question.

It is a commonplace that music and the visual media played a huge role in medieval liturgy. The mass and the Divine office were all mainly sung, and the same is true for most other church celebrations, including processions and special ceremonies as for instance the so-called liturgical dramas. In addition, the choreography of ceremonies was clearly of importance. The way for instance processions were planned either within a monastery or a cathedral, along processional routes inside and outside of a monastic building complex, or a city, for example around a cathedral. Visual markers as crucifixes played a basic role in processions and, obviously, images, architectural features of various kinds used or related to in ceremonies, thuribles, banners, and other artefacts used in processions belong in this context.[5] Also tactile, gustatory, and olfactory senses come into the picture, not least in connection with the various sacraments, and especially in the cases of baptism and the Eucharist, which involved washing as well as eating and drinking. Altogether, any ceremony would include some or many of the following elements involving different senses: words recited or sung, the use of particular architectural settings (in or around a church), natural ingredients as water (also for sprinkling in various cleansing ceremonies), processed material elements such as bread and wine, but also particular artefacts for certain ceremonies, the font for baptism, the cup for the Eucharist, vestments, crucifixes, thuribles and incense and also, in some cases, relics. All such elements addressing various human senses in addition to the overall planning of the performance, involving the senses of seeing and hearing as well as the intellect, played together in various ways and contributed to the understanding and the atmosphere (see further below concerning this term) of a given ceremony, obviously in various ways for different ceremonies.

I shall pursue this intersensorial significance more specifically for the so-called *mandatum* ceremonies: the washing of the feet. In the Middle Ages this involved singing as well as the carrying out of an act of washing the feet of a certain group of persons, i.e. a tactile experience, taking place in a specially chosen place. The term 'mandatum' refers to John 13:34 where Jesus, after having washed the feet of his disciples as an exemplary act (John 13:14-15), formulates as his new commandment (mandatum in Latin) that they shall love each other as he has loved them. The word 'maundy' (Maundy Thursday) derives from the Latin term.

The Mandatum Ceremonies

In this section I shall present various performative, liturgical representations of Jesus washing the feet of the disciples, primarily in connection with Easter celebrations, and as mentioned based on a unique narrative in John 13:1-17. A brief historical sketch will take me from Milan in the fourth century, over important tenth-century liturgical centres, and up to houses of regular canons in the twelfth century, even taking up documents of the Teutonic Order in the fifteenth century. These are examples and must be treated as such: they do not provide a full historical narrative concerning ritual representations of this biblical story.

The first to be considered here is a reference to a ceremony by Bishop Ambrose of Milan (c. 340-397) in *De sacramentis* and *De mysteriis*.[6] He described a feet-washing ceremony as part of the post-baptismal rites, which in Antiquity and the early Middle Ages were primarily performed during Easter night. Here the feet of the neophytes were washed by the bishop *after* baptism, but before the signing of the forehead of the newly baptised with chrism. In his *De sacramentis*, Ambrose refers to the biblical exchange between Peter and Jesus (John 13:6-10), Peter refusing to have his feet washed by his master, but changing his mind when told that he would otherwise have no share in Jesus. Then he wants Jesus to wash not only his feet but even his hands and head. However, Jesus responds that, "One who has bathed does not need to wash, except for the feet, but is entirely clean." For Ambrose this was a fitting measure for the newly baptised. Apparently he interpreted the ceremony as an extra help against falling out of the grace of baptism (*De sacramentis*):

> Therefore you wash your feet, so that in each part where the serpent has laid traps the greater help is near through which it will no longer be possible for you to stumble. Therefore, you wash the feet so that you will clean the serpent's poison.[7]

Ambrose notes that the practice to which he refers was not in accordance with Roman practice.[8] From letters of Augustine, we further know that the mandatum was carried out on Maundy Thursday in Hippo,[9] just as this later – considering the biblical account – obviously seems to have been a particularly favored place for it. Later Ambrosian documents still refer to the Washing of the Feet after baptism and *after* the signing with chrism.[10] Some documents, which seemingly reflect Roman customs, the *Ordo XI* and the *Gelasian Sacramentary*, do not have a Washing of the Feet in connection with baptism. Documents of Gallican rites from around 700, however, such as the *Missale Gothicum* and the *Bobbio Missal*, have short references to the washing of feet after baptism. As in the later Ambrosian documents this also happened *after* the signing of the forehead.[11]

On the other hand, the canons of the Council of Toledo (694) refer to a ceremony of foot washing on Maundy Thursday,[12] and it is found in important and influential Carolingian liturgical documents as a special ceremony on Maundy Thursday. It is for instance mentioned by Amalarius of Metz in his *Liber officialis* (written in the 820s).[13] From the ninth century onwards such a ceremony seems to have found a fairly stable position on Maundy Thursday,[14] reflected also in manuscripts, which have been implemented in the so-called *Roman German Pontifical* of the tenth century (from Mainz), as well as in the English monastic rule *Regularis Concordia*. Whereas earlier references do not mention songs for the ceremony (which does not necessarily mean that there were none), the first of the mentioned tenth-century ceremonies does. It specifies that the ceremony may be held before or after the evening meal. The bishop proceeds with priests and other clerics *ad locum ubi mandatum perficere vult*, "to the place where he wants to hold the mandatum," with candles, censers, Gospel books etc:

> And the deacon begins the Gospel, "Now before the festival of the Passover" (John 13:1), just as at mass. After the reading of the Gospel, the bishop says this prayer: God, whose meal, as above. After he has given the prayer, the bishop vests and girds himself with a linen cloth and prepares to wash the feet of his disciples. And first, with the pontiff beginning, they shall mutually wash their feet and dry them while singing the antiphon *Mandatum novum* (A new commandment; John 13:34). Psalm: *Beati immaculati* (Psalm 118:1), "Happy are those whose way is blameless"; (English Bible, Psalm 119:1).

A large quantity of antiphons and psalms follow, the antiphons mainly rephrasing various parts of the Gospel narrative of the washing of the feet, but also incorporating texts referring to the betrayal of Judas and more general statements about being a disciple. After these the text goes on as follows:

After having finished the antiphons the deacon or reader whose task it is begins the Gospel of John reading the lesson from the place where it says: "Very truly, I tell you, servants are not greater than their master (John 13:16) [...]".

It thus takes up the Gospel recitation at the end of the narrative of the washing of the feet. Thereafter follows post-mandatum prayers.[15]

Sequences of antiphons for mandatum ceremonies are very normal in such ceremonies, generally featuring texts reflecting sentences from the narrative, but also sometimes paraphrasing other New Testament narratives or statements deemed relevant, as for instance a quotation concerning the woman who washed Jesus' hair (Luke 7:36-50). The songs vary substantially between ceremonies, although in each version they roughly represent the Gospel narrative from John 13 with some additional contextualising antiphons. The following is a list of the antiphons from an eleventh-century Aquitanian fragment, one folio from a Gradual. The Gradual (choir book for the mass liturgy) seems to have been a favorite place to note antiphons for mandatum ceremonies, although occasionally such antiphons are also found in office antiphonaries (choir books for the Divine office). As such, the *mandatum* belongs neither to the mass liturgy nor to the standard ceremonies of the Divine office. A number of the antiphons contain substantial melismas (melodic configurations on a single syllable; see ill. 25), but it is also noteworthy when comparing ceremonies, that melismas were not generally placed in the same place in antiphons based on the same text in different manuscripts. The mentioned fragment lists the following antiphons:

Ad Mandatum

a. Postquam surrexit dominus ad cenam misit aquam in peluem coepit lavare pedes discipulorum hoc exemplum relinquid suis. (John 13:5).

Ps. Audite haec omnes gentes auribus percipite omnes qui habitatis orbem.
[Ps. 48 (49 in English Bibles)].

a. Mandatum novum do vobis ut diligatis invicem sicut dilexi vos dicit dominus. (John 13:34).

v. Dixit Ihesus discipulis suis. Mandatum (John 13:34).

a. Vos vocatis me magister et domine et benedicite (sic!), sum [etenim]. si ego lavi vestros pedes dominus et magister et vos debetis alter alterius lavare pedes. (John 13:13-14).

a. Surgit ihesus ad caenam et ponit vestimenta sua et cum accepisse linteum precincxit se dixit que discipulis suis. Vos vocatis. (John 13:4).

a. Misit denique aquam in pelvem et cepit lavare pedes discipulorum et extergere linteo quo erat precinctus dixit que discipulis suis. Si ego. (John 13:5).

a. Postquam ego lavi [sic!] pedes eorum et accepit vestimenta sua cum recubuisset iterum dixit eis. Et vos. (John 13:12).

a. Si ego dominus et magister vester lavi vobis pedes quanto magis vos debetis al[ter] alterius lavare pedes. (John 13:14).

v. Exemplum enim dedi vobis [ut] quemadmodum ego feci vobis ut et vos ita fa[cia]tis. Si ego. (John 13:15).

a. Si dilexeris me et verba mea in vobis manser[o] [et] vere discipuli mei eri[ti]s et cognoscetis veritatem et veritas liberabit vos dicit dominus. (John 8:31-32).

a. Cena facta sciens dominus ihesus quia omnia dedit ei pater et quia ad [deum] exivit et ad deum vadit surgit ad cenam et ponit vestimenta sua et cum accepisset linteum deinde misit aquam in pelvem [*NB melisma*] cepit lavare pedes discipulorum suorum et extergere linte[o] in quo erat precinctus et ait qui lotus est non indiget nisi ut pedes lavet sed mundus totus. [*NB melisma*] (John 13:2-5 & 10).

v. Venit autem ad simonem petrum et dixit ei petrus domine tu michi lavas pedes non lavabis michi pedes in eternum. [*NB melisma*] (John 13:8 a). Respondit ei ihesus qui lo.

a. Domine tu michi lavas pedes respondit ihesus et dixit ei et si non lavero tibi pedes non habebis partem mecum. (John 13:8 b).

v. Venit autem ad simonem petrum et dixit eis petrus. Domine. (John 13:9).

v. Domine non tantum pedes set et manus et capud. Respondit.

a. In hoc cognoscent omnes quia mei estis discipuli si dileccionem [h]abueritis ininvicem. (John 13:35).

v. Dixit ihesus discipulis suis. In hoc. (John 13:35).

a. Maneat in vobis spes fides caritas tria haec maior autem his est caritas. (1 Cor 13:13).

v. Nunc autem manent fides spes caritas. Maior. (1 Cor 13:13).

a. In diebus illis mulier que erat in civitatem peccatrix ut cognovit quod ihesus recubuit in domo simonis lep[ro]si atulit alabaustrum unguenti et stans retro secus pedes domini ihesu lacrimis coepit rigare pedes eius et capillis capiti sui tergebat [...] (Luke 7:37-38).[16]

In the tenth-century monastic agreement from the Winchester synod (970s), *Regularis Concordia*, the mandatum had a double course:

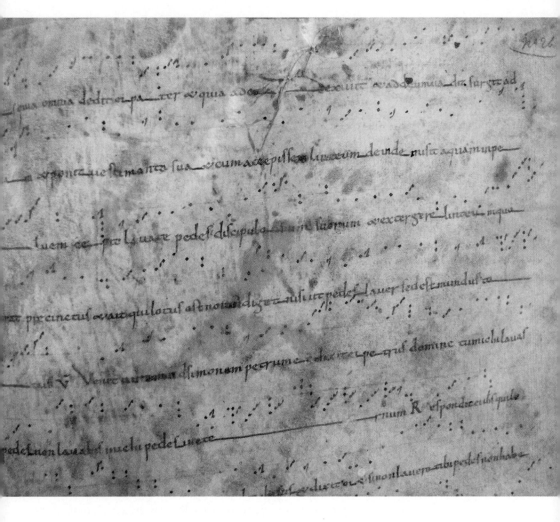

[III. 25] Toulouse, Archives Départmentales de la Haute-Garonne, H 121, fragment 26, verso, top part of page. Note the long melisma on "eter--num."

When Mass has been celebrated, all the brethren shall partake of the *mixtum*, after which the abbot shall carry out his own Maundy, taking with him those of the brethren whom he wishes. When this is finished Vespers shall be celebrated; the brethren shall then have their meal and thereafter, at the proper time, their Maundy shall take place; but they must wash their feet carefully beforehand. When the ministers of the week, preceding the abbot as is their wont, come to the Maundy, they shall perform their part in it, and after them the abbot shall wash the feet of all in his own basin, drying and kissing them, being assisted by those whom he has chosen for this service.[17]

There is no reference to the singing of antiphons in the description of this ceremony, only to the reading of the gospel text. It seems surprising, however, in view of the general liturgy of the *Regularis Concordia* and the emphasis on singing in most contexts, that the ceremony would not have included singing. The double mandatum in itself, however, is not unusual.[18]

In Cluniac customs as well as in certain rules for Augustinian canons there seems, at least in a number of cases, to have been a massive focus on mandatum ceremonies, which were basically of two different types. Two early twelfth-century customaries (*consuetudines*) for houses of canons both contain two (related) types of mandatum ceremonies. This documentation comes from the regular canons in German Marbach and the canons of the cathedral of Lund in medieval Denmark. The Lund consuetudines have been preserved in the *Necrologium lundense*. The document is to some extent dependent on the Marbach consuetudines, quoting the Marbach text verbatim in some parts of the descriptions of mandatum ceremonies.[19]

The Marbach *consuetudines* themselves are dependent on earlier Augustinian sources, taking over much from Cluniac and Hirsau reforms, not least concerning the *mandatum*.[20] The Marbach book has four chapters devoted to the mandatum, giving also information about when and when not to perform the rite. The much shorter consuetudines in Lund spend 3 out of 35 chapters on this particular ceremony and its various uses for poor people or guests or among the canons themselves. The regulations are not identical at all, but certain passages from the Marbach consuetudines were quoted verbatim in the book from the Lund cathedral. The main structure of the ceremonies is roughly the same as one finds in almost all of these ceremonies, but the ceremony is used in two different contexts: there is the action of washing the feet of the brethren, but also the washing of feet is performed on a number of poor people invited into the house of the canons. In the Marbach consuetudines, chapters 118-20 and 122 are devoted to these ceremonies: mostly they take place on Saturdays (with some exceptions detailed in chapter 118). There is the internal mandatum (chapter 119) and the mandatum pauperum (chapter 120) and then the mandatum pauperum on Maundy Thursday (chapter 122). For the Lund consuetudines, there is the daily mandatum (chapter XXIV), the mandatum pauperum on Maundy Thursday (chapter XXV), and the general mandatum (also on Maundy Thursday, chapter XXVI). All of these washing ceremonies were framed by the reading of the Gospel narrative from John 13 and accompanied by antiphons mainly based on the Gospel text, very much in similarity with what was noted for other mandatum ceremonies above. The books do not provide musical notation, and thus the use of melismas cannot be explored.

Discussion

The point here is not to discuss the degree of interdependency or the differences be-tween the documents. Many other manuscripts and variants of the ceremony could have been chosen and would indeed be necessary in order to even approach discussing the transmission of these ceremonies.[21] It is also not the point to discuss the genre of the ceremony. In his monumental study of medieval church drama Karl Young discussed the mandatum considering it to be "an observance [...] perfectly adapted for transformation into drama" but also remarking that, "of such a transformation the available records make no mention."[22] Young's understanding of drama in relation to medieval liturgy has been challenged by numerous scholars and must now be regarded as outdated.[23] In any case, this is not the question I am pursuing here. Karl Young is obviously right stating there is no sign that the abbot or the bishop or whoever officiates and leads the washing of the feet is trying in any way to be or, in Young's formulation, to "impersonate Christ."

There is, of course, as observed by Young, a strong aspect of mimesis involved, but no identification as such. The biblical narrative accompanies and sheds light on the action that goes on simultaneously with the readings and the song. It may be said to define the action, to put it into perspective. Each of the mandatum ceremonies in the texts cited here transposes the biblical narrative into an action that explicitly concerns the community in which they are carried out. All participants represent themselves at the same time as they in some way re-enact (the basic action of) the biblical narrative. For this reason, the ceremony can be said to rather stage a self-understanding in the light of Christian communal ideals which constitute an important element, not least in the construction of monastic identity or, similarly, in houses of the Augustinian reform. The first point I want to make concerns the great importance this particular (type of) ceremony seems to have had in the two Augustinian places considered above, since so much space was devoted to its regulation in the documents and since it was held with such a frequency (and in different contexts). Although the Marbach consuetudines had taken over a Hirsau ceremony for the most traditional Maundy Thursday mandatum, the mandatum observances in Marbach were not merely taken over from Hirsau, but were closely related to those of another early Augustinian house, namely that of Saint Ruf near Avignon and also similar to contemporary practices in the Lateran.[24]

It not only seems possible to point to particular emphases of these liturgical observances, but also to point out how these can be understood in relation to the theological reform ideology among Augustinians. A number of common traditional practices for Holy Week and Easter Sunday are not mentioned in the cited customaries, as for instance the representational liturgy for the burial and Resurrection of Christ for Holy Week and Easter, also quite common in Augustinian houses.[25] That does not mean that they were not practiced in Marbach or in Lund, but it raises the question, why there was such an emphasis on precisely the mandatum ceremonies in the customaries?

The mandatum was not, as has been made clear, in any way unique to the canons regular. The mandatum was seemingly celebrated in all branches of the church during the Middle Ages, also for instance, and quite frequently, in Cistercian houses.[26] Still, the strong focus in the mentioned Augustinian documents requires an explanation. Indeed, I believe that the foot washing ceremonies may be seen as a ritual particularly suited to confirm Gregorian priestly ideals and canonical reforms. They emphasise the priestly community and sanctity by way of an exemplary act by Christ; they fuse the apostolic preaching and teaching with the ecclesiastical hierarchy, since the mandatum ceremony was carried out among the canons themselves as well as for external, lay, poor people.[27] Few of the many medieval representational practices would seem better suited to efficaciously reinforce the theological and ecclesiological ideals of the reform movement of the eleventh and twelfth centuries than the mandatum.

The same is also true in a more general way for all the contexts in which the mandatum was performed, including monastic as well as cathedral contexts. What stands out is how the mandatum emphasised not only the communality of priestly and monastic communities, but also their (ideal) humility, since the mandatum pauperum highlighted how such communities also were to serve the poor and the sick in imitation of Christ. Although, it must parenthetically be noted, in Marbach and Lund there are also (identical) remarks excluding those "who should not be allowed to enter the claustrum, i.e. those with unhealthy feet or the young" (what exactly is meant by *iuvenes*, the young, in this context seems unclear).[28]

These rituals of communality and brotherhood as well as of humility and service to the poor were brought into a liturgical sphere by way of the singing about what one was about to do, underlining (sometimes, and more or less) by way of melismas different parts of the songs, probably according to local sensibilities, traditions, and stylistic ideals. The combination of the bodily act of washing feet with the act of singing, two types of actions which do not usually belong together, would seem to manifest a multimedia ritual, which crosses dividing lines between the domestic and practical on the one hand and the liturgical and elevated on the other.

The mandatum ritual thus manifests not only humility and brotherhood but also a link between everyday necessities, the restraints of sensory earthly life, and liturgical, spiritual freedom through the redemption and salvation of Christ. It is thus a ritual, which is able to express and thus confirm a general Christian understanding of life, which encompasses earthly secular life as well as the heavenly sanctification of human life. It thus embraces basic Christian ideals found not least in the letters of Paul. The sanctification of the priestly and religious life, however, occurred particularly from the tenth century onwards through Cluniac ideals and from there was taken further by the Gregorian reform movement including the Augustinians.

The mandatum manifests a community between the high and the low, between the spirit and the senses, between the head of the community and the feet, that is, between all the limbs of Christ. It is noticeable that this is expressed by the involvement of the senses, through water, bodily movements including mutual touching, sometimes including a kiss (as in the Regularis Concordia ceremony) between the clergy and others, as well as through sophisticated liturgical chant. The intellectual contents are expressed precisely through the sensory materiality and the bodily acts involved in the ritual.

The Notion of Ritual and Medieval Church Ceremonies

I have already used the (modern) term 'ritual' in my discussion; heuristically, it seems to work well in connection with the mandatum ceremonies, not least since these ceremonies seem to perform mental or spiritual transitions by way of material action and multisensory appeal. At the outset of this article, however, I promised to return to the less straightforward problem of using the modern notion of ritual to medieval church ceremonies. However, just as for ceremonies within court culture, the application of a modern anthropological term such as 'ritual' is a recent development in scholarship. The term *rituale* has been commonly used in scholarship to designate medieval handbooks for priestly use containing primarily the rites for baptism, penitential ceremonies, funerals, and (mainly from the thirteenth century onwards) also marriage. Historically, however, the term only came into use as a title of this type of book since the sixteenth century.[29] Completely independent of the terminology for the mentioned liturgical books, the modern anthropological term ritual was applied to medieval liturgy by some scholars in the late twentieth century in order to bring new, social, and anthropological perspectives to bear on the field.

One of the pioneers in this regard was C. Clifford Flanigan, whose studies of the so-called "liturgical drama" in the 1970s and 1980s were able to point to a social and ritual function of these ceremonies which in previous scholarship mainly had been discussed as religious drama, frequently in isolation from their liturgical context and rarely addressing their function within that context.[30] More recently, other scholars have also taken up such broader social perspectives within liturgical studies.[31]

Philippe Buc has pointed to the dangers in applying modern social theory on medieval culture, explicitly discussing the use of notions such as 'ritual' within the context of medieval, political culture. Buc emphasises the danger of reductionism in using the "too-often vague, and essentially alien concept of 'ritual'."[32] Indeed, the diversity of a concept of ritual in modern scholarship, which has not resulted in any general scholarly consensus, must in themselves give rise to caution.[33] Flanigan, in his work, mainly referred to Clifford Geertz and Victor Turner, and specifically to Geertz' understanding of a ritual as an event in which the participants' general understanding of the world would be reinforced through the experience of symbolic actions. Geertz' famous formulation, quoted by Flanigan, "in a ritual, the world as lived and the world as imagined [...] turn out to be the same world,"[34] provided a perspective on medieval liturgy which was not meant to reduce or simplify interpretations but rather to address questions of function in addition to multilevel interpretations, also taking the interdisciplinary construction of the ceremonies seriously. Thus the theoretical level in Flanigan's work was always given as an added perspective in a critical dialogue with historical interpretations of the texts and media involved.[35] Precisely, this understanding of 'ritual' fits in extremely well with the mandatum ceremony in clerical communities, a ceremony consisting in a symbolic act: the washing of feet which in some cases were even made clear to have been cleaned in advance, underlining the ceremonial act to be symbolic; participants were obviously not meant to actually clean dirty feet. This symbolic act emphasised the imitation of Christ's action in John 13:1-17, the response to his commandment to do so, and constituted at the same time a sensory sign of brotherhood and charity, fundamental ideals for the religious identity of the groups carrying out this ceremony. The *mandatum* enacted a sensory gesture of community, a tactile 'communion' of feet and hands touching each other as limbs of one communal body in Christ.

Even so, Buc's questions concerning the relevance of employing modern theory to medieval texts must be taken seriously. On the one hand, modern theories correspond to the questions modern scholars (necessarily) bring to bear on the medieval materials they investigate. On the other hand, these materials must be allowed their potential resistance to such questions and categorisations. One must – in principle – always be prepared to question the methodology with which a scholar approaches historical materials, as well as the questions posed by the scholar. In the case of medieval liturgical ceremonies, it is important to note that a parallel to the Geertzian understanding seemingly appears in a widely acknowledged medieval understanding, albeit of course differently formulated. A traditional tag concerning the agreement between Christian doctrine and church services goes back to the fifth century and implies at least partly what Geertz' statement – more generally – pointed out as the meaning of rituals, "lex credendi, lex orandi:"[36] the rule of belief must be in agreement with the rule of praying. In our context, the Geertzian phrase only seems to reformulate – in a modern scholarly language – a traditional claim that there must be agreement between what is experienced during the ritual and the general understanding of the participants, the doctrines of their religion.

Further, the wider perspective in Geertz' characterisation of ritual, the efficacy, in the sense that the ritual is thought to bring about a confirmation or reinforcement of the general beliefs of participants, also seems to have been part of how liturgical ceremonies were viewed in the Middle Ages. The notion of a sacrament is important in this context. The well-known, late-medieval understanding of a sacrament – defined by the list of seven sacraments (of the New Testament), as listed in Book IV of Peter Lombard's influential *Sententiae* from the second half of the twelfth century – was preceded by a more general understanding, according to which a sacrament was a sign pointing to something sacred. This general understanding had been promoted by St. Augustine, especially in *De Doctrina Christiana*, III, 13, where he pointed out how Christ's Resurrection had led to the existence of some few sacred signs for the Christian. Ultimately this replaced the complexity of all previous signs (notably signs from the Old Testament typologically prefiguring Christ). In spite of the generality of his theory of sacraments, Augustine only mentioned baptism and "the celebration of the Lord's body and blood."[37]

Even so, in theory the notion of sacrament was very broad. In principle it incorporated any sign pointing to God's grace, and no definitive list of sacraments was (or could have been) given at this time and for centuries after. Theologians would – with some individual nuances – understand the notion of a sacrament in a similar way.

This was summarised by Hugh of St. Victor in *De sacramentis christianae fidei* (written in the 1130s): "the doctors have designated with a brief description what a sacrament is: 'A sacrament is the sign of a sacred thing'."[38] Hugh's own modified definition takes its point of departure in the traditional understanding, narrowing it and making it clear that he would not consider, for instance, imagery to be included among sacraments. He demanded firstly that sacraments had a divine institution and secondly that they were given a particular sanctification. The latter, as it becomes clear, especially during Hugh's discussion of the example of baptism, must be understood as referring to the ceremonies through which the Church, as God's instrument for the restoration of man, effectuates the sacraments through words of sanctification added to the material element. In this, of course, Hugh drew on St. Augustine's famous formulation about baptism. Hugh gave his definition of a sacrament in these words:

> A sacrament is a corporeal or material element set before the senses outwardly, representing by similitude and signifying by institution and containing by sanctification some invisible and spiritual grace.[39]

In some respects Hugh's sacramental understanding constitutes a narrowing of the older notion of sacrament, introduced so as to make it clear that sacraments were salvific means provided by God's grace for the restoration of man and administered by the Church. The title of Hugh's work, *De sacramentis christianae fidei*, does not refer to his new understanding of sacraments, but to the very broad earlier meaning of *sacramentum* as *mysterium*, mystery or secret, i.e. a general account of the depths of Christian faith as the contents of the work demonstrates. The sacraments in Hugh's more specific understanding are introduced precisely at the point where Hugh needs to discuss God's means for the restoration of individual persons, fundamentally, of course, by reference to Christ's incarnation and his reconciliatory death and Resurrection.

Although Hugh's understanding represents a narrowing of earlier ways of talking about sacraments as signs pointing in particular to God's grace, this is still a very broad notion, which is not restricted to a particular number of sacraments. Hugh discusses examples of sacraments with obvious focus on baptism and the Eucharist, but admits the use of the term sacrament, for instance for the sign of the cross and for gestures by which sacred signs are expressed and, particularly important in this context, the liturgical songs and the liturgical devotions altogether. In this connection it must also be stated that Hugh's demands concerning his mentioned notion of the sanctification of a sacrament are not clearly defined, as the last mentioned examples demonstrate.[40]

What is of particular interest here is to see the briefly mentioned elements of Hugh's theology in a wider context where the notion of sacrament is in the process of being negotiated between a very broad and early understanding of signs pointing toward God's grace in Christ, and Hugh's more specifically ecclesiastical understanding, pointing out that such means of grace are and must be administered by the Church for the restoration of man. The changes in the understanding of the notion of sacrament during this process of negotiation must be seen also in the context of the Gregorian reform movement and was reflected not only in theoretical understandings, but also in the musico-liturgical practices of the Augustinian canons, as emphasised and demonstrated by Margot Fassler especially concerning the Victorines.[41]

Thus, still at this point in time, just as earlier, it was possible to consider many kinds of ceremonies as sacraments, aside from the later seven sacraments. Through the Carolingian reforms around 800, music had been awarded a very central place in liturgical ceremonies, expressed among other things through the rise of musical writing and thus the possibility to have music represented in authoritative books. Statements by Carolingian authors, among these Alcuin and Amalar of Metz, may be understood to underline the sacramental significance of liturgical song through the very tangible quality of sweetness (*suavitas*, *dulcedo*) of the voices used to attract the faithful. Writing in the 820s Amalar seems to connect the efficacy of liturgical song to what may be understood as its sacramental 'sweetness'.[42]

Regardless then of whether we insist on using a modern terminology of 'ritual', it seems that the basic understanding brought about by Flanigan's approach is indeed corroborated by theoretical considerations by medieval theologians and commentators of the liturgy itself, albeit in a sacramental terminology, which during the crucial centuries from the Carolingians to the High Middle Ages was not entirely stable.[43] The efficacy of the liturgical ceremonies in question at the time of Hugh of St. Victor depended on their correspondence with ecclesiastically defined doctrines and the particular divine institutions and ecclesiastical sanctifications. The sacraments, as ecclesiastical means of restoration for the faithful, would help them on their way to salvation and confirm their affiliation with the Church. This was true for all priests and monks including the canons regular, they would all be reinforced by the sacraments in their overall Christian beliefs and identity. It would seem that the mandatum, instituted by Christ in the Gospel of John, and sanctified through the ceremonial staging in the religious communities, should be seen as a sacrament in such an understanding of the notion – not least in its capacity to reinforce the religious communities in their identity as such. By signifying a holy community in Christ and giving it a highly sensible expression, the washing ceremony in reality re-instituted this very community by sanctifying it. The rinsing water and the ritualised gesture of human touch constituted a real act of grace – a grace bestowed through the sensory communication of hands and feet, of cleansing liquid, and touchable skin.

Atmosphere and the Senses

In recent years, the German theatre historian Erika Fischer-Lichte has presented a theory on aesthetic experience based on the notion of performativity.[44] The theory is clearly inspired by theatrical practices, as two of the most important terms, *Inszenierung* (staging) and *Performativität* (performativity) make clear. However, this is relevant to much wider categories of cultural phenomena than theatre, for instance various rituals and other public performative practices.[45] Four main terms are of particular significance in Fischer-Lichte's theory and for the application I want to make in pre-modern liturgical contexts.[46] In addition to the two already mentioned, we also find the notion of *Atmosphäre* (atmosphere), which depends on the notion of *Verkörperung* (embodiment).[47] What I need to note here about these terms is that staging regards that in a performative event, which can be rehearsed or planned prior to the event, i.e. the controllable part. In contrast, performativity marks that which is dependent on the actual event – that, which cannot be planned or controlled. This has to do with what occurs in a unique way at the very performance under consideration and is not repeatable. For instance, in a liturgical ceremony, what is written in the liturgical documents and is carried out every time belongs to the staging; but spontaneous movements, gestures or additional words said on the spur of a moment's inspiration belong to the performativity of the event.

This may include inadvertent errors, but more importantly, especially for planned performances, as were at least the historical liturgical ceremonies of which records have been preserved in liturgical books, the performativity comes to the fore by way of atmosphere. For Erika Fischer-Lichte atmosphere is connected to the embodiment of those who take part in the performance; in the case of a liturgical ceremony this may be priests, other parts of the clergy, singers, etc. but also the congregation, the – seemingly – passive partakers of the performance. Through presence, more or less noisy participation, through movements, as well as through visual appearance, all these persons influence the atmosphere and thus the uniqueness of a specific performance of a liturgical event. In addition, we find that the architectural frame, the particular light at that specific time and day, the weather, as well as other individual factors, influence the atmosphere and thus the uniqueness of a specific performance of a liturgical event.

The change in sacramental thought, as discussed above, brought important devotional performative acts into a higher degree of liturgical and ecclesiastical staging. Other confrontations with the sacred, including individual sensory experiences of what had earlier been considered as sacraments, experiences of signs pointing to God's grace beyond ecclesiastical control, were relegated to be considered less important with regard to their salvific function.

The application of Fischer-Lichte's terminology on medieval liturgy, and specifically on the mandatum ceremonies, helps to clarify the extent to which the impact of these rituals on the senses was staged, planned, foreseen, and how much was open to individual and local decisions in the moment. Texts, music, and action were all planned in great detail. But it is noteworthy how little rubrics say about the coordination and relation between the song and the action, and the requirements for the place. The latter would probably mostly have been decided locally including how the room would have been furnished and decorated. How was the interaction between the participants in the actual washing of the feet? Was the water heated, how much water did they actually use? How much did they actually touch each other and in what ways? What kind of kisses would they have exchanged? How regulated were such kisses? Although the singing as such was staged in most cases, the way the songs were sung, the sound of them, as it were, is not commented on in most liturgical documents (however, with a fair amount of exceptions). Were there pauses between the songs, did they sing one antiphon straight after the other? How much was up to local tradition, how much to the individual cantor leading the song? Did they all sing or was there a group of singers singing without taking part in the actual washing of the feet? It seems hard to imagine singers coping with long complicated melismas while washing the feet of another. Possibly, as in some liturgical situations, antiphons may have been sung by one participant at a time.

Similar questions can be asked about many medieval, liturgical ceremonies. Asking such questions may help make us aware of the huge impact the involved media would have had on the experience of the ceremony, but also how little we actually know about that experience and even about its material basis. Still, becoming aware of our ignorance and the seeming impossibility of overcoming it underlines how important the multisensory stimuli must have been for the atmosphere of the ritual and ultimately also for the individual interpretation of the devotional act. This would very likely not have been the same for all; especially one would imagine that the invited poor people might have had rather different experiences than the canons in the *mandatum pauperum*. The staging would, of course, have gone further than the documents tell us, in terms of traditions and oral instructions by the abbot, bishop, or who else was in charge.

What stands out, in any case, is that the ritual was staged as a multisensory event, which depended on words, music, physical action, and interaction between the participants and between the participants and the materiality of water. The ritual of the mandatum, centering on brotherhood and community, more than most liturgical ceremonies, seems to have put this idea of community into practice by way of actually making it felt through the senses, as did Jesus with his disciples in the narrative basis of the devotion. One may say that the ritual insists on the bodily basis of the spiritual community, i.e. a tangible manifestation of sensory and spiritual communion.

A Sacrament of Christian Sacraments

By way of conclusion, I shall mention two more examples from yet another context: that of the Teutonic Order, originally established in Acre in the early 1190s as a military hospital order during the third crusade. To my knowledge, scholars have only recently begun to study liturgical manuscripts in the State of the Teutonic Order (bordering on medieval Livonia). This has for instance been done through a collection of manuscripts in the Church of St. Mary in Gdansk, which was taken over by the Teutonic knights in 1308 and recently explored by Anette Löffler.[48] The two mandatum ceremonies I shall mention here are both from the fifteenth century, one from a missal printed before 1499 in Nürnberg for the Teutonic knights, the other from a manuscript of a missal from the early fifteenth century, which is kept in Gdansk.[49] These two mandatum ceremonies are clearly related, although one is much longer than the other, presumably written for a larger congregation. They are both solely concerned with an 'internal' mandatum. At least there is no mention of a mandatum ceremony for the *pauperum* or the sick, as in the orders for the Augustinian houses. This seems surprising considering that the Teutonic Order was originally founded as a hospital order. The general outline is very much like the other ceremonies consid-

ered here: combining chants, which broadly represent the narrative from John 13:1-
17, while also drawing on other contextually relevant stichs from the New Testament.
The shorter of the two ceremonies seems like a contraction of the longer. Possibly,
there was a particular Teutonic tradition of the mandatum.

However, what appears important is to underline how this ritual, which was carried out in individually localised ways in different monastic and clerical contexts at
the same time, seems to have the same fundamental character, at least from the tenth
to the sixteenth centuries, as in the other examples considered here. This also seems
to be so for the ritual character, understood as shorthand for a sacramentally efficacious ceremony as discussed previously. As pointed out already, the sacramental efficacy of the mandatum is in agreement with Hugh of St. Victor's notion of sacrament as expressed through the action and the materiality of the ceremony in washing,
drying, and singing. We only know the staging, and then only to some extent, since
we do not have specific knowledge of the architectural setting and the imagery connected to that. Also, in many cases even the music has not been preserved. Yet, we
still know that there was, in all these mandatum ceremonies from the high Middle
Ages onward, music, and in some of the texts we are informed that there seems to
have been a conscious use of specific rooms, "the place where the mandatum is meant
to take place." We do not know the details of the choreography, but we do know that
there was at least an overall scheme for how to do the ritual, and we can also conclude
that there would have been a very important role for atmosphere, as discussed above.
How the poor, who were drawn into the *mandatum pauperum* as described in the
consuetudines of the canons, experienced the ceremony, is impossible to say. But from
the point of view of the clergy, the canons, or the monks who were part of the mandatum ceremonies, the atmosphere of the ceremony would seem to have been simple, solemn, and ritualised, i.e. in a formal, stable, and repetitive form confirming the
interconnectedness and cohesion of the priestly brotherhood or monastic community. The attitudes toward the poor (which one may query based on the restrictive
comment in Marbach and Lund as mentioned above) may have made themselves felt
in the atmosphere, and maybe the atmosphere would in some places or depending
on some agents at various times have been genuinely embracing and loving as the
general intention of the ritual clearly supposes. Also, it seems possible to say that if
that was achieved, it would have been so through the bodily senses, the feeling of a
genuinely friendly, brotherly interaction between human bodies in the mutual washing of feet, combined with the audible experience of spiritual song referring to exactly such an experience as told in the biblical narrative.

199

The ritual and its meaning(s) may have been perceived in very different ways even within the same well-defined staging. In any case, its complex combination of sensory means and narrative references would seem to have manifested at least in some way a confirmation of a fundamental Christian understanding of life. This was done by joining together basic conditions of the poor, of earthly needs, and sacramental prefiguration of a heavenly brotherhood, as embodied in the service of the highest to the lowest clergy, or even to poor laymen. One may assume that the music might have pulled out the ritual from a sphere of moralistic teaching and condescending attitudes toward the lowly people (or clerics/monks) partaking in the event. This, however, can only be a speculative assumption.

The biblical account, John 13:1-17, tells that a performative act by Jesus was meant as a sign with an explicit morale: "So if I, your Lord and Teacher, have washed your feet, you also ought to wash one another's feet. For I have set you an example, that you also should do as I have done to you" (John 13:14-15).

What is described in the biblical mandatum narrative must, in the context of the early medieval Church, clearly have been understood as a sacrament. As already stated, any of the mandatum versions noticed here would have been possible to understand as a sacrament up until (and including) Hugh of St. Victor's definition of a sacrament. They were clearly acts with a material basis set before the faithful and instituted by Jesus in the Gospel text. In each individual version sanctified by the church through the ecclesiastical authority responsible for carrying out the ritual with words, actions, and materiality including song, this combined in an efficacious ritual manifesting religious community. It is obvious that the significance of the ritual is to point to the meaning of Christ's life with his disciples as an example for the life of any Christian, and even more specifically those who follow the example of Christ through their monastic or priestly calling.

All this comes to the fore in the interpretation of the double mandatum by the Benedictine Rupert of Deutz, who incidentally also seems to have been a staunch supporter of Gregorianism.[50] In his early twelfth-century *Liber de divinis officiis* he makes it clear that the *mandatum pauperum* corresponds to the grateful actions of the sinful woman from Luke 7 who anointed Jesus' feet with oil, pointing out that what is done toward the poor is done toward Christ (Matt 25:40). The *mandatum fratrum*, on the other hand, conveys what Christ did to his disciples, to the brethren, through the abbot. So, Rupert says, this latter one is a moral act, the other allegorical. Rupert even combines the mandatum with the Eucharist claiming it to be a sign to explain the meaning of the sacrament of Christ's body and blood:

In order that we may know with what love and humility he gives us this sacrament of his body and blood, he first washed the feet, as already stated, commending through this parallel this cleansing in the most appropriate way.[51]

In Rupert of Deutz' understanding we thus have a description of the mandatum as a sacrament of the sacrament of the altar. The mandatum is a ritual that combines the solemn sacraments in the liturgy with the bodily and basic life conditions of humans, as Jesus did in his ritual with his disciples according to John 13. The representation of Christ washing the feet of the disciples in Duccio di Buoninsegna's famous altarpiece commissioned in 1308 and set up in Siena Cathedral in 1311 exemplifies this, insisting on ritual skin contact between the members and bodies of the community [ill. 26].

[**III. 26**] Panel of Christ washing the feet of the disciples from the back of Duccio di Buoninsegna's *Maestà* (1311), now in Opera Duomo di Siena (Opera della Metropolitana). By permission of the Opera della Metropolitana.

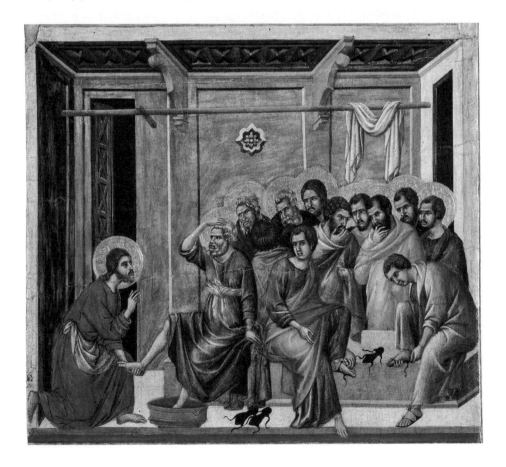

Here, the sensorially charged washing scene is placed among numerous passion panels right on top of the last supper at the back of the altarpiece, which was placed at the high altar of the cathedral where the Eucharist at the main masses would be celebrated. Apparently, the altarpiece had been placed in such a position that these images faced the community of canons who were seated behind the altar whereas the front of the altarpiece featuring a Madonna and Child faced the congregation in the nave.[52]

In the terminology of performative aesthetics, the ritual is performative, depending on the very individual act at the time and place where it takes place. In its staging, it presents the Christian disciplehood of those who take part in it; at the same time, it also stages their relation to the world, manifesting in its multimedia construction the complexity of human life in a Christian perspective.

A mandatum ceremony therefore manifests – in sensory terms – what all Christian rituals are about. It is, as Rupert pointed out, a sacrament of the Christian sacraments. This comes to the fore in the very materiality and bodily acts of the ritual, through its multimediality and the sensory appeal of its construction. It is a sacrament of efficacious touch, a sacrament of the senses more than any other of the known medieval sacraments, even baptism.

Notes

1 John Caldwell 2001, esp. pp. 586 & 588. Petersen 2007A, esp. pp. 332-36, Petersen 2007B, esp. pp. 89-92 and 99-106.

2 Heffernan & Matter 2001, p. 1.

3 See Flanigan, Ashley and Sheingorn 2001 & Petersen 2007A, pp. 332-36.

4 For a critical comment on the use of the term 'para-liturgy', see Flanigan 1996, pp. 15-16. For a late use of 'para-liturgical', see Stevens 1986, p. 80. An example of the use of 'extra-liturgical' can be seen in Young 1933, vol. I, p. 182.

5 The literature on medieval liturgical music, on the relationship between architecture and liturgy, and on the liturgical meanings of visual imagery is huge. Here, I also point to the relevant chapters in this volume containing further references.

6 Ambroise de Milan, ed. & trans. Dom Bernard Botte, 2007.

7 Ambroise de Milan, ed. & trans. (into French) Dom Bernard Botte, 2007, pp. 92-97 (quotation, p. 96): "Ideo lauas pedes, ut in ea parte in qua insidiatus est serpens maius subsidium sanctificationis accedat, quo postea te subplantare non possit. Lauas ergo pedes ut laues uenena serpentis."

8 Ambroise de Milan, ed. and translated by Dom Bernard Botte, 2007, p. 94. See English translation (by Edward Yarnold) of such a statement by Ambrosius in Whitaker 2003, p. 180.

9 Augustine, epistles 54 & 55, see Whitaker 2003, p. 147.

10 Whitaker 2003, pp. 192 & 203, see altogether pp. 183-203.

11 Whitaker 2003, pp. 261 & 273, and see pp. 212-51.

12 Leclercq 1931, col. 1388.

13 Amalarius of Metz, ed. Hanssens 1948, p. 80.

14 Leclercq 1931, col. 1388.

15 *Le pontifical romano-germanique du dixième siècle*, ed. Vogel & Elze 1963-72, II, pp. 77-78: Latin text : "Et diaconus imponat evangelium: *Ante diem festum paschae*, sicut ad missam. Lecto evangelio, dicat episcopus hanc orationem: *Deus cuius cenam*, ut supra. Data oratione, episcopus ponat vestimenta sua et precinctus linteo, preparet se ad lavandos pedes discipulorum suorum. Et primum, incipiente pontifice, mutuatim pedes lavent et distergant, canentes antiphona: *Mandatum novum. Psalmus Beati immaculati* [...] Finitis antiphonis, diaconus aut lector cui mandatum fuerit, imponat evangelium secundum Iohannem, quasi lectionem legens ab eo loco ubi scriptum est: Amen, amen dico vobis, non est servus maior domino suo [...]."

16 Toulouse, Archives Départementales de la Haute-Garonne, H 121, fragment 26, recto et verso. There are no rubrics in the fragment. I thank Dr Eduardo H. Aubert for showing this manuscript to me, for providing images for me to study as well as help with the transcription. The fragment breaks off at this point. Compare also Hesbert 1963-79, II, pp. 310-11, listing antiphons for a *mandatum* ceremony from the Hartker antiphonary (c. 1000).

17 *Regularis Concordia*, ed. and translated by Dom Thomas Symons 1953, pp. 40-41 (40). Latin text: "Peracta Missae celebratione omnes ad mixtum pergant; post mixtum quos uoluerit abbas ex fratribus secum assumens suum peragat Mandatum, quo peracta Vesperas celebrent. Dehinc refectionem fratrum agant post quam tempore congruo eorundem agatur Mandatum; qui tamen fratres prius pedes suos diligenter emundent; uenientesque ad Mandatum hebdomadarii ministri,

secundum morem suum abbatem antecedentes, Mandatum agant, quos subsequitur abbas in concha sua singulorum pedes lauans, ministrantibus sibi quos uoluerit ad hoc obsequium, quos extergat et osculetur."

18   *Regularis Concordia*, ed. & trans Dom Thomas Symons 1953, p. 40, n. 2. See the ceremonies in *Ælfric's Letter*, ed. & trans. Christopher A. Jones 1998, pp. 130-31 (sections 40 and 42) and see the commentary, p. 195.

19   *Die Consuetudines des Augustiner-Chorherrenstiftes Marbach*, ed. by Josef Siegwart 1965, pp. 101-261. *Necrologium Lundense*, ed. Lauritz Weibull 1923, pp. 14-45. *Consuetudines lundenses*, ed. by Erik Buus 1978, pp. 110-78. For the relationship between the documents, see Siegwart's "Einleitung," pp. 30-31. Swedish translation of the *consuetudines canonice* from Lund in Ciardi 2003. See also Møller and Buus 1987. The manuscript is preserved at Lund University Library, ms. 6; it is also published on the internet at http://laurentius.ub.lu.se/volumes/Mh_6/detailed/.

20   *Die Consuetudines des Augustiner-Chorherrenstiftes Marbach*, ed. Josef Siegwart 1965, "Einleitung," pp. 57, 59-60.

21   Just to mention a few others, rather randomly chosen: mandatum ceremonies fairly similar to the one from the fragment cited above (at n. 16) are found in two graduals kept in the Bibliothèque Nationale de Paris, BN lat 903 (early eleventh century, from St. Yrieix), f. 65v-68r, and BN lat 780 (late eleventh century, from Narbonne), f. 58r-59v. A sixteenth-century manuscript containing a processional from Châlons-en-Champagne, Bibliothèque Nationale, Paris, MS lat. 541 (previously 756), dated 1544 contains antiphons for a mandatum ceremony. All the songs are transcribed in *The Manuscript 541 of Bibliothèque Mazarine, Paris: The Processional of Châlons-en-Champagne*, ed. by Orsolya Csomó 2010, pp. 126-33, see also the introduction, pp. 1-87, where the mandatum is commented on pp. 72-73. All the ceremonies referred to here and above have elements in common but also many differences. The antiphons in the MS 541 have very few and only short melismas (except for the antiphon *Ante diem festum*, p. 131) distinguishing them from the early musical manuscripts mentioned. This seems rather to be due to a general stylistic development than to a particular musical interpretation of the mandatum.

22   Young 1933 (repr. 1967), vol. I, p. 99.

23   See Petersen 2012B & Petersen 2007A.

24   *Die Consuetudines des Augustiner-Chorherrenstiftes Marbach*, ed. Josef Siegwart 1965, "Einleitung," pp. 57, 59-60.

25   Norton 1983, pp. 156-57.

26   In spite of their polemics against Cluniac observances. See *Les Ecclesiastica Officia, Cisterciens du XIIème siècle* ed. by Danièle Choisselet and Placide Vernet 1989, 21.12; 23; 28; 31-45 and 23.30, pp. 102-105 and 108-109, indicating the practice of mandatum on Maundy Thursday as well as Holy Saturday. I thank Prof. Mette Birkedal Bruun for providing me with this information.

27   See the discussion of the ideology of regular canons in Fassler 1993 & 2011 pp. 264-65.

28   *Die Consuetudines des Augustiner-Chorherrenstiftes Marbach*, ed. by Josef Siegwart 1965, p. 223 (ch. 122): Qui tamen pauperes prius a camerario et elemosinario electi sunt, ne tales sint aliquomodo, qui claustrum non debeant intrare, id est non sanis pedibus vel iuvenes. See the same text verba-

tim – except for a changed order of a few of the words – in *Consuetudines lundenses*, ed. Erik Buus 1978, p. 157 (ch. XXV).

29   Palazzo 1993, p. 203.

30   Flanigan 1996; Flanigan 1985; Kobialka 1999; Petersen 2012B.

31   See for instance Palazzo 2000; Flanigan, Ashley & Sheingorn 2001; Boynton 2006 as well as the literature cited in the previous note. For a new important investigation of liturgy and the five senses, see Palazzo 2014.

32   Buc 2001, p. 247.

33   Bell 1997, pp. 1 & 21. See also Buc's criticism of Bell's attempts to solve the problem by way of the broader notion of ritualization instead of ritual, Buc 2001, p. 248.

34   Geertz 1966, p. 28 & Flanigan 1996, pp. 10-11, see also Petersen 2004, pp. 18-20.

35   Flanigan 1996, pp. 11-17. Flanigan 1991, pp. 21-23.

36   Wainwright 1980, pp. 218-83; see also the discussion in Petersen 2007B, pp. 91-92.

37   Augustine, ed. & trans. R.P.H. Green 1995, p. 147.

38   Hugh of St. Victor, trans. Roy J Deferrari 1951, p. 154. Latin text, PL 176, col. 317B: "Quid sit sacramentum, doctores brevi descriptione designaverunt: 'Sacramentum est sacrae rei signum'."

39   Hugh of St. Victor, trans. Roy J. Deferrari 1951, p. 155 (slightly modified). Latin text, PL 176, col. 317D: "sacramentum est corporale vel materiate elementum foris sensibiliter propositum ex similitudine repraesentans, et ex institutione significans, et ex sanctificatione continens aliquam invisibilem et spiritalem gratiam." For Hugh's understanding of the sacraments see also Fassler 2011, pp. 227-33, Coolman 2010, pp. 113-21.

40   Hugh of St. Victor, translated by Roy J Deferrari 1951, pp. 158 & 164. Latin text in PL 176, col. 321C-D, 322A & 326C-D.

41   Fassler 2011; see also Coolman 2010, pp. 103-4.

42   Petersen 2004, pp. 20-25; see also Ekenberg 1987, pp. 28-29.

43   On the discussions of liturgical drama and the changes in Eucharistic thought in the same period, see Kobialka 1999 & Petersen 2009.

44   The following brief points are based on Fischer-Lichte 2001.

45   Fischer-Lichte 2001, "Einleitung: Zwischen 'Text' und 'Performance'", pp. 9-23, and also pp. 299-300.

46   Petersen 2010 & Petersen 2012A.

47   For definitions and discussions of these terms, see Fischer-Lichte 2001, pp. 291-343.

48   Löffler 1998 & 2006.

49   *Liturgiczne aciskie dramatyzacje*, ed. Julian Lewaski 1999, pp. 218-22.

50   See Engen 1983, pp. 11-55.

51   Deutz, ed. and translated (German) by Helmut and Ilse Deutz 2001, II, p. 738-39, and see the full discussion, pp. 732-39. Latin text: "Quod quanta caritate et humilitate faciat, ut sciremus, illud nobis sui corporis et sanguinis sacramentum traditurus prius pedes lavit, sicut iam dictum est, per hoc simile purificationem illam decentissime commendans."

52   See Henk van Os 1988, vol. I, pp. 39-62, esp. pp. 39-43.

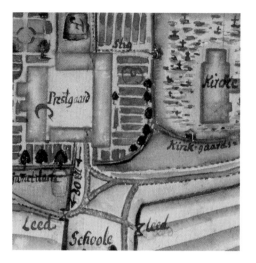

206

[**ENVIRONMENT**] This chapter addresses the role of the senses and material culture in understanding early medieval church environment in southern Scandinavia (i.e. eleventh to thirteenth centuries in this context). While emphasis is on the normative power of liturgy, theology, and text in the interpretation of medieval churches, this chapter argues that the senses and bodily movement are formative in the human appreciation of abstract phenomena. The chapter therefore includes considerations on the landscape and the churchyard in defining what constituted the early medieval church environment. It is suggested that the significance of events and action inside the church was already beginning to form in the movement towards the church and across the burial ground. The formative power of this journey unfolded further inside the church through a host of embodiments, materialisations, and sensory experiences. Together these worked towards the formation of particular ecclesiastical concepts and ideals of which the presence of the immaterial God was essential.

ENVIRONMENT

Embodiment and Senses in Eleventh- to Thirteenth-Century Churches in Southern Scandinavia

[Mads Dengsø Jessen & Tim Flohr Sørensen]

Environment as Sensory Landscape

Over the past millennium, the Christian church in Denmark has equipped the landscape with a very clear staging of religious worship and devotion through its position in the physical environment. However, the physical and spiritual construction of church and churchyard are not only grounded in discursive theological and liturgical principles, but also contains a number of sensory and material qualities. These materialities, we argue, are central to understanding the church environment and appreciating its social and spiritual functions in the Middle Ages as well as today.

In this chapter, we will therefore focus on the physical organisation of the church environment in relation to the churchgoers' location and movement, as we seek to explore what we hold to be an intrinsic dialectic between physical location, material qualities, and the cognitive space of the church environment. Introducing the notion of the 'church environment', we seek to address the overall sensory and ideological *milieu* that connects the wider church landscape, churchyard, church institutions and functions, and of course the users of the church and churchyard.

Pursuing the themes of environmental influence, we attempt to illustrate how material and sensuous experiences interact and influence each other. We suggest it is through such reciprocal and continuous dialectics that sociality, politics, religious practice, and performativity are put into play and that the product of this interaction is the physical, social and cognitive organisation of both the internal and external church environment. The interaction between the material and the sensory are conditioned by physical acts, or embodiments, which we consider to be co-creative for a multimodal surface of signification, which produces both discursive as well as pre-reflexive references, as will be explored below.

We address these issues by focusing first on the phenomenological and cognitive aspects of the church environment. We then briefly outline some of the key sensory similarities and material structures that can be identified at medieval cemeteries and in churches, and then discuss the perspectives that can be drawn by combining material observations with the multimodal meanings that arise at the intersection of body, movement, and cognition.

Re-orienting Religious Experience: Materiality and the Senses

There has often been a tendency to apply unidirectional interpretation models in the analysis of churchly activities and religious life. This directionality transfers general theological principles to particular physical spaces, which means that a 'top-down' analysis of liturgy and architecture framed by discursive formulations has been prevailing.[1]

Offering an expanded interpretative framework, we seek to actualise a 'bottom-up' approach to these issues, thus focusing on the tangible sensations that the church and its immediate environment demanded of and offered the perceiver. Through the bottom-up approach, we therefore seek to trace the phenomenological qualities that may materialise near and in churches, and which affect the conceptualisation one may generate from use of the medieval church. The phenomenological basis emphasises the importance of understanding the bodily situatedness and attunement of human experience.[2] The intersection of situatedness and shifting attention, we hold, are part and parcel of the constitution of the medieval church environment. This contention will form the interpretative frame of reference for the present chapter. We do not claim that a bottom-up approach should be understood as giving access to a more 'true' or 'authentic' image of the church environment than other approaches. We simply hold that it offers a complementary view on the use and perception of the medieval church that emphasises the role and perspective of the ordinary churchgoer and their engagement with the church environment through the intersecting sensory modalities. This also includes an appreciation of the congregation's appropriation of structural (or 'top-down') schemata.

To enable this perspective, there are certain premises one must keep in mind.

Firstly, *sensing* can and must pass through the physical body and be absorbed through the sense modalities that humans are biologically equipped with. This simply implies that they can smell, feel, see, taste and hear.[3] Secondly, bodily experiences are grounded in a *pre-linguistic* understanding of the world. This means that any linguistic formulation of a given ritual situation can not only create meaning in a particular religious act, but are also very likely to include an abstraction of a bodily experience. Thirdly, impressions from the individual sense modalities will often combine, reinforce, and underpin the particular meaning-context one is situated within – that is, meaning is constructed on *multimodal* experiences. The latter, however, we choose to denote as the 'recursive' or 'replicative' tendency, which cognitive studies have shown to be deeply embedded in human thinking and meaning construction.[4]

209

A central challenge to the church environment is the fact that part of its *raison d'être* is accessing the sacred and the holy, which within Christianity includes an immaterial and un-embodied transcendental and omnipotent entity. Perhaps the incorporation of material objects into the religious structure will offer scaffolding for the otherwise negligible stimuli of the transcendental, or even constitutes the basis of such stimuli. Without incorporation of the material world, the experience of a religious world would be severely impaired or perhaps even impossible.[5] Therefore, to put religious information into the material environment will inevitably lead to a tangible and sensuous grounding of religion itself. Such entities can only be presented as objects or bodily activities. With this in mind, we regard the bottom-up channel of sensing as providing a sort of framing function for religious sensing, within which top-down cultural influences can operate.

For these reasons, we choose to adopt a fundamentally material and bodily approach to the church environment, but expand this frame of analysis by pointing out the potentially universal human sensory inclinations that underlie the particular expression that the ritual space in the southern Scandinavian Middle Ages articulates. But because human experience of bodily dispositions is – at least in part – culturally variable we need to scrutinise the particulars of the medieval church environment and their cultural context in order to transcend the interpretative frameworks that are based solely on contemporary perspectives. We will therefore look at the sensory interaction and exchange that can be expressed by assuming a bodily basis for the research on space and action, and how bodily experiences ground abstract meaning. In doing this, we also allow intentions, emotions, experiences, and actions in the world to become meaningful in themselves and constitutive for the human understanding of the world. The consequence of such a view upon human ontology is the renunciation of any rationalistic view, separating subject and object. The mind and body organisation can be seen as embracing both outer and inner structures, between which a constant circulation and mutual elaboration unfolds, which in effect breaks down any simplistic dualism, conforming to a clichéd Cartesian separation of mind and matter. That is, a dialectic system, which integrates material as well as mental structures, and defines both spheres as generative and necessary for the construction of meaning.[6]

The Physical Environment

Nowadays the church tower often exhibits a prominent visual expression in a parish, and especially in rural parishes. The church tower can be seen from afar and has been even more visible in more treeless eras of Danish history.[7] In the dark winter around the time of Christmas, we see how spotlights illuminate the church and church tower in many parishes throughout Denmark. This accentuates the visual and topographical fix point that church towers have formed since their development from the previous bell towers (from ca. 1200 onwards), especially as a result of Gothic modifications.[8] Herein lies another aspect of the tower's reach, which not only relates to its visual effects, but also the aural embrace of the landscape. The church is a centre of experience, or a target for movement towards mass, wedding or funeral, and it is a focal point in the parish, which can be either seen or heard far and wide. On most locations where Romanesque churches were erected they radiated a very obvious physical presence and authority as a result of their innovative and unconventional design principles. This is especially evident in southern Scandinavia, where the earliest churches offered a particularly distinctive quality as they were among the first stone-built buildings (we here deliberately omit the few wooden churches, which are registered among the earliest church buildings as their number and dating leave more questions than answers).[9] Stone is a sturdy building material, which means that churches often outlived other nearby structures, and held a deep biography in comparison to other structures. The churches therefore dominated the landscape and were visually compelling when one approached them. Moreover, stone also exhibits certain immanent properties: permanence, stability and non-earthly power which may appear to be particularly suitable for religious buildings. In addition, a stone-built church forms a palpable contrast to the ordinary, surrounding buildings and hereby underlines the specific functions pertaining to this particular structure.

Presence and Proximity

In numerous religions burial grounds are usually placed in seclusion from the temples and in many cases also from the ordinary settlements. The traditional layout of the ritual environment within Latin Christianity places graves in a specified area around churches, and even places the churches inside profane settlements, and therefore marks a radical opposition to this pervasive trend (we here focus on burial and the churchyard as the vast majority of the congregation was excluded from intramural burial).[10] The theological background for the nomination of the area around the church as the 'natural' place to lay devout believers to rest has deep historical roots within the Latin Christian Church and is tightly connected to the founding of Christian cult sites. Originally the cult around the Christian martyr graves (in Rome from the third century onwards) dominated the ritual environment, as these were places of great veneration. Here the mass also took place to commemorate the martyr's date of death. Gradually such graves became equipped with altars and cult houses were built to protect these. In combination with the advent of detailed cultic practices, the Christian teachings became more elaborate as did the theological position of the saints and martyrs, which resulted in increasing investments into the cult houses, making them what we might call 'churchlike'.[11] In these new teachings the martyrs are believed to be the first to rise at the Second Coming of Christ. They will assist him in separating the pious from the doomed and in guiding the awakened believers to the eternal kingdom. An unintended consequence of this teaching was that it became desirable to be buried contiguously with martyrs: physically and palpably near them, in order to be guaranteed a qualified guidance to eternal salvation.[12] In the mid fourth century, following Emperor Gratian's eager intentions to complete the introduction of Christendom as the official ideology of the Roman State, there occurred a transfer of relics from different martyr-graves to the Roman temples which were being converted into Christian churches (particularly in Rome and Milan). This was a process, which strengthened the bond between ritual building and ritual burial. For this reason, Latin Christian churches and funerary practices came to accompany each other intimately, and the first steps to regular churchyards were taken. Hereby a bond was formed, which has existed ever since.[13]

A tangible effect of this intimacy between the component parts of the church environment was that being buried close to the church was desired and contested. Eventually, at least for the Scandinavian churchyards, the organisation of the burials necessitated legal management, and different charters designating who were allowed to be buried in the more attractive zones were prepared.[14] An interesting feature of the proximity parameter can be recognised in the otherwise rather insignificant graves of the royal family during the period under investigation. Inside St. Bendt's church in Ringsted, Zealand, a series of royal graves dating from Earl Knud Lavard (dead 1131) to queen Margrethe I (dead 1341) all follow the same principle: the deceased were interred closely around the altar.[15] Seemingly, the grave itself becomes a symbolic extension of the deceased's social heritage and functions as a locational agent in the revering of the 'eternal home' of the royal family. The position of a grave therefore related to the religious as well as social propriety of the deceased, and the normative directions for the positioning of graves rested on ideological and sensory principles for how the dead, awaiting doomsday, should be positioned in relation to God.[16]

This implies that, in the course of movement across the burial space towards the church, the churchyard is the physical locality that binds the sacred and the profane together in more than one sense. Demarcation of the graveyard was a ritual imperative for Latin Christians and being buried in unholy ground was virtually unthinkable. Great measures were therefore often taken to fulfil these ideological and material requirements.[17] Thus, the physical churchyard was consecrated, but it was not a holy place in the same sense as the church, although the churchyard was bounded from its profane exterior by, for example, dikes or small embankments. Still, the churchyard did not contain an absolute holiness in itself, but framed the dead matter, which in a theological sense, was (and is) the germ and promise of eternal life for humankind. In the churchyard, and according to tradition, the dead usually lie buried with their heads to the west and feet to the east,[18] so they can sit up at the last day and face the light of resurrection coming with the Redeemer.[19] When medieval churchgoers moved across the churchyard, they therefore travelled from the profane sphere into the sacred. In this respect the churchyard was a kind of intermediary space, which connected the earthly life of the congregation with holiness and eternity.

In medieval times, the physical frame for movement over the churchyard was characterised by some of the same elements, which we also meet at contemporary cemeteries. Churchyard walls (or ditches) defined the extent of the consecrated space, where doors and gates presented transitions between the interior and the exterior. In addition, gratings were installed in the gates to prevent domestic animals in the rural parishes from entering the churchyard.[20] There were, however, obvious differences in the aesthetic qualities of the medieval churchyard, and only very seldom

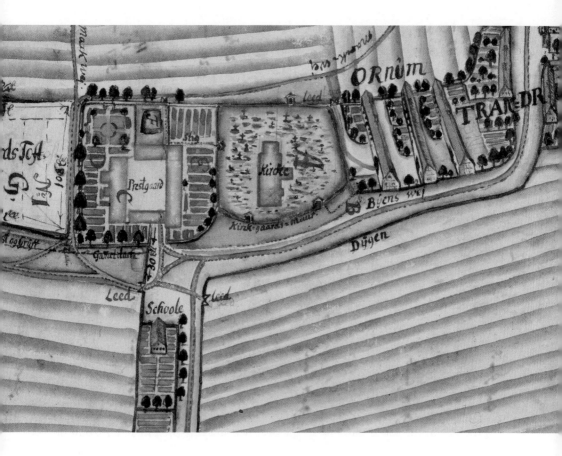

[**Ill. 27**] In the "Cadastre over the Churches and Vicarages on Ærø – 1734" the Tranderup church, third parcel from the left, is illustrated in detail. In the picture the small grave tufts with the occasional wooden cross are clearly visible, and the difference in appearance in comparison with the ordinary parcels on either side of the churchyard is evident. At the churchyard trees are absent and the parcel is, as the only one, demarcated by a low wall with four roofed gates. (North is towards left). Photo courtesy of N.J. Poulsen.

do plants, trees and hedges form part of the portrayal in the few drawings and pictorial representations of graveyards that we know of from that time [see ill. 27 for a later *albeit* telling depiction].[21] Inevitably, the churchyard would appear as a monotonous and lifeless parcel and such a sensory austerity would have comprised an environment in stark contrast to the surrounding village with its small farming plots and their diverse buildings and constellations. The surrounding cultivated landscape characterised by crop rotation and longer periods where the fields would lie fallow,[22] would, however, mirror the 'inactive' churchyard. In a way, this expressive similarity can be seen as highly appropriate for accommodating graves, which were conceived of as sensory arid and intermediate places of rest for the human corpse, while awaiting the Second Coming. Accordingly, inside the graveyard the visitor would have encountered little more than the graves themselves, and the immediate appearance of the graveyard was almost completely defined by the small graves. Medieval graves assumed the form of low, grassy elevations of the soil that was turned over each grave, called grave tufts. Among common people, memorial markers usually consisted in a wooden cross, whose durability roughly corresponded to the life of the grave, i.e. the time until the earthen mound had collapsed and become level with the surface around it.[23] There was thus an apparent service-life built into the graves of the commoners, standing in stark contrast to the graves that the higher strata of society could expect with elaborate naming and memorial texts carved in stone, or burial under the floor of the nave of the church.

Moreover, individuals, who were not interred inside the very church, would often later have their memorial stones transferred to the church. The material qualities of the grave demarcation were thus meaningful as a social marker of the deceased; some were defined by permanence, while others decomposed in the organic sense as well as in social memory. The sensory qualities of the memorials were thus also expressions of the social morality of the deceased, playing on a hierarchisation of the decomposable (i.e. forgettable) versus the permanent (i.e. worthy of preservation). Here, it is worth keeping in mind that the majority of the rural population was less affluent. They would not have financial access to building permanent memorials for themselves or their beloved. In this sense, the penetrable and perishable organic materials in the earthen grave would imply a humane and mundane death, while the graves built in stone suggested an eternal existence, resembling the alterity of the divine.

It has also been suggested that the construction of the earliest cemeteries can be interpreted as a micro-cosmic replication of an idealised cityscape.[24] The concentric structure prevailing in the early medieval townscape, i.e. with the cathedral and/or other ecclesiastical buildings as visual and physical focal point, is echoed in the churchyards with the church as an absolute centre and with the graves almost presenting themselves as small houses inhabited by individuals or families. As mentioned, the Christian ritual locales also have a profound urban genesis, and in some regions it was not until after AD 1000 that the rural areas started seeing Christian temples – exactly the period when the Danish parish churches were being built. For this reason, the sensory experience generated by movement through this ritual space became a replication of the idealised urban space or maybe *vice versa*.

Formalised paths did not always define the movement across the churchyard from the gate to the church as in the contemporary urban environment, and as we know from today's cemeteries.[25] In addition, new graves were arranged where there was room for them, with certain areas of the churchyard being considered more de- sirable than others. This valorisation of the churchyard was not only based on the above mentioned proximity or distance from the church building, but also revolved around a fusion of sensory experiences and elements of folklore. Here, the sensory and symbolic perception of daylight plays an important role, because luminosity and the sun's heat were considered to add specific benevolent attributes to certain locations in the churchyard. The eastern and southern parts of the cemeteries have traditionally – at least in certain parts of Denmark – been the more popular places of burial, while the cooler and darker areas in the churchyard's northern and western parts rarely contain as many graves.[26]

The activities taking place inside the churchyard not only generated a certain atmosphere, but likewise affected the environment beyond the consecrated area. Already in the eighth century it was common, as in continental cloisters, to initiate the funerary rite by sounding the church-bell. In the beginning, bell-ringing announced that a member of the convent had passed away, and intercession should therefore commence. In time, bell-ringing itself became an autonomous, ritual component, as it was believed that the sound of the bell was particularly efficient in keeping at bay demons pursuing the soul of the deceased. This practice is, for example, described in Scandinavian texts as being part of the mortuary procession, where the ringing of small bells could accompany the deceased from his deathbed to his grave. When the procession came closer to the church and entered the churchyard, the church-bell would start ringing and call the parishioners to join the *requiem*.[27] During the Middle Ages it was believed that the dead body was both vulnerable and possessed potentially destructive powers, wherefore the journey with the corpse was not taken lightly. Through timely prayer, the relatives (or the priest) would thus keep a vigil over the body until it was properly buried, and protect it during the mortuary procession. During these prayers, the sound of the bell was perceived as an aural defence against the diabolic – a prophylactic, auditory effect that could cleanse the surroundings through its tangible sonic presence in the sensory environment.

Consequently, even if the use of bells can be regarded as a rather late introduction, it had a profound influence on the Christian environment. Not only were special buildings erected to accommodate large church-bells, but also the sound itself would alter the soundscape of the affected areas. Bell-ringing, especially with regards to the church-bells, would comprise the perhaps most pervasive contact between the church environment and the congregation. The sound-waves would reach far and even pass through walls and be heard inside other buildings. Such auditory experience would have begun at the first sound of the church bells, through which the churchgoer would attune to the emotional context of participating in the *requiem* or the mass and priming a sensation of holy presence.[28]

Altogether, the valorisation of the grave as a location at the churchyard was thus not simply a matter of schematic geography, but also revolved around the qualitative constitution of bodily sensations that in turn were decoded with reference to religious and cultural top-down perceptions of benevolence and malevolence.

Between Matter and Metaphor

Moving into the church, the organisation and appreciation of sacredness continues to build on sensory effects, yet it is also transferred to different modalities. Many of the sacred manifestations that the churchgoer would encounter would therefore entail sensory experiences, which were both very familiar to the churchgoer, but at the same time appeared out of place or with at special quality attached to them. How the comprehension of such multimodal experiences came about, can be related to more habitual activities encountered outside the church environment.

For instance, a central ritual phenomenon, such as the Eucharist, seems to be based on a replication of ordinary, domestic events, since the consumption of the particular food items has historically been a re-enactment of the Last Supper and thus refers to a well-known situation.[29] Thus, what is normally considered a logical problem can become mediated: the dead and absent God is made present and is no longer just an indexical reference, but assumes concrete and sensory presence. The body of Christ is concretised through what in an anthropological sense must be considered a 'magical' transubstantiation, which takes place by the unification of the priest's speech acts and the material-cultural dimension in the form of the consecrated sacramental bread and wine. The actual sensory qualities of the food items are not changed in comparison with ordinary wine and bread, but still under the influence of the physical laws and will *de facto* provide exactly the same sensory stimuli. However, the recurring theological instruction that bread and wine in the Eucharist are manifestations of the flesh and blood of Christ influences the sensual understanding and perception of the ritual. Therefore, the transubstantiation is a replication of a familiar sensory experience that is played out during the sacrament, but in the magical context inside the church becomes elevated to sacred significance.

Religious references often occur in direct relation to conceptual categories, which are inaccessible to the human sensory apparatus; i.e. abstract, theological formulations of religious concepts. That is why the Latin Christian world order was simulated through the manipulation of materials in the typical Romanesque church. For example, the easternmost section of the church consisting of the chancel, often with an apse as the easternmost marker, contains several simulative elements. The chancel constitutes the place where the priest performs the majority of and most significant liturgical activities and where direct contact with the divine takes place, while the apse functions as a prototype of the sacred tomb in Jerusalem.[30] On the border between these two spatial demarcations, the main altar is established and is theologically conceptualised as the tomb of Jesus Christ. Altogether the easternmost area therefore connotes the complex conception of the physical presence of God on earth, the absence of God and the promise of resurrection, or in other words simultaneity of past, present, and future. Inevitably, such a palimpsest of holy prowess also reaches outside the walls of the church, and contributes to the particular distribution of graves on the churchyard (see above). In this fashion, the organisation of the churchyard becomes a tangible extension of the sacred architecture of the church-building itself.

Moreover, the easternmost part of the church forms the scene for the most significant religious rituals, and functions as a fixed point for the congregation's attention during the service. The eastern part of the church is explicitly designated as the most sacrosanct area, while also implicitly experienced as particularly essential, because the congregation is oriented towards this area. The lighting too accentuates the eastern end, and only rarely, at specific ritual events, do the churchgoers set foot in this area.

In this way, imagined space and physical space is fused into a particular materiality, which anchors the theological abstraction in the sensory locale.[31] This fusion plays on a constant distance between the churchgoer and the holy; not, however, as an unambiguous and distinct separation as the worshipper is within visual and auditory proximity of the holy, but instead as a distance that stimulates a constant necessity for focal attention towards the holy. Returning to the Eucharist, we may see the element of 'attending towards' highlighted in this sacrament, which emphasises that "this is my body" and "this is my blood" (Matt. 26:26-28). In other words, it determines that the divine is unquestionably present, yet the divine is at the same time conceived as immaterial and absent.[32] Consequently, the senses are not simply directed towards a tangible object of attention, but towards being in the presence of the immaterial god.[33]

The same situation applies to the use of incense during the mass, where incense makes reference to sweet and high-flying smoke that burns through God's love and emits the scent of Christ (2 Cor. 2:14-16). Moreover, the point is that incense has a prophylactic effect, if not medically then spiritually. And of course the burning of incense is seen as an integral part of the liturgy as a form of prayer. Importantly, this draws our attention not to what the substance *is* or what it *represents*, but what it *does* and how it *works*.

In other words, the use of incense in the medieval church provides the opportunity for attending to its effects as a material agent. As sensory elements, odours are unique, because the olfactory sense is the only sense that functions 'nominally' and does not already possess an intrinsic valorisation. No smell will therefore naturally be perceived as more pleasant than others, wherefore the significance of incense can only be understood through experience and context.[34]

This means that incense will not only be detected and observed empirically, but that incense will be experienced in relation to the expectations that one has learned. Friction between the body's sense modalities and the church's materiality, in this case emissions of smoke particles, will, in other words, generate a reciprocal and dialectical framework for the way churchgoers are affected by the aromatic sensorium of the church environment in a particular manner. For most of us the medieval references to "the sweet stench of the grave" must seem as a misleading description of decay.[35] However, the use of censers in the sub-floor graves mixed the smell of incense and putrefaction, and thus gave meaning to the people who were exposed to the smell of the decomposing corpses under the church floor.

We may also suggest that the smell of a putrefying corpse was not only bringing back the memory of the deceased, but offered a sensible and affective propinquity[36] in addition to expressing her or his moral righteousness.[37] Religious buildings, in this case the medieval church, can thus be seen as theological catalysts that link technological innovation, architectural qualities and divine presence into a concrete earthly manifestation. The church building can be considered an extra-somatic and sensuous religious concept, incorporating the heavenly kingdom on earth – it thus forms a religious phenomenon, which can be experienced, i.e. sensed.[38] It may, in fact, be shared by the entire congregation, despite potential differences in the intellectual access to particular meaning contents of the ideological and theoretical foundation of the church.

The Church Interior: Sound and the Resonance of God

Moreover, the sensory effects of a stone building are particularly notable with regard to the acoustic conditions that prevail here. Such structures provide a significant reverberation, sometimes echoing, depending on the number of parishioners present. Here, the congregation's recitations and iterations can be experienced as powerful, but also the utterances of individuals are easily captured, such as the priest's silent prayers without the words being recognisable – a fact which we will return to.

It is likely that these auditory sensations are, to a large extent, unique to the church, due to the fact that stone-built buildings did not become common until later in history. By its very nature the unique acoustics were therefore also generative of the particular form of religious belief unfolding in the church building. This does not necessarily have to concern the memorisation of utterances in the church in the form of statements, instructions, and messages. Referring to the multimodalities of sensory experience, we might just as well expect the churchgoers to build a memory of a less distinct impression of one's presence in the church, summing up the total sensory landscape of the church interior. In this regard, speech and singing could have been appreciated for their affective agency on the body, such as the rumble of bass sounds, the way in which sound fills the room and the vibrato of one's own voice.

In Latin Christian liturgy the ritual semantics of most of the mass are nonsense, literally, for the vast majority of the congregation in the medieval church. As a consequence, the presence of meaning is not based on the actual *understanding* of language, but on the *performance* of speech.[39] In this context it is therefore possible to consider the liturgical Latin as an essential material-cultural element, which does not differ fundamentally from other conventional, physical components appearing in the medieval church environment. This means that the theological properties in the ritual language are projected into the ritual frame and cause a specific type of speech act. Hence, only the audible elements – i.e. the material properties of spoken or recited words, the reverberation of sound waves – will offer the listener an extension of her religious understanding. This prompts three major aspects of medieval ecclesiastical language: Firstly, the word has an indexical or iconic connection to the ritual object it presents. Secondly, it implies the emergence of a pragmatic context defined by the beginning and ending of the ritual (i.e. a liturgically definite sequence often involving the manipulation of objects), which distinguishes the hieratic aura of this specific wording from the milieu of everyday life. And finally, there is a social and authority-based differentiation between the consecrated clergy, who can use and understand Latin, and the congregation that predominantly senses the language as a pre-textual experience. So, the priest performs a ritual, which, to a certain extent, contains a kind of 'sacred knowledge' and the congregation experiences a special presence through the auditory resonance and sonic impact of the 'Word of God', not belonging to ordinary people's language.[40]

The linguistic factors used in Latin Christian liturgy become a sort of 'underdetermined signs' without completely resolved meaning content for the recipient, but rather attaining meaning through the context of usage.[41] While this normally would be devastating for ordinary, everyday verbal relations, it is not necessarily the case in a ritual context. The possible meanings of words are loosely demarcated by the schematic structure that is inherent to their iconic and indexical properties (i.e. the liturgical reiterations), as well as the symbolic elements that are present in their immediate context (i.e. the church environment).

This means that the words' sensory – or *aesthetic* – qualities dominate over their semantic references. One can almost talk about an objectification of the linguistic sign relation, with the result that the liturgy becomes a register of 'free-floating signifiers', which merely present aural significance.[42] That is, a collection of indices for the listener, which find their place not in relation to syntax or semantics, but in relation to the pragmatic dimension, i.e. in relation to the context, namely the church.

The important thing is therefore to acknowledge that the intersection of spiritual, liturgical, and ideological elements on the one hand, and on the other hand the tangible, sensuous and corporeal aspects is not just a metaphorical paraphrase of an underlying narrative and discursive program, but equally serves as an instrument of actualisation. The friction between conceptual meaning and actual church environment works to the extent that it has an ability to make the abstract present and accessible. This lies beyond the discursive understanding of materialised liturgy, and one cannot, for example, exclusively understand the rituals taking place during mass as the communication of semantic knowledge in a linguistic form, but must rather see the rituals as the process of embedding the believer in the physical here and now, being near and moving towards the divine. Here, the body and the sensuous take centre stage, thus unfolding as a pre-linguistic relationship of sensory meaning consigned by an organised atmosphere of significance.[43]

Embodying the Holy in the Medieval Church

We may sum up the main point of our argument as emphasising a pre-reflective mode of comprehension as the primary relationship between church architecture and churchgoer in the medieval religious environment. In the examples mentioned above, movement, positioning, and bodily interaction with the physical environment – the landscape, the churchyard, and the church – are essential factors: moving in physical space internalises the understanding of the transcendental and abstract dimensions of the holy.[44] The sacred is found at the end of movement, in the heart of the labyrinth that is constituted by the organisation of the parish, churchyard, church, choir, and altar. These dimensions also imply that there is a difference between interior/exterior, near/distant, high/low and up/down in the structuring of the sacred space, suggesting to the churchgoer that the structure takes place in all three dimensions.

Moreover, we have identified the specific auditory space in relation to the experience of architecture and landscape, the haptic experience of walking across the churchyard as a cognitive journey from the domestic to the sacred sphere, and we have identified the importance of the Eucharist by associating symbolic and practical consumption, furthermore intensifying the complex theological friction between that which is present and that which is absent, and the material and the immaterial aspects of the divine. The contrasts to the secular world are, in other words, generated through movement and sensation, and not so much via rational communication.

It is therefore important to keep in mind that replications of the secular in the sacred space are often grounded in replicating ordinary worldly experience, but one which at the same time is orchestrated in contrasting contexts. Such a situatedness saturated with contrasts may greatly help to intensify the experience of being in the church, producing the effect that the ritual is better remembered and thus better internalised by the congregation. In general, the experience of the original and the peculiar makes a clearer trace in the mind of the perceiver than would every day, ordinary sensations. From a ritual perspective, it is essential that the ritual environment and the performative content differ from secular life – that it seems to stand in contrast to what one experiences outside the church walls.

One of the effects of this contrast is to stage the ritual locale as a place with a particular potential for experiencing the *presence* of the divine. Recently, the predominant focus within the 'linguistic turn' on meaning and semantic value[45] has been challenged by research that observes how meaning and discourse do not always take centre stage in human experience of the world, neither in human social life nor in the formulation or performance of cultural ideas and values.[46] This critique challenges us to draw attention to aspects of human experience that exceed meaning, whether as a result of sensory saturation, lack of knowledge, ignorance, confusion, altered states of consciousness, or by the simple fact that some experiences can be felt as 'meaningless' or conversely 'incomprehensible'. Such experiences, we maintain, were indeed part of the medieval religious practice conducted in the church environment, and we suggest that the passage from a *sphere of meaning* to a *sphere of presence* was orchestrated through the movement from the domestic, profane landscape, over the consecrated churchyard to the interiority of the house of God.

Discussing a Late Antique context and thus a rather different religious environment, Peter Brown describes how early Latin Christian pilgrimage was centred on the movement that brought the worshipper into the presence of relics and saints, or within the *praesentia* of the holy.[47] This movement, Brown contends, is to be understood as a "therapy of distance" within which the pilgrim remained at all times. Even upon arriving at the goal of the pilgrimage after a long and strenuous journey, the relic or the saint remained hidden, out of sight. The relics of saints were shrouded in their confusing and ambiguous *potentia*, i.e. their invisible and ideal existence that was always characterised by possibility and potentiality, rather than fact or revelation. This signifies how the journey must go on within the pilgrim: the journey towards the holy is a perpetual journey as s/he is always divided from the object of the journey. Pilgrimage would thus not be undertaken for the sake of achieving knowledge or understanding of a religious concept, but in order to obtain a sense of nearness towards the holy.[48]

Even though we do not suggest that attending mass in the medieval Danish churches were the equivalent of a pilgrimage, we would like to suggest that certain aspects of *praesentia* and *potentia* were offered in different forms by the medieval church environment. In particular, the immediacy of a *milieu*, different to the senses from the everyday domestic context would have stimulated a perceptual mode of engaging in the mass, which drew on the experience of being present in the church. Attending to the sensory stimulus of the architectural environment and the sounds, smells, images, illumination, and the very feel of the church space and its props, would have taken away attention from the churchgoer's conscious awareness of the intellectual and semantic *meaning* of the service. Instead, the churchgoer would have experienced the drama of one's presence before God as an emotionally immediate experience grounded in sensory stimuli. In this light, the church environment thus turns out to be a sensory place that stirred affective encounters with the holy through its multimodal aesthetics (here we use 'aesthetics' in the classical sense of the sensory, that which stirs a feeling). Through the aesthetics of the church environment, the worshipper could achieve a sense of being in touch[49] and of being touched.[50]

In conclusion, God's house, together with its surrounding environment is a **223** physical fact, which is very hard to overlook. This ritual building provides a steady and very substantial physical presence in people's immediate environment. The obvious physical dominance, the sense of stability, the pioneering architectural principles, and the striking design would have affected anyone. The variety of sensory influences provided by this building would have played a crucial role in the formation and shaping of religious messages and not least the churchgoers feeling of belonging to a more or less bounded social unit.

We are tempted to claim that theological significance might not have been the sole or even primary reason to go to church, but rather that an entry into the congregation is action-based and grounded in participation within the emotive rituals, characterised by powerful, sensory influences. Experience and perception seem to be a fundamental premise for the constitution of a ritual reality. The power of the senses dominated, meaning that rational interpretations of the world – and the exegesis of the Bible – would yield to pre-reflective experiences.

Altogether, we argue that the movement through the church environment – signified by the connection between the landscape of the parish and the micro *milieu* inside the church – is to be seen as one unified train of environmental cognition. The resonance of the church in the wider landscape (visually and aurally), the historicity of the churchyard (involving both the pastness of the graves and the futurity of resurrection) and the immediacy of the religious actions undertaken within the 'house of God' itself (setting the human being in touch – literally and figuratively – with the divine) should be appreciated as one, multi-layered ideational trajectory. Through the sensory dialectics between the human and the environment, we contend, the churchgoer would be offered a non-literary and non-verbal access to the cosmological construction of medieval Christianity.

Notes

1 Ousterhout 1998; Liebgott 1994; see Holmberg 1990 for a more holistic attitude towards church architecture and function.

2 E.g. Heidegger 1962; Leder 1990; Merleau-Ponty 2002.

3 To stick to the classical senses; for ethnographic alternatives see e.g. Gell 1995; Howes 2009B; Kensinger 1995.

4 Barsalou et al. 2005.

5 See e.g. Engelke 2012, p. 209, who argues that "all religion is material religion".

6 Jessen 2013.

7 Fritzbøger 2004; Odsgaard & Nielsen 2009.

8 Bertelsen 2006.

9 Thaastrup-Leth 2004.

10 Andrén 2000, p. 8.

11 Christie 2006; Dyggve 1952; Vinzent 2006.

12 Nilsson 1989, p. 37 f.

13 Dyggve 1952, p. 153; Madsen 1990, p. 113 f.

14 Nilsson 1989.

15 Engberg 1996.

16 Andrén 2000, p. 9.

17 Brendalsmo 2000; Madsen 1991.

18 Kornerup 1973.

19 Møller 1929, p. 279.

20 Engberg & Kieffer-Olsen 1992.

21 Johannson 1993, p. 11.

22 Poulsen 2003, p. 458 ff.; Porsmose 1988.

23 Poulsen 2003.

24 Andrén 1999.

25 Kragh 2003; Sommer 2003; Sørensen 2009, 2010.

26 Kieffer-Olsen 1993; Kragh 2003, p. 172.

27 The first historical example in southern Scandinavia is from the eleventh century Lund in Scania; Nilsson 1987, p. 136.

28 For the notion of *attunement* see Heidegger 1962; see also Harris & Sørensen 2010; Ratcliffe 2002.

29 See also Jette Linaa's chapter on *Consumption* in this volume.

30 Krautheimer 1969.

31 Bille & Sørensen (in press).

32 See also Buchli 2010, pp. 193-194.

33 See also Engelke 2007.

34 Howes 2002, p. 75 f.; Köster 2002.

35 Durandus 1966; Kragh 2003; Madsen 1981.

36 See Kus 1992; Metcalf 1987.

37 Durandus 1966.

38 Jessen 2012A, 2012B.

39 Searle 1974.

40 See also McGuire 2008.

41 Levi-Strauss 1987.

42 As n. 41.

43 See also Bille, Bjerregaard & Sørensen (in press) for staged atmospheres.

44 Also known as the "process of objectification", see Miller 1987, 1998.

45 E.g. Clark 2004; Pálsson 1995.

46 E.g. Bille, Hastrup & Sørensen 2010; Engelke 2007; Engelke & Tomlinson 2007; Gumbrecht 2004, 2006; Runia 2006; but see also Armstrong 1971; Ong 1967 for earlier examples of this point.

47 Brown 1981.

48 See also Buchli 2010 & Jørgensen 2010 for similar descriptions.

49 Runia 2006, p. 5.

50 Dufrenne 1987, p. 29.

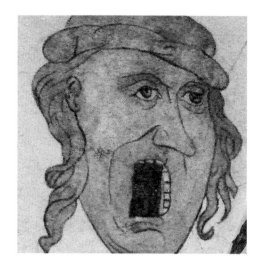

[CONSUMPTION] Medieval perceptions of the senses have been dealt with previously in great detail by numerous other authors, but in the context of the present volume the aim of this chapter is to focus on the medieval practise of sensory *media* and perceptual *mediation.* The chapter addresses the sensorial activity of *consumption* and how this was embedded in the senses and transmitted through a range of media inside and outside the church. It is argued that the paradigmatic model of perception constituted by the integration of senses and media was the same both inside and outside the physical boundaries of the church, leading to the construction of one world of perception to be expressed in real and ritual meals across the medieval world. In every church and village, monastery and manor, actual or ritualised consumption of food and drink constituted a centre for transformation, incarnation, embodiment, and negotiation, constantly fluctuating between excess and restraint, gluttony and abstinence. At the very foundation of this consumption were, of course, the senses and especially the sense of taste – *gustus.*

CONSUMPTION

Meals, Miracles, and Material Culture in the Later Middle Ages

[Jette Linaa]

The Medieval Sense of Consumption

Consumption lies at the very heart of medieval, sensorial perception. Many sensuous experiences were expressed in consummative terms: Christ was the fruit of the Tree of Life, his body was partaken of in the Eucharist, and his words were consumed during mass. However, this emphasis on consumption was not a medieval invention. Communal consumption of food and drink in ritual or actual meals had previously acted not only as a source of bodily nourishment, but also as spiritual nourishment as well as a scene for offerings, celebrations, transformations and elevations, at occasions and events ranging from the Greek symposium to the Roman bacchanal, or the Last Supper and Viking Age yuletide.

In the Middle Ages consumption played an equally important role. Every church and village, monastery and manor, were arenas for actual or ritualised consumption of food and drink constituting, as it were, processes of transformation, incarnation, embodiment, and negotiation. It constantly balanced on the edge of excess and repression, gluttony and abstinence. At the very foundation of all these different forms of consumption were the senses, and in particular the sense of taste: *gustus*.

This chapter does not restrict itself to a particular place or space. Although – or perhaps because – many of the other chapters in this book have focused on the ecclesiastical world, emphasis will not only be on consumption within the church, but also on the actions and events that took place outside it. It will be demonstrated that the model of perception and its mediation were similar both inside and outside the spatial boundaries of the church. The integration of the senses and their appertaining media were the same in both contexts. However, although this study aims to transgress thematic and spatial boundaries, it in no way lacks boundaries in terms of time and space: It is written from a Scandinavian perspective and draws on Scandinavian examples dating primarily from around 1500.

This analysis is driven by an interest in interpreting interactions between materiality and human perceptions both in the past and in the present. Our perception is profoundly different from that of medieval times. Thomas Aquinas stated that taste is a touch of the tongue and thus that the gustatory act was fundamentally intersensorial, linking taste and touch, thereby exposing the multisensory dimensions inherent in corporeal and perceptual processes.[1]

Consumption is an embodying activity, which allows an ideology to be literally integrated into the body.[2] A well-documented historical example of such practise in so-called primitive societies is the physical consumption of ancestors or enemies, in order to incorporate their strength. Although such examples represent an extreme, the practise of embodying ideology through less taboo-ridden consumption was in no way unknown in a medieval context, as will be demonstrated below.

The aim of this study is therefore to analyse how consumption through the involvement of the five senses: sight, hearing, touch, smell, and taste – *visus, auditus, tactus, olfactus,* and *gustus* – simultaneously transmitted through many media, was transformed from simple nourishment of the body to provision of food for the soul – from bodily need to a communal confirmation of a divine order and an integration of the past into the present.

However, the senses were not for pleasure alone. In the heart of medieval epistemology lurked the paradox of the senses: that the senses were the source of both knowledge and evil, and this dual nature of medieval perception is clearly visible in the medieval praxis of consumption.[3] Moreover, the very character of medieval materiality must also be taken into account. Many late medieval objects seem almost insistent in their materiality: dazzling gold and silver on tables and altars, coloured gems in jewellery and on religious objects, bright colours and soft silks employed in dress and equipment or shining glazes on tiles and tableware. Of course, this materiality had various prerequisites in terms of technical developments, production techniques, and access to new resources. However, the scope of this study does not extend to manufacturing techniques, theatrical effects, or illusory paintings.[4] Was medieval consumption equally insistent in its materiality, equally opulent in its display, equally theatrical in its sensuality?

Consumption studies are nothing new: Studies of material culture over time have provided a wealth of information on food and drink, vessels and glasses.[5] We speak of conspicuous, conservative, aesthetic, or sumptuous consumption among burghers, conservative consumption among the nobility, ascetic or restrained consumption in monasteries, religious consumption among women or mystics and sumptuous display among princes.[6] But this chapter takes its lead from recent works on medieval consumption, senses, and materiality. The religious role of consumption among medieval women has been dealt with by Caroline Walker Bynum,[7] and the same author has recently conducted an in-depth analysis of Christian materiality, while the senses have been addressed in the context of medieval households by Christopher Woolgar.

Ours is a time often thought to be particularly media-dependent, but the Middle Ages were just as defined by the communicative media, although these took a very different form from those of today.[8] It seems that miraculous divine intervention directed at materiality was perceived as a physical, if sometimes debatable or even unwished for, reality in the Middle Ages – a divine mediation. The Bible has an abundance of references to central events involving consumption and food-related miracles, all rooted in the transfer of divinity through materiality – through touch. Matter was seen as being able to possess spiritual qualities, as exemplified by relics, or to be transformed through miracles. At the core of this lies a biblical miracle, whereby the woman with the bloodflow was cured by touching the rim of Jesus' garment and he felt some of his powers being transferred at her touch (Luke 8:40-48). As such, sensing, and the senses thereby transferred or even incorporated, are not only the tangible qualities in objects, but also their intangible or spiritual properties. These were embedded in materiality, changing the nature of things and blurring the boundary between materiality and spirituality. This explains why holiness could be transferred or incorporated by touch, sight, hearing, smell, and taste, i.e. by touching relics, seeing the holy light, hearing the holy words, smelling the sweet smell of holiness, and indeed by consuming the holy.[9] Even the inevitable decay of matter could be transformed or halted through divine intervention, as seen in notions of a sweet smell arising from graves containing bodies untouched by decomposition.[10] And miracles were an abundant phenomenon in the later Middle Ages. Statues wept, relics bled, images came to life and the wounds of Christ marked the bodies of the chosen few.[11]

Consumption played a major part in many of these miracles: The best known are mentioned in the New Testament: Turning water into wine (John 2:1-12), or the five loaves and two fish feeding the five thousand (Matt 14:13-21). Following the pattern of the Scripture, consumption-related miracles were numerous in the later Middle

Ages: Bread turned into roses, saints fed by the Eucharist alone, the host turned to flesh and the chalice never ran empty.

This chapter deals with both the secular and the ecclesiastical world. In dealing with the latter, consumption is seen from the point of view of medieval laymen in its most literal sense. In the former, consumption is addressed from the point of view of noblemen, burghers, and villagers, and differences in the nature and quantity of the sources available must be taken into account. Most sources are clerical in origin and an analysis of the religious/spiritual sensorium of the laity during mass rests on a firm foundation.[12] The very lack of sources dictates that the media and social frameworks of consumption outside the church are less well known.

Consumption and Holy Communion

Consumption in its many incarnations played a fundamental role in medieval society. Inside the architectural space of the church, an analysis of the religious/spiritual experience of consumption, internally and externally, arrived at through the integration of many diverse media, is solidly founded. We know of the involvement of elements of *visus*, *auditus*, *tactus*, *olfactus*, and *gustus* in the performance of the Sacrament of the Eucharist during mass. The liturgy performed in Latin during mass must have been incomprehensible to most attendants and the words of hymns and prayers almost inaudible, reflected, distorted or bestowed with heavenly presence in the resonant acoustics of the nave. Burning incense added a sweet smell of holiness and the faint daylight and flickering candles created a 'chiaroscuro' in the dimly lit room. All of this stimulated the senses and created a physical background for the worshippers' spiritual perception of religious magic: the Eucharist. Holy Communion was a ritual mode of communication that was not aimed at teaching, but at an intense experience of inclusion and participation, creating an emotional response, which transcended the individual and the congregation, forging intense bonds between the worshippers.[13] Inside the church, consumption was linked to the Sacrament, the Eucharist, whereby bread and wine were transformed into the blood and body of Christ, i.e. the host.

The Eucharist was thereby perceived as a sacrificial meal at each mass, symbolically consumed by the congregation or their clerical representative. The bread and wine did not *represent* the body and blood of Christ – they *were* the body and blood of Christ in the medieval epistemology after 1200.[14] The body and blood of *Jesus Christ are truly contained in the sacrament of the altar under the forms of bread and wine; the bread being changed (transsubstantiatis) by divine power into the body, and the wine into the blood.*[15] This transubstantiation is underlined by the well-known motif of St. Gregory's mass, where Christ reveals himself during the Eucharist, his open wounds bleeding into the chalice. This scene is depicted on the high altar in Aarhus Cathedral in Denmark, establishing a dialectic of *visus* and *gustus*, of the Eucharist performed in the medieval era in Aarhus in 1479 and Gregory's revelation, which demonstrated and proved Christ's actual presence during the Sacrament.[16] The depiction of St. Gregory's revelation was no coincidence, as miracles relating to the host appear often in the later Middle Ages. A bleeding host in Brussels and one that turned into flesh in Flanders are just two examples of these miraculous transformations, which sparked off mass pilgrimages. Closer to the geographical focus of this chapter, a host in the church of Kippinge in Northern Falster began to bleed, prompting mass pilgrimage and even attracting royal attention. To us, these may seem like very convenient miracles providing Northern Europe with appropriate pilgrimage sites and probably also with alternative places of devotion. However, the medieval political use of miracles lies beyond the scope of this chapter. What is relevant here is that medieval churchgoers perceived the transformation of the host (the bread) into the body of Christ, and medieval consumers embodied Christ at every mass through consumption, either by *gustus* or by *visus*.[17] But this placing of matter in the hagiosensorium did not go unchallenged. During the later Middle Ages, religious dissidents questioned the divine presence in religious objects and even the doctrine of the physical presence of Christ in the Eucharist. Transubstantiation never ceased to engender suspicion.[18] Nevertheless, consumption of Christ remained the focal point. Christ himself is frequently mentioned in consummative terms outside the Sacrament of the Eucharist, as the fruit of the Tree of Life.[19] How much the layman understood of the more refined theological discussions surrounding transubstantiation is difficult to know, but through the medium of spoken words, altarpieces, and murals depicting St. Gregory's Mass, most laymen were probably aware that Christ was present in the Eucharist. As a consequence, consumption of the host re-established the divine order lost in the partaking of another meal, when Adam and Eve consumed the fruit from the Tree of Knowledge, leading to the fall of man and banishment from the Garden of Eden. This spiritual connection between Christ and consumption, the fall of man and Holy Communion/the Eucharist was commonly reinforced and underpinned through *visus*, as evident in the carefully planned program of murals. In the church at Sødring, an axis of consumption links the apple that led to the fall of man with the fruit of atonement, Mary's breast, by which she asks forgiveness for man on Judgment Day. Here, the temptation was clearly visible to worshippers during the Elevation of the Host, linking this sacrificial meal to the former act of consumption that lead to the fall of man. It is suggested that the involvement of *visus* during mass activated the memory of the worshippers and stressed the link between the two meals, adding visual strength, depth, and meaning to these two interlinked sets of transformation and consumption. The aforementioned altarpiece in Aarhus and the murals in Søodring were both donated by the Bishop of Aarhus, Jens Iversen Lange, in 1479 and 1491. They show us an influential cleric taking a firm stand among believers in the late medieval debate on the holiness of matter.

232

Secular Consumption: Senses and Media

A similar ritualisation of the senses is evident in the secular sphere, with consumption playing a comparable and equally important role in its organisation, mirroring the order of the church. The church lay at the centre of the medieval world, and the physical and spiritual organisation of secular dwellings mirrored its physical layout and cognitive space. This is clearly evident in medieval Scandinavian laws, where fines for assault were defined according to a very precise ranking of space: From the outfield, where fines were modest, through meadows and barns to the farm itself, and finally to the actual dwelling, where fines were much higher. This demonstrates a clear link between the ordering of domestic and ecclesiastical space, expressing a similar ranking of degrees of holiness, from farm to graveyard, to church and altar.[20] As stated by Anders Andrén, these two spheres can be seen in conjunction, as a coherent world view of settlement and landscape surrounding the church, a Christian spatial hierarchy organised around the altar.

Looking at the secular sphere, considerable research has been carried out in recent years into the food traditions of Northern Europe, mostly within the fields of archaeobotany and archaeozoology.[21] However, in order to focus on materiality, we have to concentrate primarily on combining this data with the spatial organisation of the meal. Domestic houses, large or small, were dominated by a single room or hall where the family or household gathered. Information on the arrangement and decoration of these domestic rooms and halls in Denmark is sparse, as very few middle and lower class dwellings have survived.[22] Much more information is available on manors and castles, where preserved decorations, mainly in the form of murals and tapestries, are largely dominated by hunting scenes. At the manor of

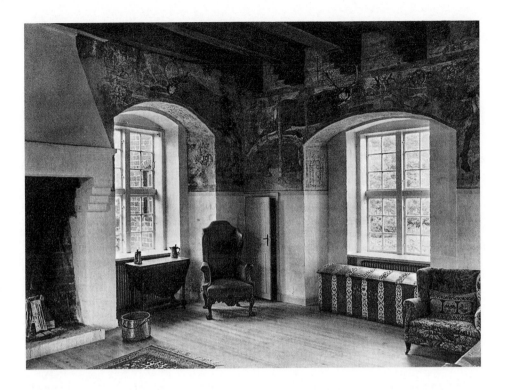

[Ill. 28] Deer frieze on the walls of the hunting trophy hall in Hesselagergaard manor on Funen, belonging to the chancellor Johan Friis, c. 1550.
Photo: The National Museum of Denmark, Copenhagen. Egmont Lind, 1964.

Hesselagergaard on Funen, built in 1538 by Johan Friis, who was chancellor to King Christian III, the representative hall is located on the ground floor with direct access through an entrance hall. The walls are covered in murals, the main motif of which comprises deer in forest and meadow landscapes. However, the deer is not only depicted in paint, but also represented through other mixed media; the heads of the animals are small plaques, clearly intended to hold trophies, probably skulls [ill. 28].

The furnishing of these halls with hunting scenes is no coincidence. Hunting was a much-loved sport – a leisure activity and privilege of noblemen and princes. Commoners were not permitted to hunt and poaching was severely punished. Furthermore, the consumption of game, particularly venison, was strictly reserved for the privileged few, being monopolised by the nobility in a way that resembles the widespread sumptuary laws of the eighteenth century: the consumption of venison linked cultural and social stratification – the incorporation of noblesse itself.[23] We must imagine the nobility engaging in communal consumption of elaborate venison dishes both at feasts, such as those associated with weddings, funerals, and marriages, and in their everyday meals. The venison provided nourishment for the body as well as food for the soul – confirmation of their nobility through *gustus* – permitting them to enjoy the taste of privilege. Taste was interlinked with sight, via the trophies and paintings of deer on the walls, and sometimes even with touch, through eating with utensils, especially knives bearing figurines of deer and hunters, thereby depicting the actual activity of hunting in the great hall itself.[24] These knives are often found in pairs, which allowed the nobleman to engage in the noble activity of sharing them with his fellow men at the table. Even the ritual washing of hands in the mass was mirrored in the secular sphere. The washing ceremony, a significant element in the medieval dining ritual, is described in courtesy books, and special vessels for this purpose are not uncommon either as archaeological finds or as images from the Middle Ages. The spout of the vessel was commonly shaped to resemble a horse's head and metal examples were even cast to resemble knights in armour, musicians, or noblemen and ladies on horseback, clearly linking the ritual of hand-washing with idealised noble perceptions of knights, troubadours and courtly love.[25]

The seating of participants at banquets was of huge importance. Documentary and pictorial sources, such as the aforementioned depiction of the rich man's meal in the Carmelite monastery in Elsinore, show us the arrangement of tables and benches: Guests/participants were ordered by rank along the bench behind the high table, while the servants walked from the kitchen to the table and dresser and back, serving the meal and pouring wine for the diners. As the participants were not regarded as social equals, their physical distance to the host and guest of honour reflected their social position, resembling the spheres of holiness in church, with laymen in the nave and priests in the choir. However, the stratification went further than this: Not everyone seated at the table was in a position to taste all of the dishes. Several regulations relating to meals in larger households reveal that it was the privilege of the lord of the house to receive all the dishes. Thereafter, the remains from his table were distributed to the other members of the household in a highly regulated and ritualised order, overruled solely by the lord's random grace.[26] By such means the order of the household was displayed and maintained, establishing the lord as master of his household and ranking its subordinate members on a scale directed by distance from him: his wife, guests, children, apprentices, and servants. Through such examples, of which only a few have so far been presented, the parallel between what we might call noble and divine matter appears obvious. The similarity may lie at the centre of this materiality, the many rules, the privileges, the careful seating arrangements, and even the fact that not all participants were in a position to receive all dishes. The elaborate ceremonies surrounding the eating of venison may reflect unease with respect to the transformative powers of the meat, and establish the lord of the household as the individual controlling who was to be transformed and who was not; who was to be included and who was to be excluded. Thus far, consumption appears routinised, lacking the intense emotional involvement evident in the religious experiences.[27] Emotional involvement in secular consumption comes with the intake of alcohol and this will be dealt with later.

Memory and Media:
Eating, Touching and Living the Past

But the meal did not only take place in the present of the past, it represented an integration of past and present and an activation of memory through the senses both in the secular and ecclesiastical sphere.[28] Memory of ancestors is short when confined to the human mind, but is seems that medieval individuals attempted to secure an afterlife in the memory of their descendants through a variety of tangible and intangible means.[29] The past was made present through manifest buildings with halls and gates of stone or wood, extending decades or even centuries back in time in a landscape where most secular buildings were short-lived. The heraldic symbol of the nobleman and his ancestors was clearly visible everywhere, carved on stone and in wood, woven into tapestries, cast on spoons and cups of gold and silver, constantly reminding the nobleman of his descent. But these items were not only symbols of nobility and ancestry by virtue of the coat of arms they bore, they were frequently also heirlooms in their own right, as evident from medieval inventories and testaments.[30] The actual items became the living past, enabling an integration of the noble past into the present, restoring the dead to the memory of the living by the most direct means: the touch of the metal, the sight of the gold emblems, the taste of the wine, thereby transforming the act of eating into a process of integration of past and present, of nobility and ancestry. For us today, our ontological perspective, developed to its full potential since the eighteenth century, has forged a modern tradition, in which matter comprises systems of signs and codes and expressions of inner values, inspired by semiotics, the study of signifier and signified. This perspective has mainly been criticised for being Eurocentric and very modern in its character.[31] Medieval ontology may have been somewhat different: There does not seem to have been such a marked perception in most secular circles of the superiority of in-ternal values over matter, as this volume clearly demonstrates. If the ontology of medieval nobility is viewed in this light then objects and the body – or the outer surface, one could say – did not reflect or express an inner core of nobility – they actually *were* nobility and performed nobility. This may be the reason why display, in terms of objects, furnishings and the behaviour of nobility, appear to have been so very important.

This observation also sheds new light on the value of heirlooms and the senti-ments associated with such noble objects that are clearly expressed in documentary records. For example, in an inventory from 1534, Ide Lunge lists a family drinking horn and adds "from which we used to drink at Christmas".[32] Through this qualifica-tion, the drinking horn itself, a very archaic vessel type at that time, is presented as a mediator between past and present, living and dead. Clear parallels to this can be found in the church, where objects of very different age, such as chalices, religious sculptures, murals and even the actual buildings, acted as integrators of past and present, bridging the gap between then and now.

The Rituals of Consumption:
a Materialising Process

One of the best known and most influential works on worldly sensing is *The Civiliz-ing Process* by Norbert Elias. Here, Elias claims that a gradual movement away from an authenticity of the senses in the earlier Middle Ages gained momentum in the sixteenth century and continued up through modern times, with a foundation in court culture.[33] At first glance, the obvious diversification of the material records, especially in the later Middle Ages and early post-medieval period (fifteenth to six-teenth century), appears to support Elias' view: The archaeological record reveals marked differentiation and specialisation with respect to the phenomenon of the meal, apparently lending support to the idea that a civilisation of the senses began at this time.[34] This differentiation and specialisation is visible not only in the introduc-tion of the fork, but also in the appearance of a range of specialised tableware: cups, pans, jugs, mugs, and sets of plates – forms that were gradually introduced in the later Middle Ages and early Renaissance. These innovations appear to mirror the development of a complex meal, with many sets and courses served at the same time: A complicated and refined cuisine with starters and appetisers, sets of fish and vege-table dishes, meats and fowl involved in complicated preparation. These developments appear to support the idea of a disciplined etiquette of consumption in the later Middle Ages.

However, there has been some – perhaps rather controversial – criticism of this view by the German sociologist Hans Peter Duerr. Duerr points out that so-called primitive cultures were and are anything but primitive, simple, or authentic in their sensorial behaviour, but demand quite advanced rituals involving a discipline of the senses, controlling sight, hearing, and touch.[35] There are few available sources relating to human behaviour in the Viking Age and early medieval times, but those that do exist do not provide any indication of spontaneity of the senses and seem therefore to counteract the perception of progressive disciplining in this respect. Instead, they indicate an existing, but immaterial, discipline of the senses and, in particular, a preference for cleanliness. English medieval sources mention elaborate rules for socialising with neighbours that are aimed at avoiding gazing upon them in private situations, thereby demanding disciplined *visus* and *auditus*, as well as *gustus* and *tactus*.[36] The development of separate sleeping and dwelling chambers, away from the public eye, did of course make some of these customs redundant, thereby representing a materialisation of the disciplined gaze that should not be confused with the invention of the concept of privacy.[37] Returning to consumption, introduction of the fork, plate, and mug in the sixteenth century provides obvious and rather familiar examples of similar materialisations of a disciplined *tactus*: Detailed accounts of how to behave at the table while eating with the fingers from common plates show the latter to be neither easy nor straightforward.[38] Therefore, it seems apt to perceive the integration of fork, plate and mug as a materialisation process whereby manners involving discipline of *tactus* and *gustus* were transformed into tangible matter, rather than as a civilising process.

The Dangers of Sensing:
Gluttony and Mortal Sin

Consumption was a double-edged sword that could lead to the holy or to the Fall. This suspicious dual nature of *gustus* and, consequently, of consumption, leading either to divine order or to ruin, is stressed by the apostle Paul in his letter to the Corinthians: "Therefore, whoever eats the bread or drinks the cup of the Lord in an unworthy manner will be guilty of sinning against the body and blood of the Lord" (1 Cor. 1:27). So, at the very roots of Christianity, the discipline of the senses is stressed as a prerequisite for unification with God through the Eucharist. Undisci-

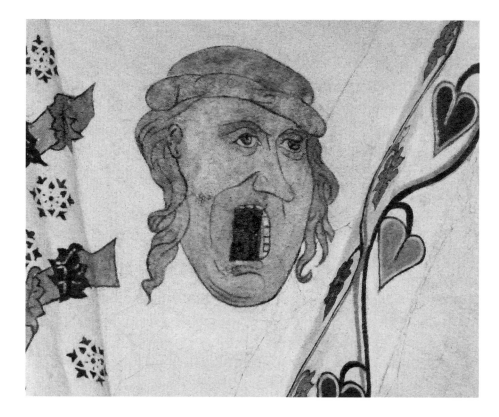

[**Ill. 29**] Grotesque mask from c. 1500, Carmelite Priory in Elsinore.
Photo: Tommy Olofsson.

plined sensuality in consumption thereby became the cardinal sin of *gula* (gluttony), a wilful violation of God's laws and, as such, a direct route to perdition and eternal damnation if not confessed and atoned for. Gluttony was the sin most commonly mentioned in church sermons, and not without reason. Medieval and post-medieval records provide numerous examples of ecclesiastical condemnation of gluttony, especially of excessive drinking, in every layer of society from kings to peasants and priests.[39] Well-known examples are the secular and religious guilds of late medieval Denmark that acted as a social and spiritual framework for the life of many townspeople. A number of laws regulated the behaviour of the members of these guilds, with frequent mention of fines to be paid for disorderly conduct during excessive drunkenness, thereby putting pressure on the individual in order to discipline gusto.[40] Gluttony lay at the heart of everyday medieval devotional praxis. Medieval prayer books include several examples of prayers intended to keep and protect individuals from gluttony.[41]

[**Ill. 30**] Baltic jug with grotesque mask, c. 1425 – found at Rosborg castle near Vejle.
Moesgaard Photo / Media-lab.
Photo: Søren Christensen, 2005.

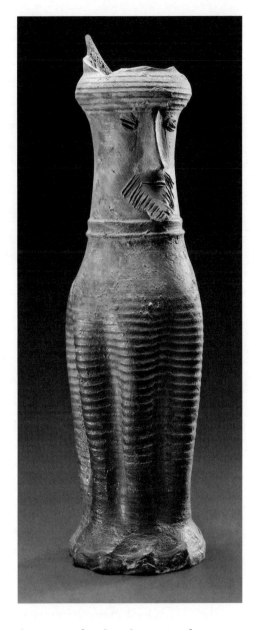

What can be interpreted as images or renditions of gluttony, as well as other mortal sins, are quite commonly depicted in the Scandinavian medieval churches: masks of vomiting men and women fill out the marginal areas of the western vaults and walls, close to the laymen occupying the western part of the church, towards whom their message was directed [ill. 29].

Their spatial distance to the holy men and women situated in the higher parts of vaults and walls seems to be a visual reflection of their moral distance: a very clear statement in a medieval world where contrasts lay at the very heart of perceptions and arguments. This included the moral contrast between holy men and women, who moderated their consumption, and sinners, who did not.[42] However, these grotesque figures were also integrated in worldly culture. Grotesque masks were a familiar decorative feature on wine tankards, commonly found both in secular and religious dwellings in the fourteenth, fifteenth and sixteenth centuries.[43] These vessels were popular and have been found at many urban sites, manors, and even villages all over Scandinavia. They are clearly bodily representations, with the mask situated at the neck and the body of the vessel obviously representing the torso of a man, sometimes marked by belts or replicas of limbs [ill. 30].

The vessels are predominantly globular in shape, making the man appear obese or even pregnant. Interpretations of the origin and symbolism of these masks show considerable diversity, being sometimes linked to the fauns and satyrs of Roman culture, sometimes to medieval Central European myths of wild men or to theatrical figures, or even to the medieval mummers and morality plays, with their buffoons and masquerades.[44] Whatever they represent, both written and archaeological sources clearly demonstrate their use in a masculine sphere.[45] The vessels are of Hanseatic origin, produced in the Rhineland and around the River Oder in the fourteenth and fifteenth centuries: from here they were traded by members of the Hanseatic League to Flanders, England, and Scandinavia, together with wine and hopped beer in barrels and casks.[46] The Hanseatic wine consumed from these Hanseatic vessels may have served to embody the Hanseatic culture in the consumer in the most direct way possible: by taste, sight, and touch. We have very little written evidence relating to the specific symbolic significance of these face masks, but wine and beer were certainly believed to have the ability to transform the character of those who drank it, even when partaken of in moderation, but leading to bad behaviour when consumed to excess.[47] This transformative nature of alcoholic consumption is clearly evident from Danish court rolls. These state that fines imposed on members by the village council were paid in beer that was then consumed immediately by all the men of the village, thereby settling the conflict and allowing the transgressor to transform himself back into an accepted member of the community through common consumption. In towns, any transfer of ownership of goods or services was confirmed in similar way: by the sharing of a flagon, beaker or glass of wine, or beer in the local tavern. Many additional examples of this use of alcohol can be found associated with village fairs, the courts, public houses, the town hall, or the guild hall.[48] This consumption of alcohol was predominately a male phenomenon, as medieval court rolls tell us that drunken males were excused of their drunkenness, while drunken women were severely condemned.[49]

These examples demonstrate a medieval perception of the consumption of alcoholic beverages as a transformative and moderating medium, able to re-establish or confirm order in the private or public sphere; either in the house or the family. If this point is valid, then the grotesque mask mediated a sense of alcohol as a warning about gluttony, thereby employing the vessel as a means to a moderated and therefore pious lifestyle.[50]

Reversed Consumption

Moving from communion to banquet to gluttony, the final aspect we must address is reversed consumption. In the medieval world of contrasts, it was only logical that opposition to order, established and negotiated through consumption, was expressed through a reversal of consumption.[51] In this, emphasis was placed not on the pleasing of the senses, but on the unpleasant – on the sticky, the ugly, the dissonant and the repulsive. This reversed consumption had its own media in late medieval theatrical traditions involving parodies, grotesques, chaos, disharmony and a general upside-down attitude and protest against nobility and authorities.[52] This aspect is also evident from written documents, which state that reversed consumption, mostly in the form of public exposure of bodily orifices was regarded as a social or even devilish protest, shaming and shocking to onlookers. Figures indicating or signifying reversed consumption are quite common in Scandinavian medieval churches, where images of buttock-baring and vomiting men and women occupy the marginal areas of the vaults and walls, suspiciously close to the congregation in the western part of the church. Neither are these figures uncommon in the few surviving examples of pictorial programs in secular architecture. One of the more notable examples is in the so-called Adam's House in Angers, a merchant's dwelling from the fifteenth century, which is a magnificent example of secular architecture that is far too complex to be dealt with within the framework of this paper. Whether the presence of these figures was intended to be a protest against established order, or a warning against gluttony and excess, the graphic images appear in harsh contrast to the divine figures, occupying their position on the periphery of the medieval hagiosensorium.

The Social and Sensory Community of Consumption

This chapter takes as its foundation two distinct modes of consumption: the Eucharist and the secular banquet. It has been argued that late medieval consumption was not purely a matter of fulfilling bodily needs, but a carefully planned sensuous experience with transformative powers. Ecclesiastical and secular ritual praxis, pictorial programmes, music, space, and sensory experience were interlinked through the practice of consumption, while at the same time it created a fundamental sense of participation and community. Inside the church, consumption of the Eucharist created bonds between the members of the congregation; bonds that were also useful in day-to-day social interactions within the community. Outside the physical boundaries of the church, ritualised consumption involving alcohol and restricted food, such as venison, acted as a spiritual and social mediator, establishing and re-establishing order in the daily life of communities. The parallel between what could be referred to as two sets of rituals, two sets of miraculous transformations, is marked in the need for physical and spiritual purity of the participants. Ritual washing of hands is familiar from both spheres, as is the rule of harmony: In order to take Holy Communion in church, the individuals had to confess their sins and repent, and in order to participate in the meals outside church, individuals had to confess their crimes and make amends. Consumption in the church and in the secular world constituted a major part of almost every aspect of the medieval world. Transitional points in human life were marked by events that involved consumption: Funerals were celebrated with a feast, as were weddings and baptisms.[53] This gives the impression that communal consumption was an act of acceptance or transformation of individuals from one social or spiritual position to another, conferring on the trinity of *gustus*, *visus*, and *tactus* the role of mediator, with the power to transport individuals from one social and spiritual stage to another, implementing the order of things among the living in all parts of society.[54] This took place among people who may have had a perception of reality very different from that of today, assessing sensory matter not only as expressions or indications of inner values, but as the actual values themselves. In this sense, matter was not a surface – matter was the substance. Matter embedded agency, it implemented practice and it changed forever through growth or decay. Matter was consistent only in its inconsistency in a world, where God was the only constant. The intense debates between elite scholars in the late Middle Ages on the degradation or durability of holy matter may also have had an influence on laymen.

A mundane, but well-documented example is the widespread shift from pottery to metal tableware in the later Middle Ages. Although this clearly had its cultural, technical, and economical prerequisites, it can still be considered as a very practical attempt to halt time and control matter, just like brick houses and stone epitaphs. Numerous other examples of practices aimed at halting or slowing down the speed of decay, and even of time itself, are evident in the later Middle Ages. At the same time as pottery was replaced by metal, stone houses began to be built by burghers, craftsmen and the nobility, both in towns and in the country, replacing the previous, highly ephemeral and flammable wooden and half-timbered buildings. As a consequence, consumption became surrounded by stone churches, stone manors, stone houses, metal vessels and gemstones, as well as that eternal metal – gold. Apparently immutable materials framed consumers and conferred on them a sense of stability, organising their senses into a hagiosensorium, in which God was the only constant.[55]

This materiality of consumption became embedded within a specific late medieval historical and cultural context, shared by people of very different educational, social, cultural and economic backgrounds, across both the ecclesiastical and secular spheres. Materiality and the senses appear to have been in focus everywhere, from advanced theological discussions among leading scholars, to the lives of lay people, of whom we know so very little. The notion of what might be called an extended materiality or material turn of the later Middle Ages has already been touched upon, drawing parallels between the increasing emphasis on variation and degree of materiality in churches and halls, hopefully pinpointing that matter and the senses were of major concern and importance both inside and outside the walls of the church. However, it is still important to stress the dynamic, interactive character of this mediated sensuousness and to stress the ambiguous nature of medieval consumption, because consumption could lead to good as well as to evil. Consequently, medieval consumers appear to navigate between an acceptance and a rejection of materiality, between fear and desire, Heaven and Hell.[56] This dual nature of consumption is visualised in the fall of man through the consumption of the apple from the Tree of the Knowledge, which is placed in opposition to the wonder of the Eucharist depicted in the murals painted in many churches. The masks, wild men, beasts and monsters in these same paintings pointed out the dangers of consumption and the need for order. Order was fundamental to everything. Besides from being a devotional fix-point, Holy Communion had a clear social function relative to the congregation, establishing trust and social equilibrium and defining the congregation relative to outsiders. Likewise, the aim of secular consumption was primarily bodily nourishment. Even so, consumption was still organised in order to promote a desired or pious lifestyle. The hagiosensorium was permeated by consumption of sensuous experiences in order to secure salvation of the soul. It marked a social and spiritual framework for mediations, negotiations, transformations and incarnations, regardless of whether these took place in the ecclesiastical or the secular sphere. Consumption did not only apply to the food and drink itself, nor to a special place or space, but to a medieval perception of embodied sensuality. The act of consuming referred to experiences integrating senses and media, transgressing boundaries, opening a space outside time, where divine order could be re-established, the past integrated into the present and all conflicts resolved.

Notes

1   For a further treatment of Aquinas' view on taste and touch, see Hans Henrik Lohfert Jørgensen's chapter on the *Sensorium* in this volume; Woolgar 2006, p. 102.

2   Fischer & DiPaolo Loren 2003, p. 238.

3   The paradox of the senses is dealt with in Kristin B. Aavitsland's chapter on *Incarnation* and Laura Katrine Skinnebach's chapter on *Devotion*, both in this volume. See also Spiegel 2008 & Bynum 1987.

4   Poulsen & Hybel 2007.

5   E.g.: Bartels 1999; Burke 2009; Gaimster 1997; Gaimster & Stamper 1997; Linaa 2006; Linaa (in press); Poulsen 2000A, 2000B, 2004, 2011.

6   Bynum 1987; Dyer 1998; Poulsen 1999; Unger 2004; Woolgar 2001, 2006, 2010.

7   Bynum 2011; Woolgar 2001, 2006, 2010.

8   Faulstich 1996, p. 9.

9   Woolgar 2006, p. 2.

10   Mads Dengsø Jessen & Tim Flohr Sørensen deal with the sensory aspects of medieval burial grounds in their chapter on *Environment* in this volume; see also Woolgar 2006, p. 119.

11   Bynum 2011, pp. 128-130.

12   Bisgaard 1994, pp. 359-362, 2004, pp. 55-100; Dinshaw 1999; Dinzelbacher 1996, 2002; Le Goff 1982; Le Roy Ladurie 1975.

13   Whitehouse 2002, pp. 293-295.

14   Bynum 2011, pp. 125-130.

15   Bynum 2011, p. 160.

16   Moltke 1970.

17   Bynum 2011, pp. 143-150.

18   Bynum 2011, pp. 163-165.

19   Bonaventure's treatise on the Tree of Life, *Lignum Vitae*, is investigated in detail in Henning Laugerud's chapter on *Memory* in this volume.

20   Andersson & Hållands 1997, pp. 583-586; Andrén 1999, pp. 385-386.

21   Karg 1998; Isaksson 2000.

22   Linaa & Skov 2004; Poulsen 1999; Ganshorn 1999.

23   Miller 1995, pp. 134-136.

24   Stiesdal 1956.

25   Chambers 1914, p. 15; Linaa 2000, 2006.

26   Isaksson 2000, pp. 21-27; Mulryne 2004; Olden-Jørgensen 2000; Poulsen 2010; Wade 1996.

27   Whitehouse 2002, pp. 293-295.

28   Scholliers 2001.

29   Whitehouse 2002, pp. 293-294.

30   *Danske Samlinger*, 2; R; 6, 1877-79, pp. 170-188.

31   Keane 2005, p. 184.

32   *Danske Magazin*, 4; R; II, 1873, pp. 3-16.

33   Elias 1994.

34 Linaa 2006.

35 Duerr 1988; Duerr 1994.

36 Duerr 1994, pp. 158-160; Wright 1862, p. 276.

37 Poulsen 1999, pp. 195-201; Poulsen 2003.

38 Larson 1917, p. 228; Cooper 1996; Elias 1994, p. 48; Wright 1862, pp. 366-367.

39 Woolgar 2006, p. 112.

40 Nyrop 1895-1904; Bisgaard 1994; Poulsen 1999, pp. 201-202.

41 Nielsen 1946, p. 19; the author wishes to thank Laura Katrine Skinnebach for providing this information.

42 Jaritz 2000; Simon-Muscheid 2000, pp. 37-44.

43 Gaimster 1997, p. 209; Gaimster 2007; Linaa 2006; Reineking-von Bock 1975; Stephan 1988, 1996.

44 Burke 2009; Faulstich 1996, pp. 205 ff.

45 Linaa 2006.

46 Unger 2004, pp. 67-69.

47 Examples derived from a translation of *Secreta Secretorum* from c. 1300; Steele 1898, pp. 79-80; Woolgar 2006, p. III.

48 Appel 1999, pp. 284-286; Nyrop 1895-1904; Poulsen 1999, pp. 200-201; Simon-Muscheid 2000, p. 54; Andersen & Pajung 2014.

49 Simon-Muscheid 2000.

50 Cumberpatch 2006.

51 Jaritz 2000, p. 10.

52 Faulstich 1996, pp. 221-222.

53 Bisgaard 2004, p. 252; Poulsen 1999, pp. 201-202.

54 Buc 2001, pp. 164-166.

55 Bynum 2011, p. 285.

56 Bynum 2011, p. 269.

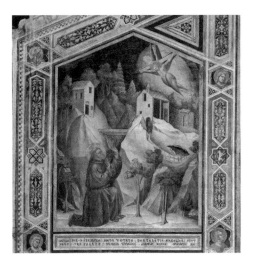

[**MEMORY**] This chapter addresses the sensorial aspect of memory and the question of its intermedial and multisensorial manifestations, but also whether it can be seen as a place for intermedial and intersensorial expressions, experiences, and forms of understanding. The point of departure is a close study of a medieval meditation motif conveyed both by St. Bonaventure's *Lignum Vitae,* dating from c. 1260, and its pictorial 'mirror-image' in Taddeo Gaddi's frescoes in Santa Croce at Florence, executed c. 1350. Through comparison, the chapter discusses the sensorial and material aspects of memory, showing how it may be perceived as an intermedial component of the working mind. It is argued that memory was understood as being inherently sensuous and corporeal, which was crucial in order to establish a connection between the inner and the outer sensorium. This perceptual and cognitive interchange also substantiates the implication that the senses were comprehended as mutually interlaced and not separated into closed compartments.

MEMORY

The Sensory Materiality of Belief and Understanding in Late Medieval Europe

[Henning Laugerud]

The Medium of Memory:
A Place in the Senses

Memory can be seen as a *topos* – a place or medium – for intermedial and multi-sensorial expressions, experiences, and forms of understanding. This understanding of memory can already be found in St. Augustine (354-430), who declared that memory is based on all kinds of sensorial impressions and experiences that entered memory each in their own particular way, 'by its own door', but the things themselves did not enter: "[…] only the images of things perceived are there for the thought to remember."[1] Memory is both material and immaterial in its character. It is in a sense visible both as a physical and as a mental image, but these mental images are more than just pictures in an optical visual sense. They have other sensorial characteristics as well. Memory is at the same time creative and conserving – something to be stored and reactivated – and has its foundations in both sensory perception and abstraction. Memory is interpreted reality; it is not a passive act of 'mechanical' registration.[2]

The art of memory was a central component of the classical and the medieval traditions of learning. The treatment of memory was therefore not restricted to psychological aspects, but covered understanding, knowledge, communication, and cognition. Memory concerned the construction, or the very fabric, of thinking. The classical recommendations pertaining to the art of memory were full of symbols, personifications, and prominent figures and pictures; all systematically ordered and located in some kind of space: a building, a city, or a landscape. These memory images, or visual representations, were all of a mental or para-visual kind, which are visual phenomena not seen by the physical eye but with the inner eye. These are nevertheless related to optical visual 'pictures' and figurations seen with the physical eye.[3] The boundaries between mental pictures and physical ones must have over-lapped, as was already noted by Francis Yates in her classic study of the art of mem-ory from 1966.[4] Images of all kinds, symbols and allegories are, where memory is concerned, *effective* for many reasons. One of them is their aptitude for *rhetorical concentration*, of being able to compress a large amount of content into one expres-sion. This is an expression that is syntagmatic, in the sense that its references are a selection of several elements that belong together or are joined together.

Memory is also a place – or places – where physical sense perceptions and mental activities are stored, united, and combined. St. Augustine writes about the: "fields and spacious halls of memory."[5] In the classical art of memory the *placing* of *images* was one of the basic components and rules of mnemotechnics.[6] Furthermore, it is a *temporal activity* in the sense that something of the past is activated in the present with a prospective perspective. Memory takes place in time. In the medieval reflec-tions and understanding regarding memory we can clearly detect these multi-spatial and multi-temporal perspectives. Memory was both of the past, the present, and the future: "to remember the eternal joys of Paradise and the pains of Hell", as Boncom-pagno da Signa (c. 1170-1240) states in his *Rhetorica Novissima* from 1235.[7]

At the same time, this concept and this perspective open up to other 'vistas' of the mind, as memory was integrated into the existential foundation of medieval man. Memory related to knowledge of the World as well as of the Self, but more importantly, it related to the knowledge of God and the Ultimate Reality: "If I find thee without memory, then I shall have no memory of thee; and how could I find thee at all, if I do not remember thee?" as St. Augustine formulates it.[8] This is an-other angle from which to view the understanding of sensing and perception, which perhaps dislocates the concept somewhat, yet it shows that the medieval Christian tradition(s) of sensing and perception was a multifaceted phenomenon at the core of an integrated yet polysemous and complex worldview.[9] Here the body, sensuality, and the senses were understood in what we today might perceive as paradoxical rela-tions to the mind, the spirit, and God.[10]

My point of departure will be the *Lignum Vitae* by St. Bonaventure (c. 1221-1274).[11] This is a text that manifests the role of memory's sensory and sensual founda-tion and its spiritual implications in an exceptionally profound and illuminating way. This text also has its 'mirror-image' in a concrete painted mnemonic device in Taddao Gaddis large fresco in Santa Croce in Florence, which manifests the relation between memory and sensing in an energetic way. Through a close reading of these two text images, I hope to bring to light these 'vistas' of the combined understanding of the mind and body during the medieval period. We shall start with St. Bonaventure's treatise.

The *Lignum vitae* of St. Bonaventure

In the prologue to the *Lignum vitae*, St. Bonaventure emphasises that the true believer should try; "always to carry about, in soul and body, the Cross of Christ" until he himself could feel the truth of St. Paul's words; "With Christ I am nailed to the cross."[12] This defines the primary or ultimate goal of the meditation: to internalise and imitate the life and sufferings of Christ. Already in the first part of the prologue, he connects this meditation to *memory*:

> Now, in order to enkindle an affection of this sort, *to assist the mind and stamp the memory [imprimatur memoria]* [my emphasis], I have attempted to gather this bundle of myrrh from the groves of the Gospels, which deal throughout with the life, passion and glorification of Jesus Christ. I have tied it together with words that are few, orderly, and parallel for easy grasping; that are common, simple, and plain enough to avoid the effect of extravagance – and to foster devotion and faith.[13]

He continues to say that he has chosen to arrange the meditation in the form of an imaginary tree, "because imagination assists understanding".[14] Already at the outset of this meditation, St. Bonaventure has established the connection between *meditation* and *memory* and he links it all up to the sensorial, and particularly, but not exclusively, to the visual. Furthermore, the meditation is carefully arranged according to the classical recommendations pertaining to the art of memory; order and symmetry. Everything centred on a powerful image of a syntagmatic character. It is an imagined visual *representation* of the 'Tree of Life', presented to us as a meditative object, as an instrument of devotion, and as a mnemotechnic device. This image becomes a medium for memory. But as we shall see, the sense of *visus* is not the only one in play, and the connection between the different parts of the inner and outer human sensorium is complex.

St. Bonaventure starts the meditation, and the text, with this mental image of a tree: "Picture in your imagination a tree."[15] Trees and tree structures were quite common mnemotechnic figures or means of organising memory. We can find this figure used within a similar context by Hugh of St. Victor (c. 1096-1142) in his *De arca Noe Morali*, which was written for monks and meant to be read aloud during the their communal meals. Hugh introduces the image of the *arbour*, or *lignum sapientiae*, to organise his sermon.[16] Just as Ramón Lull (c. 1232-1316) makes frequent use of similar images and figures both in writing and illustrations and as a mental figure or image.[17] However, it was particularly compelling within a Christian cultural framework. There are several trees of great moral and symbolic significance in the Bible, which are associated with knowledge of the ultimate truth.[18] As the title of the meditation states, this is the Tree of Life, the *Lignum Vitae*.

The Tree of Life is the tree God allowed to grow in the Garden of Eden, and whose fruits God denied Adam and Eve after they had eaten the forbidden fruit of the Tree of Knowledge.[19] What was once denied man after the act of Original Sin has now been made possible by the Redemptive suffering for our sins by Our Lord Jesus Christ. In Revelation, Chapter 22, we can read that between the new heaven and new earth stands The Tree of Life: "with its twelve kinds of fruit".[20] This well-known figure of Redemption is, of course, in itself a well-suited ordering principle for the meditations on the Life, Death, and Resurrection of Christ. The image or motif would be familiar to most people, and in this way already in itself contain the core message of the meditations of St. Bonaventure. The Tree of Life is also a *memoriale*, a reminder of Paradise and of the past. It evokes what was lost and what shall be attained again through the suffering, Death, and Resurrection of Christ, the New Adam. Past and future are amalgamated in this one life-giving tree where Christ is identified as the source of life in a fallen world.

St. Bonaventure asks the reader or listener to imagine a tree with four roots from which four rivers are gushing forth.[21] These rivers irrigate the garden, not of Paradise, but of the Church. The next step is to imagine a trunk with twelve branches adorned with leaves, flowers, and fruits. These branches are numerically and symmetrical arranged in three parts containing four branches each, all ending in a fruit of true knowledge. Each of these branches contains four points. He uses striking metaphors meant to produce vivid images that are easy to remember. This is a classical mnemotechnic arrangement, and can be seen illustrated almost in every detail in Taddeo Gaddis fresco, making it a nearly perfect picture of the mnemonic and mental image in St. Bonaventure's writing.

The inner picture, the mnemotechnic picture of the 'tree', is not only an inner representation of another picture; it is also a representation of St. Bonaventure's *text* of the *Lignum Vitae* with all its references, connotations, and meaningful associations. His meditations may be seen as an image, and one does not *necessarily* have priority over the other. A reception of the 'text', then, is an inner sensual representation of both this 'image' and the writing of St. Bonaventure, in all of its sensual expressions and impressions. The memorisation of the 'text' is a relation between the 'image' of the writing of St. Bonaventure and its reception by both the outer and inner senses of the recipient, and here all the human *sensoria* are activated. He invites the reader to imagine:

> […] that the flowers glow with a many-hued splendour and are *fragrant with the sweetest perfumes* [*odoris suavitate*] [my emphasis], awakening and drawing on the longing hearts of men of desire. Let there be twelve fruits, *endowed with all the delights and conforming to every taste*, offered to God's servants as a food they may eat forever, being fed but never sated.[22]

The 'fruits' to be eaten is off course both the body and the truth and knowledge of Christ:

> These instances I call fruits, because their full flavour refreshes and their rich substances strengthen the soul who meditates upon them carefully considering each one; abhorring the example of unfaithful Adam, who preferred *the tree of knowledge of good and evil* to the Tree of life. […] Give us Your Fruit as our food.[23]

Hearing, *auditus*, is also activated in this meditative sensuality. St. Bonaventure writes in the first 'fruit', the illustrious ancestry of Christ, that: "[…] if you could hear the Virgin singing in her delight, […] together with the Blessed Virgin you would most sweetly sing this holy canticle […]."[24] In the last paragraph in this chapter he concludes:

> And now, my soul, embrace the sacred manger; press your lips upon the Child's feet in a devout kiss; follow in the mind the shepherds' vigil; contemplate with wonder the assisting host of angels; join in the heavenly hymn, and sing with all your heart and soul: *"Glory to God in the highest, and on earth peace among men of good will."*[25]

Hearing is also intrinsically activated through reading itself, because reading in the Middle Ages was not only done with the eyes, but also with the lips: "[…] pronouncing what they saw, and with the ears, listening to the words pronounced, hearing what is called the 'voices of the pages'. It is a real acoustical reading."[26] Smell, taste, hearing, and nourishment are all central metaphors and devices for creating memorial 'hooks' or sensual images. As we see, they are also combined with poetic metaphors, such as to "sweetly sing" with the Virgin.[27] The crucial aspect of this memory, however, is never a simplistic 'storing' of static information or 'rote' learning; its vital essence is the *internalising* of knowledge, truth, and belief, which transforms *the Self* into a living image of Christ through memory. The reading of the pages is a sensory and emotional, as well as intellectual or rational experience. This is emphasised in the prologue and several other places in the meditation, that one shall feel the physical pain of Christ in his suffering; feel it in one's own body. These *mental scenes* are *places* to be inhabited by the believer.

St. Bonaventure demands emotional engagement and compassion from his fellow believers, readers, listeners, or beholders.[28] This is the ideal of discipleship, which has a long tradition dating back to the origins of Christianity, modelled on Jewish ideals, as Yves Congar has formulated it: "The disciple not only received oral lessons from his master, to be memorised – a most effective practice for including 'tradition', and one that Jesus certainly applied to his disciples – he also learned from his master's actions and personal way of life."[29] This is a memory that is active and practical, connected to actions as well as mere abstract activities. It is also an orthopraxis that involves both body and soul. Can one find any better or more appropriate metaphors or 'images' than tasting and eating for this ideal of internalising and of transforming the Self? By 'ruminating' on this presentation of the mysteries of faith, the viewer, reader, and listener would take sustenance from its 'fruits', hoping one day to 'taste' the prophesied life-giving fruits in the hereafter. This interlacing of physical and mental sense impressions finds an almost literal expression in Taddeo Gaddi's 'mirror-image' in Santa Croce.

The *Lignum Vitae* of Taddeo Gaddi

Taddeo Gaddi (c. 1300-1366) painted a large fresco around 1350 in what was then the refectory in the Franciscan convent of Santa Croce in Florence, with a striking depiction of the *Lignum Vitae*.[30] The picture painted on the rear wall of the refectory

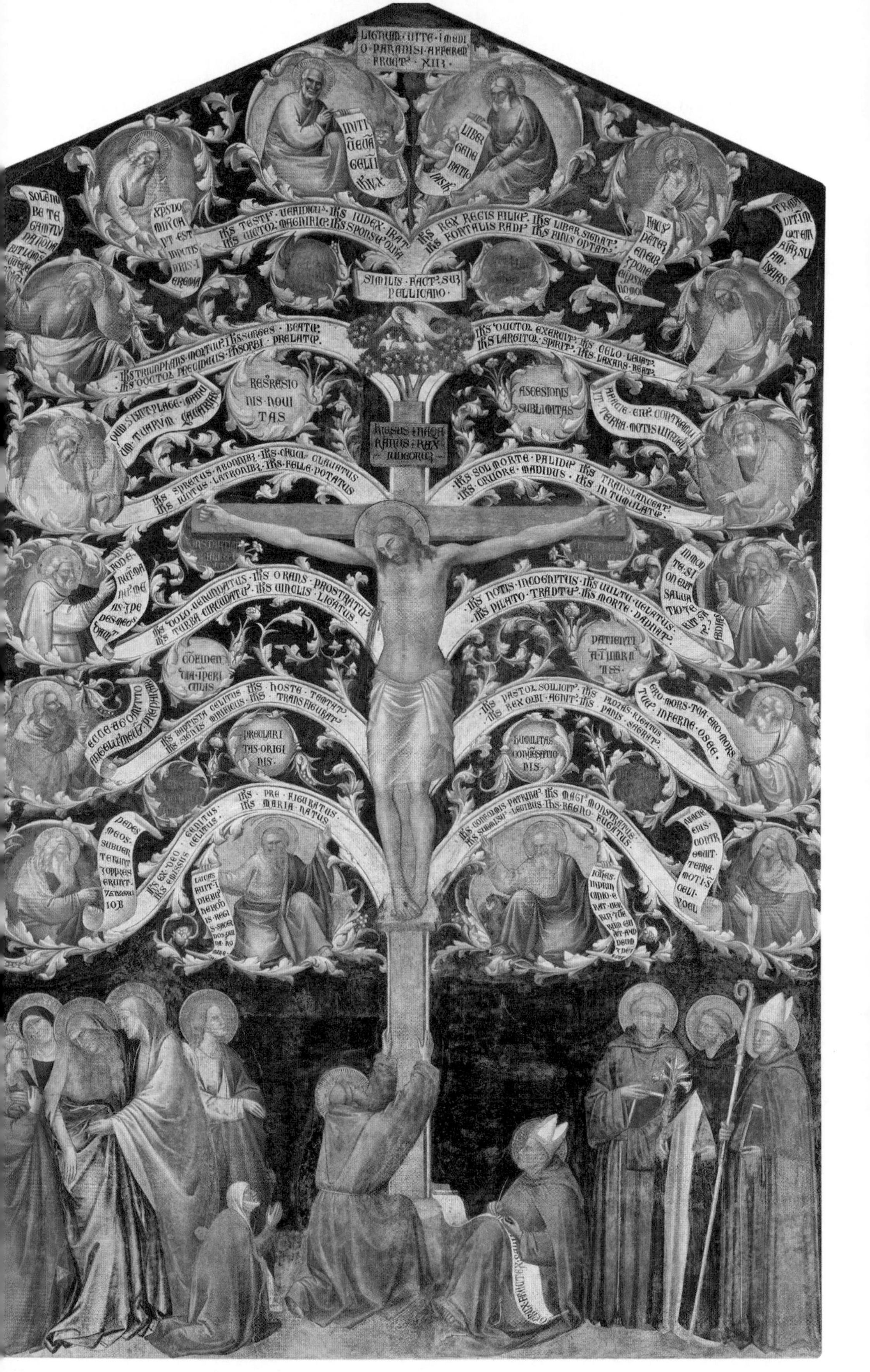
LIGNUM · UITE · I MEDI
O · PARADISI · AFFERENS
FRUCT⁹ · XII ·
SIMILIS · FACT⁹ · SUB
PELLICANO ·
IHESUS · NAZA
RENUS · REX
IUDEORUM

shows Christ crucified on the *Tree of Life*, framed by five other scenes [ill. 31 & 32]. The main motif depicts the Tree of Life in the form of a cross with twelve floral branches symmetrically divided, with six on either side. Each branch ends in a flowery medallion with an Old Testament prophet identified by a scroll inscribed with a text prefiguring Christ. Written images or references to Christ's life are inscribed on the branches, and each branch has a 'fruit' hanging from it. Each of these 'fruits' represent either an abstract characteristic of His life or one of His virtues. The motif is also a Crucifixion scene, and below the Cross we can see the swooning Virgin supported by the three Marias, a contemporary female patron and the Saints John the Evangelist, Dominic, Anthony of Padua, Louis of Toulouse, Bonaventure and Francis, who is embracing the foot of the Cross.

Below the main motif we find a depiction of the Last Supper, a common motif in refectories, yet which also has symbolic and theological significance for the main motif above. The other four scenes 'framing' the *Lignum Vitae* are on the right side from top to bottom as follows: The stigmatisation of St. Francis and St. Louis feeding the poor and sick of Toulouse. On the top left side, a scene from the life of St. Benedict; the priest at his Easter meal receiving word from an angel of St. Benedict's hunger in the wilderness. On the lower left side there is also a depiction of St. Mary Magdalene washing the feet of Christ.[31]

The main motif, the Tree of Life, does not exactly grow out of the Last Supper below, but is directly connected to it visually. It is also related to it symbolically, because the image of Christ as 'the Word become Flesh' was from the earliest times likened and linked to the 'Tree of Life', the fruits of which represent the body and blood of Christ in the sacrament of the Eucharist, as already discussed.[32] This particular version of this well-known Biblical, theological, and iconographic motif, is directly related to, or 'pictorially' derived from the mystical and contemplative text *Lignum Vitae* of St. Bonaventure, who is depicted at the foot of the Cross, writing on a scroll.[33] The text is fully legible and we can read the opening words of a poem from the prologue of the meditation: "O crux, fructex salvi[ficus]".[34] The motif of the 'Tree of Life' that St. Bonaventure uses to organise *his* text and Gaddi represents in his fresco, has in itself meanings and references that would have been familiar to all

[Ill. 32] Taddeo Gaddi (c. 1300-1366): The entire rear wall fresco of the refectory with the *Lignum Vitae,* or 'Tree of Life', framed by five other scenes. Santa Croce, Florence, c. 1350. Photo: Scala.

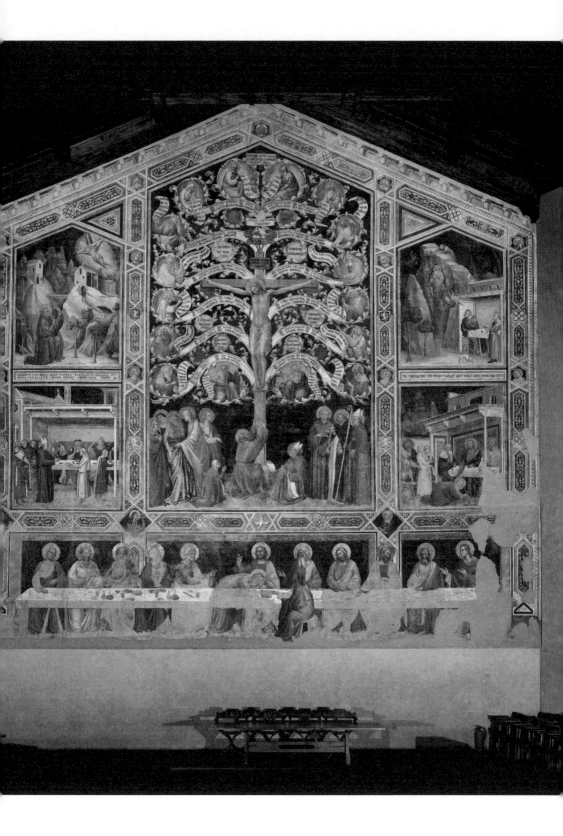

MEMORY

those who saw the fresco, or read or heard the meditations of St. Bonaventure. The iconography of this motif, in its different variations, dates back to at least the fourth or fifth centuries.[35]

Seen spiritually, the *Lignum vitae* in Eden was a prefiguration of the cross, the restorative tree of life.[36] This connection is emphasised in the fresco version with its Old Testament references in the medallions, which does not appear in St. Bonaventure's writings. These passages are references prefiguring Christ; The Old Testament prefiguring the New in a typological manner. "The *Lignum vitae* aspect of the Cross is part of the meta-historical and historical economy of salvation, which has its beginning in the *felix culpa* that occurred in Paradise and will end in redemption."[37] Even if these additions deviate from St. Bonaventure's meditations, they are in keeping with its spirit and can be found in several other illustrations of it. This is a typical example of the medieval way of thinking, in layers upon layers of meaning and intertextual references in an almost never-ending chain of significance. Here the 'medium is the message' in a complex and multimedial manner, in the sense that medium and message are interlaced.

This is both a *reflection of* and a *reflection over* St. Bonaventure's meditations. Not in the sense that the *written text* is the necessarily privileged original; it is but a part of an elaboration of it and a continuous mediated *meditation* on the 'meditation'. Reading is, after all, a remedial technique in itself. The ultimate remedy for the Fall of Man is God and his merciful wisdom, and all human intellectual strivings and practices are remedies, *remedium*, remediating this wisdom.[38] St. Bonaventure's intermedial text is full of images and visual references, and Taddeo Gaddi's intermedial frescoes are full of writing. Moreover, there are a lot of cross-references in the two and new associative references in each of the two that refer to a larger (con)text or web of thoughts. This can also be described with the term *nesting*, which was coined by visual studies theorist W.J.T. Mitchell as a form of intermediality where one medium appears inside another.[39] There is no sharply defined boundary between the two expressions. The relationship between these two manifest expressions is not one of translation from one primary medium (the written text) to a secondary medium (the fresco), but one of intermediality. They are both part of the same and yet different 'texts'.[40] There is constant movement revolving around *images* in the memory, moving from one materialisation to another, where the media are interlaced or mixed. This calls for a closer look at the context of the 'pictures' in the refectory.

The *Textus:* The 'Text' and the 'Painting' in the Refectory

The fresco covers the entire rear wall of the refectory. We do not know how the room was furnished, but the 'high table' – for the convent's superior and others of certain rank – was presumably placed directly below the Last Supper and the other tables against the two adjacent walls, as was the common arrangement. The refectory was the place where the monks or conventuals took their meals, but it was also a place for spiritual nourishment. It was common practice to read aloud to the monks while they ate, and it was often the abbot or superior himself who read. Both the texts for this kind of use – sermons, florilegiae, meditations, Bible commentaries etc. – and the reading session itself were often referred to as *collatio*, collecting.[41] The term collation retained the idea of collecting or gathering together in its many senses. It might refer to texts, including other texts by masters and students; and of nuns, monks, or friars gathered over their readings during a meal. Collation was also a part of composition.[42] Meditations and other intellectual activities were often metaphorically described as spiritual nourishment.[43] This is evident in the *Lignum Vitae*. As we can see there is a connection between composition, reading, and food, but also its consumption, and these readings were conducted at different monastic *collations*.[44] This was a spiritual meal that was meant to accompany the physical meal in communal consumption. St. Bonaventure's meditations on The Tree of Life were most likely read aloud during the communal meal – conceivably directly below the fresco – by the prior himself or by some other person appointed to the task.

St. Bonaventure uses several metaphors related to the senses and nourishment in particular, as when he for instance talks about the fruits of the knowledge of Faith, which of course is juxtaposed with the fruit chosen by the faithless Adam. He is very explicit in his references to both smell and taste. The Fruit of the Tree of Life that grows on the twelve separate branches has 'twelve different flavours'.[45] In the poem from the prologue, sensorial metaphors such as 'fruit' (*fructus*) and 'sweetly scented' (*aromaticus*) are used. In the concluding prayer of the prologue it reads: "Give us Your Fruit as our food."[46] What could be more fitting in the context of a refectory, where the listeners were actually ingesting, tasting, and smelling as they heard about and observed the Tree of Life, thus giving them a wealth of material to ruminate on, or masticate, for the benefit of their working memory, and in this way to inscribe a Faith in Christ and His salvific physical sufferings onto their own body and soul in a sensuous manner.

In this context the scenes surrounding the *Lignum Vitae* are of significance. All of the four scenes refer, among other things, to bodily or sensuous matters, matters that concern sensual or physical phenomena with a spiritual relevance, as well as a series of references to the human sensorium. *The Stigmatisation of St. Francis* refers to the physical, physiological *imprint* of Christ's suffering onto St. Francis' body; a symbol of being nailed to the Cross with Christ. The sensory experiences involve both *touch* and *sight*, on the part of both St. Francis and the beholders.

St. Louis feeding the poor and sick combines the good deeds with its spiritual and moral point of departure – and end. In a way, this is likening the ministration of bodily food with the ministration of spiritual food in the celebration of the Eucharist. As the hungry and sick of body are being helped (saved) by the food, so shall the spiritually hungry and sick be saved through the Eucharistic meal. This motif refers particularly to *sight* and *taste*.

The Priest at the Easter meal accentuates a similar idea of the good deeds and the ministering of bodily sustenance with reference to its spiritual analogy. Ministering spiritual food to the believers is what the priest does in the celebration of the Eucharist. It is interesting to note that in this motif the messenger, or arbiter, between the priest and St. Benedict is an angel, as is the case in the Eucharistic celebration between Heaven and Earth. Here the sensual references are *taste*, *hearing* and once again; *sight*.

The last image, *St. Magdalene washing the feet of Christ* and anointing them, shows how the believer may come in *touch* with Christ literally by humbling her or himself.[47] The sensual references in this picture are *touch*, *smell*, and *sight*. This can also be seen as a parallel to St. Bonaventure's encouragement to kiss the feet of the Child in the manger in the concluding paragraph in the first 'fruit' of his meditation.[48] Again St. Francis is depicted embracing the foot of the Cross.

The senses are at the centre of attention in these pictures. At the same time all have some kind of resemblance or parallel to the activities in the Refectory. This is also the case with the depiction of the last supper. In this manner the mnemotechnical elements not only connect to the inner sensorial experiences but to the outer as well. All the senses are activated, both in an inner and outer manner. The Franciscan conventuals here in Santa Croce were literally collating and ruminating both their physical and spiritual nourishment with the aim of gaining the maximum effect of remembering and internalising. This kind of collation results in what Leclercq defines as "[…] a muscular memory of the words pronounced and an aural memory of the words heard. […] It is what inscribes, so to speak, the sacred text in the body and in the soul".[49] And we might add: with a visual memory structure to bind it together into an all-embracing structure, "always to carry about, in soul and body, the Cross of Christ", as St. Bonaventure states. This is a sensorial catechesis and a kind of encoding of a monastic or contemplative sensorium where memory, among other things, is a *mediator* between the outer and inner experiences and functions. The sacred 'text' is to be inscribed in the body and in the soul. Why, then, are all these references and uses of sensual metaphors and experience so important and so powerful?

Human Knowledge Rooted in the Senses

To comprehend this, we must take a closer look at the understanding of knowledge in the medieval period. In *Summa Theologica*, concerning a discussion of how God can be known to us, St. Thomas Aquinas states: "Our natural knowledge begins from sense. Hence our natural knowledge can go as far as it can be led by sensible things."[50] He writes elsewhere that: "[…] it is natural to man to attain to intellectual truths through sensible objects, because all our knowledge originates from the senses."[51] The first things we have any kind of knowledge of are the perceptible physical objects. Our natural knowledge starts with sense experience.[52]

St. Thomas states that the senses were given to man for the purpose of knowledge, and not only for procuring the necessities of life, as in other animals. He also emphasises the central epistemological status of *visio* – vision, sight or gaze – as a metaphor for understanding and knowledge. This is not simply a metaphor though: "All science is derived from self-evident and therefore *seen* principles; wherefore all objects of science must needs be, in a fashion seen."[53] Along with all the other theologians and philosophers during the Middle Ages, St. Thomas was of the opinion that sight was exceedingly important among the senses.[54] St. Augustine had already voiced the sentiment that sight was equivalent to knowing. This theory of vision, and the understanding of sight in St. Augustine, can be found in the twelfth chapter of *De Genesi ad litteram*. Here St. Augustine takes St. Paul's reference to a visionary experience in his second letter to the Corinthians as his point of departure. He thus refers to the man who was, "caught up to the third heaven".[55] St. Augustine explains that the three heavens referred to by St. Paul are three kinds of human sight. The first is corporeal or optical vision, where one sees the incorporeal through natural optical perception, e.g. apparitions. The second is spiritual or imaginative vision, where one sees incorporeal shapes, as in dreaming. The third is intellectual vision, where one has a direct sight of incorporeal beings and the Divine truths.[56] Here we find a theory of sight, or vision, where optical and physical vision is intimately connected to spiritual sight, and ultimately to cognition. This is central to St. Augustine's thinking and is emphasised in all his writings.[57] Optical sight was part of a process of understanding, and spiritual or intellectual 'sight' was an extension of optical or physical sight.[58] All these levels of vision were modalities on the same hierarchical scale, where one moved from the lower to the higher in an anagogical manner.[59]

260

Sight was also knowledge in a psychological sense because, according to St. Thomas, man understands through inner images or *phantasms*. We think, so to speak, with images. Our intellectual concepts are images stored in our minds.[60] Bonaventure expresses the same tenets in his *Itinerarium Mentis in Deum*:

> [...] *since the creation of the world His invisible attributes are clearly seen* [...] *being understood through the things that are made* [...] *Thanks be to God* [...] *through our Lord Jesus Christ*, who has called us *out of darkness into His Marvellous light*, when through these lights externally given we are led to re-enter the mirror of our mind in which divine realities are reflected.[61]

The boundaries between seeing a physical image, and seeing a mental image – a phantasm or a memory image – or an 'enlightened' vision of a heightened understanding of the realities of the world and beyond, were blurred. This understanding of the senses and sensing, and of sight in particular, was an integrated part of the medieval understanding of mans cognitive faculties, where optical perception was seen as a revelatory process.

From this it would seem that, for medieval thinkers, sight was the most important and noble of the senses. However, their perception of the senses was more complex than as such; medieval philosophers did not separate the different senses into closed compartments as in our modern understanding.[62] One could eat by sight, *manducatio per visum*, as Alexander of Hales (c. 1185-1245) formulates it in his *Sentences*, where he discusses the Eucharist. But here the sensual complexities disclose themselves because, according to Alexander, the sacramental ingestion through taste, *manducatio per gustum*, was the only real *sacramental* one, even if this was not always that clear-cut.[63] Eamon Duffy has argued that in the late Middle Ages (after 1200): "[...] for most people, most of the time the Host was something to be seen, not to be consumed."[64] This tension between different sensorial aspects of the ritual and its form "[...] informs much of the writing, teaching, criticism, and confusion, [...]" of the late medieval discussions of the Eucharistic symbolism, as Miri Rubin has ar-

gued.[65] The Eucharist is of course a central theme in the discussions of sensory processes and the senses in the Middle Ages due to its theological and salvific importance, and its sensual and commemorative character. This sacrament does, however,
also reveal memory as being at the core of Christianity. The Sacrifice of the Mass –
the Eucharistic celebration – is a continuing recollection, *anamnesis*, of Christ's redemptive Sacrifice for Mankind. This is not a mere reminder of a past event, but a   **261**
recollection of the deepest kind of truth made real and effectively present. In this liturgical celebration all the senses are activated – smell, touch, taste, hearing and seeing – in a kind of 'memory theatre' as the one and only 'perfect memory'. It is a *recollection* of a truth that eternally *is*.[66] Knowledge had a clearly sensual side, which is
reasonable when we take into consideration that in this understanding *wisdom* was
"not something but someone", as Ivan Illich has formulated it; knowledge and wisdom *are* Christ.[67] This knowledge is rooted in the memory through the senses, like a
tree that grows. Not only as an image or on a metaphorical level, but actually and
physically, because it is *rooted* in memory and actually changing, and thereby changing the whole person.

Memory and Its Art

The memory image of the *Lignum Vitae*, both in its painted form in the fresco *and*
in the writings of St. Bonaventure, can be regarded as an example of the first and
most generally used and useful kind of rhetorical *memoria*, the *memoria rerum* or the
memory of the case or thing (itself). This consists of remembering the chief subject
matters of something, in this case the meditations of St. Bonaventure, by associating
each part or element with a summary image.[68] But what is the added significance of
this memory technique? If we go to one of the lateral motifs in this fresco we can
perhaps find a rhetorical key to help us unlock the answer to this question.

The depiction in the refectory of the Stigmatisation of St. Francis on the upper
left side of The Tree of Life may refer to several things. In its polysemy, it can refer to
the Galatians 2:19, which is also referred to in St. Bonaventure's prologue to *The Tree
of Life*; but the references are far broader and richer. It is for instance used by St.
Bonaventure as ingress to another of his meditations, the *Itinerarium Mentis in
Deum*. Here the figure of the six-winged seraph is used as a structuring and mnemonic principle, and was also a well-known medieval figure to aid memory.[69] It was
meant to serve as a model for the Franciscan brothers, but also as a *memory hook* or
marker – in the form of a picture, model and image. It is a marker that reminds one

of the purpose of the meditations of St. Bonaventure, and the purpose of the painted fresco. Both of them are to be taken in, internalised and made a part of one's own body and soul. Just as St. Francis is being nailed to the Cross and literally made into an image of Christ through his stigmatisation, the beholders of this fresco shall do the same. This is particularly potent in a Franciscan context because it establishes a direct link between St. Francis and the pious believer through this activity involving memory. The active use of memory becomes in itself a re-enactment of St. Francis' vision at Monte Alverno, and as the Seraph left a physical impression on St. Francis – the stigmata – the meditation leaves an impression on the soul of the devout; a form of mental stigmata. The painted picture presents both the content and structure of St. Bonaventure's meditations *and* how to internalise and memorise it, the message and the medium interlace.

In *Summa Theologica* St. Thomas Aquinas (c. 1225-1274) emphasises the need for using images to cultivate the memory.[70] When you wish to remember something, you must make some suitable illustration of it. The reason for this, according to St. Thomas, is that simple and spiritual impressions slip easily from the mind, unless they are tied to *corporeal images*; that is, physical pictures or envisionings of something seen by the inner or outer eye. This is so, because human knowledge has a greater hold on sensible objects.[71] He also points out the need to carefully arrange these images in a systematic order, so that you easily can pass from one memory object to another.

Internalising information or knowledge had to do with creating and storing inner or mental images, which connect envisioning and thinking. These memory images were understood as being vital for human understanding. This was acknowledged as early as in the classical understanding of memory. Cicero (106-43 BC) states that the impressions which stand out most clearly in our mind are those that are received via the senses; and that amongst all the human senses, the sense of sight is the keenest.[72] Consequently, something one wishes to remember will be retained most easily in the mind by *creating* an image of it.[73] This is important to note as it connects the acts of looking and memorising to knowledge, at the same time that it emphasises the creative aspect of this act of memorising.

It is important to note, however, that the medieval art of memory was not only something inherited from the classical past as an incomplete and imperfect memory of an older and more complex tradition. It was primarily an invention of its own, originating in meditation practices based on the needs of monastic prayer and for the memorising of theological truths. More than one sort of *ars memoria* was in existence during the Middle Ages, as Mary Carruthers has emphasised. The art of memory made use of the classical tradition, but to its own ends and with its own inventions and combinations. This art was: "[…] a primary technique of meditative invention, the monks deliberately crafted a cognitive, inventive use for the images they gathered up fictively from the materials in their memories, 'pictures' seen inwardly with the mind's eye, a technique they called 'recollection'." [74]

This reveals medieval mnemotechnics as a dynamic way of thinking: "[…] the matrix of a reminiscing cogitation, shuffling and collating 'things' stored in a random-access memory scheme, or set of schemes – a memory *architecture* and a library built up during one's lifetime with the express intention that it be used inventively." [75] Ars memoria was a craft that gave a person the means and wherewithal to invent his material, both beforehand and on the spot. It was a compositional art: "The arts of memory are among the arts of thinking, especially involved with fostering the qualities we now revere as 'imagination' and 'creativity'." [76] From this we can see that mnemonics are noticeable as something more than an instrumental technique, but rather a visual – and therefore sensual – basis for knowledge. This makes visible the intersensorial and intermedial understanding of memory as well as a crucial link between past, present, and future. Memory can in this sense be seen as the sensorium outstretched in time.

Memory and the Interlacing of the Senses

As we have seen, sense experience was at the base of all knowledge, but in this understanding the senses were interlaced, or we might perhaps talk of a kind of sensual porousness. This also means that the understanding of an 'image' was not exclusively bound up to optical sight, which also implies an impurity in the understanding of media, as W.J.T. Mitchell has observed: "[…] the heterogeneous character of media was well understood in premodern cultures". [77] This demonstrates that "all media are mixed media". [78]

In his commentary on Aristotle's *De memoria*, St. Thomas emphasises that man cannot understand without images (*phantasmata*). The image is akin to a corporeal object. [79] These inner mental images are just as real as corporeal objects and exist in their own right, but they are different. In the words of Mary Carruthers: "Thus all stages and varieties of knowledge for human beings, from their most concrete to the most abstract, occur in some way within a physical matrix." [80]

Memory and the faculty of imagination (*phantasia*) were thought to be located in the same part of the mind, or the soul. What we remember, according to St. Thomas, are images of sensible things. The images of memory and phantasms are the same 'images', and the memory is the place where concrete (sense objects) and abstract ideas are united in the intellect.[81] In the *Summa Theologica* he defines the faculty of imagination as a storeroom for the forms one has acquired through the senses, and memory as the storeroom of these forms transformed into representations and ideas.[82] *Phantasms* are created by the imagination, *imaginatio* or *vis phantasia*, which is the ability to create images. Both this and memory are a part of the intellectual capacities of the soul or mind. The ability to create images is one of the prerequisites of thinking and knowledge.[83] This is what St. Bonaventure means in his prologue to the *Lignum Vitae* when he says that imagination assists understanding. As we can see, this is not only related to an understanding of image as something more than a strictly optic-visual object of perception by the outer senses. The phantasms are mental images derived from the sensing of a physical object, but transformed through an inner sensory experience. These mental images, the *phantasms*, are in some ways more concepts – not as an abstraction, but as something with a semi-concrete or semi-physical existence.

There are several matters of importance to note here; first the idea of an inner sensorium, where inner and outer are interlaced in the same way as the senses and we find the same kind of porousness. At the same time, what goes on in the inner sensorium is also something that is *experienced* in its own right. Smelling the sweet scent of truth, hearing St. Mary's song etc. are all actual inner sensorial experiences to be stored in the memory as such. However, these sense experiences are all mediated through something else. Here the flesh itself is a medium, and man is a *compositum*, a *unity* of body and mind. With Merleau-Ponty we might say that the mind is the other side of the body.[84]

Another point of importance is the understanding of memory as crucial for both sensing and understanding, as *the* place where everything is interlaced. A third element is the complex understanding of the varieties of sight and its relation to knowledge, the Augustinian relation and analogy between physical and spiritual sight noted previously. However, this understanding is rooted in the idea of a kind of sensual interlacing or interchangeability by St. Augustine. In the *De Trinitate* he states that what one sense reports to us also holds true for the rest.[85] St. Augustine voices the opinion that memory is based on all kinds of sense impressions made into images, as we have seen.[86] In chapter IX of the tenth book of his *Confessions* he also makes clear that we have memories of odour, taste, and sound, which can all be 'sensed' in the mind through memory. What he says here is that sense-experiences are made into images for the memory to work with. So, when we recall the smell of something it is the mental image of this smell that is recalled or re-created.[87] All sense impressions are converted, so to speak, into some sort of signs by and in the memory.[88]

There is an almost synesthetic character in the medieval art of memory and, as we have seen, there are many references to other parts of the human sensorium apart from sight in the *Lignum Vitae*. Almost all the senses are in some way or another referred to in the meditation of St. Bonaventure and Gaddi's fresco. To use a Thomistic-scholastic concept, we could define it as a matter of *integritas*. The senses represented a whole, and each part could only be perfected in this wholeness, in its relationship to other and higher purposes or relations that made up its integrity.[89] Every such integrated wholeness was a realisation of a higher principle. The *Lignum Vitae* of St. Bonaventure and Taddeo Gaddi express this understanding in an almost textbook-like example of rhetorically concentrated syntagmatic expression. Syntagmatic also in the way it links together the human sensorium, both outer and inner, in this one expression.

Extrapolating from this, it seems that there was an understanding that all sense perception, including the inner, were mediated through *a kind of visuality*. In line with this we might perhaps speak of a hierarchy of the senses and sight as a sub-summation of all the senses, or as representative of all the senses.[90]

The Materiality of Memory and Knowledge

It is important to remember that St. Bonaventure treatise, *Lignum Vitae*, is a mystical contemplative text. As already discussed, many of the theories and practices of the art of memory of the Middle Ages were related to the monastic and mendicant need for meditative invention. This is precisely the task of St. Bonaventure's *Lignum Vitae*. Rosemary Hale has argued that: "Medieval mystical texts are always borne of remembered religious experience, recollections of a union with, or nearness to, God filtered through memory and embodied with an array of associated sensory imagery."[91] In one of the visions of Margaretha Ebner the voice of God tells her "I am no robber of the senses; I am the illuminator of the senses."[92] The boundaries between visions, phantasms and sensory experiences were all 'blurred' or interlaced.[93]

Meditation in this sense implies: "[…] thinking of a thing with the intent to do it; in other words to prepare oneself for it, to prefigure it in the mind, to desire it, in a way, to do it in advance – briefly, to practice it. […] To practice a thing by thinking of it, is to fix it in the memory, to learn it."[94] Knowledge was not a ghostlike mental abstraction; knowledge should lead to an alteration, a change, in the person and lead to actions. The true believer should be transformed and marked by Christ in a very concrete manner and the most striking example of this kind of physical transfiguration and embodied belief was the *stigmata* of St. Francis, fittingly depicted in the refectory fresco and in the meditation of St. Bonaventure.

With this stigmatisation, Christ has made an *impression* on and in St. Francis' body, which represents a physical and material transformation of the person. This impression is a concrete and corporeal image. Analogous to this, the *phantasms* could be understood as a kind of physical-mental impression, which has a permanent effect on the substance of the brain. The images make an *impression* and in this way have a direct effect on the mind. The *phantasm*, the image of the sense impression, thus has a kind of double nature; it is both physical and mental. The recollection in memory (*recollectio*) consists of retrieving these images stamped on the rear chamber of the brain and seeing them with the intellect in a manner that is analogous – but not identical – to seeing with the eyes. Memory was a kind of inner marking, the thing to be remembered should be impressed into or onto your mind. This mediation between the outer and the inner sensorium is a tactile operation. What you take in through your senses shall be contemplated and impressed on your mind, just like the stigmata of Christ were impressed on the body of St. Francis. Memory *is* these impressions. The materiality of memory is not only related to its content, but also to how it functions. This is a material and physical understanding of memory.

This understanding was related to the optical theories of the Middle Ages, which were founded on the concept of a kind of physical connection between the seer and the seen, the eye and what the eye was looking at. One could say that the eye in some sense *touched* the object of the gaze.[95] This of course makes what is seen less a passive object and more of an active subject, since it actively participates and communicates in the process of sensing. This is a tactile optic, and an optics of dialogue.

Sight, both miraculous and conventional optics, was thought of as a physical interaction. What one 'sees' makes an impression. Sight was embodied: "To perceive or sense […] is to be materially altered." The example of St. Francis' *stigmata* on the Monte Alverno shows how his flesh became: "[…] moulded into the image of the crucified Christ."[96] St. Bonaventure emphasises this very clearly in his biography of

St. Francis, the *Legenda maior*, when describing this incident. His flesh had become 'wax' in the hands of God: "God is the divine sculptor, fashioning the image of Christ out of flesh; but he is also the Word, writing his creation into existence." The marks of the crucifixion have been 'written' on the flesh of St. Francis. "To gaze, like Francis, at a crucifix, or to meditate the Passion, would have been to enter into this fabric of associations and expectations."[97] Viewing, in this perspective, is not just a matter of interpretation or cognition, but a transformative process where the viewer is affected directly and bodily through a sensory encounter with an object: "In effect, one becomes the image through an encounter with it."[98] This is communication as 'communion', and a corporeal rhetoric of the flesh. The sensory process was open, not only a form of transmission of information about objects:

> [...] but one which enabled tangible qualities, and indeed spiritual or intangible qualities, to be passed from one party or object to another. It was also a two-way process; the senses gave out information or affected others directly, as well as receiving information or serving as a conduit that might change the individual.[99]

The memory-image generated a realisation of the truth in Christ in the mind-body of the devotee, making it possible to inhabit the scene(s) – the place(s)/loci – of the *Lignum Vitae* and thus experience that which transcends any referential description. In this way the memory-image becomes rhetorical evidence – *evidentia* – to be witnessed with your own *inner* eye, a mental *autopsia*. When we regard this in the light of, and understanding of, familiarity between all kinds of images, it becomes clear that images of all kinds are productive rather than descriptive. The *memory-image* was a corporeal experience and memory was a *sense-memory*, and this sensuality was seen as crucial for exploiting the heuristic dimension of the *image* to stimulate memory.

Notes

1 St. Augustine: *Confessions*, X, 8, cited from Augustine 2002B, p. 179; Augustine 2006, p. 96.

2 See Laugerud 2010A, pp. 7-20.

3 This understanding is modelled on Mitchell's Wittgensteinian inspired theory of the familiarity between different kinds of what goes by the name of images, an understanding that in my opinion seems to draw heavily upon medieval theories and concepts. See Mitchell 1987, particularly pp. 1-46.

4 Yates 1994 (1966), p. 91.

5 Augustine 2002B, p. 178. "[…] campos et lata praetoria memoriae". St. Augustine: *Confessions*, X, 8; cited from Augustine 2006, p. 92.

6 Laugerud 2010B, pp. 43-68.

7 Boncompagno da Signa 1892, p. 275.

8 St. Augustine: *Confessions*, X, 17; see Augustine 2002B, p. 187; Augustine 2006, p. 122.

9 It was in the Middle Ages hermeneutically connected to the *quadriga*, the fourfold way of interpretation, a hermeneutics with an existential foundation. See Laugerud 2005.

10 This is one of the central arguments in Bynum 2011.

11 See *The Tree of Life* (*Lignum Vitae*) in: Bonaventure 1960, pp. 97-144. The standard Latin edition is: St. Bonaventurae 1898, pp. 68-87. The meditation was written c. 1259-60, after he had become the Minister General of the Franciscan order.

12 Bonaventure 1960, prologue, 1, p. 97. St. Bonaventurae 1898, p. 68. The reference is to Gal. 2:19.

13 Bonaventure 1960, prologue, 2, p. 97. St. Bonaventurae 1898, p. 68.

14 Bonaventure 1960, prologue, 2, p. 98. St. Bonaventurae 1898, p. 68: "[…] imaginatio iuvat intelligentiam […]".

15 Bonaventure 1960, prologue 3, p. 98. St. Bonaventurae 1898, p. 68.

16 See Carruthers 1996A, p. 209.

17 See Yates 1994, pp. 175-196. See also Ladner 1979, pp. 252-254.

18 See Reno 1978.

19 See Gen. 2, 9 & 3, 22-24.

20 "Lignum vite in medio paradisi afferent fructus xii". Rev. 22:2. At the very top of the tree in Taddeo Gaddi's fresco in Santa Croce there is a painted plaque with this citation. I will return to this.

21 The four rivers of Eden, Gen 2:10, but here it also signifies the Four Gospels.

22 Bonaventure 1960, p. 99. St. Bonaventurae 1898, p. 69. The citation is from Wis. 16:20.

23 Bonaventure 1960, p. 100. St. Bonaventurae 1898, p. 69.

24 Bonaventure 1960, p. 105 ff. St. Bonaventurae 1898, p. 71.

25 Bonaventure 1960, p. 106. St. Bonaventurae 1898, p. 72. Lk. 2:14.

26 Leclercq 2003, p. 15.

27 This has a parallel in the late twelfth-century treatise on reading the Scriptures by Peter of Celle, who uses the same kind of bodily language. See Carruthers 2010, pp. 193-194.

28 See for instance the chapter "On the Mystery of the Passion" and the end of the seventh fruit. Bonaventure 1960, p. 126. St. Bonaventurae 1898, p. 79.

29 Congar 2004, p. 17.

30 Ladis 1982, pp. 171-182. The refectory is today a part of the museum of Santa Croce (Museo del Opera di Santa Croce). For information regarding the refectory, Santa Croce and its history see Baldini 1985.

31 Ladis 1982, pp. 171-182.

32 This connection was established in the early Church, Reno 1978, p. 106 ff, see also Hatfield 1990 & Ladner 1979.

33 There are several examples of similar 'illustrations' of the meditation of St. Bonaventure, for instance in the so called *Speculum theologiae* (Beinecke MS 416) from the Cistercian monastery of Kampen in Germany from the late thirteenth or early fourteenth century. See: http://brbl-net. library.yale.edu/pre1600ms/. This manuscript also contains several other 'tree-schemata'. Another example is the lavishly illuminated *Psalter of Robert de Lisle*, Arundel MS 83 II, in the British Library. See Sandler 1999.

34 "O crux, fructex salvificus, Vivo fonte rigatus, Cuius flos aromaticus, Fructus desideratus." "O Cross, O tree of our salvation, Refreshed by a living stream, Your blossom is sweetly scented, Your fruit so worthy of Desire!" Bonaventure 1960, p. 99. St. Bonaventurae 1898, p. 69 & pp. 86-87. Parts of this poem might be an interpolation into the text of St. Bonaventure and exists in different forms in various manuscripts.

35 One of the best-known examples is perhaps the apse mosaic in the Basilica of San Clemente in Rome from the early twelfth century. See Boyle 1972, Hjort 1990 & Hatfield 1990.

36 Ladner 1979, p. 236.

37 This relationship is not metaphorical but metonymical: "[…] one of conceptual contiguity, mutual participation, and temporal – diachronic – sequence." This relationship is important to keep in mind. See the discussion in Ladner 1979, p. 237. The Latin expression *felix culpa* means 'fortunate fall' meaning that the Fall of Man merited so great a thing as the redeeming sacrifice of Our Lord. See the latin text of the *Exultet* of the Easter Vigil. See St. Augustine: *Enchiridion*, VIII, and St. Thomas Aquinas: *ST* III, Q. 1, art. 3, ad. 3.

38 Illich 1996, p. 11. A *remedium* is also a *remedy* in the sense of something that can heal and/or overcome shortcomings. There is an interesting etymological relation to be observed here.

39 Mitchell 2005, p. 262.

40 In this context, it is worth noting that the Latin word *textus* means something that is woven, as in textile, it is a *web*. This etymology bears evidence to an understanding of *text* as a visual, tactile and material expression. See Snyder 1981.

41 Leclercq 2003, pp. 167, 182.

42 Carruthers 1996A, p. 209.

43 Leclercq 2003, p. 73, and Illich 1993, p. 20, in particular n. 37.

44 For a more general discussion of the sensorial aspects of consumption and its social and religious significance, see Jette Linaa's chapter in this volume.

45 Bonaventure 1960, prologue 3 & 4, p. 99. St. Bonaventurae 1898, pp. 68-69.

46 Bonaventure 1960, p. 100. St. Bonaventurae 1898, p. 69.

47 Luke 7:36-38.

48 Bonaventure 1960, p. 106. St. Bonaventurae 1898, p. 72.

49 Leclercq 2003, p. 73.

50 *ST* I, Q. 12, art. 12.

51 *ST* I, Q. 1, art. 9.

52 This way of thinking was based on an Aristotelian theory of knowledge.

53 *ST* II-II, Q. 1, art. 5.

54 See for instance *De veritate*, Q. 12, art. 3, ad 2. See Thomas Aquinas 1994. See also: *ST* I, Q. 1, art. 9, and in particular: Q. 67, art. 67.

55 2 Cor. 12. pp. 2-4.

56 See St. Augustine: *De Genesi ad litteram*, XII, 7; Augustine 2002A, p. 471.

57 See Miles 1983.

58 See Erickson 1978, also Caviness 1983.

59 We find similar ideas by St. Basil of Caesarea (c. 330-379). For a discussion of this patristic understanding of sight see Eden 1997, p. 47.

60 See Kretzmann 1994 & MacDonald 1994. See also Gilson 1929.

61 Bonaventure 1960, p. 27. The references are to Rom. 1:20, 1 Cor. 15:57 & 1 Pt. 2:9. See Laura Katrine Skinnebach's chapter on *Devotion* in this volume for a further discussion of this.

62 Cognitive research and studies in neuroscience in the last 30 years or so have shown that the modern, Cartesian compartmentalisation of the senses and dualism between rationality and emotions are an insufficient and probably incorrect understanding. The Cartesian mind-body dualism still prevalent in many models of understanding is, according to contemporary neuroscience, inadequate if not outright wrong. The medieval model is probably more adequate. See for instance Damasio 1994, 1999 & 2010.

63 Rubin 1994, p. 64.

64 Duffy 1992, p. 95.

65 Rubin 1994, p. 64. In this discussion hearing was by some regarded as the only reliable sense, since all the other senses were deceived in this sacrament. The words of the priest, the words of consecration, are not deceptive because in these words Christ is actually reborn. Rubin 1994, p. 228.

66 Watts 1983, p. 95.

67 Illich 1996, p. 10.

68 The second kind is memory for words, *memoria verborum*. This was regarded as less useful and more difficult since one had to remember 'an image' for every word or group of words. It was less complicated if the written text itself was remembered as an 'image'. Carruthers 1996, pp. 80-107; Carruthers & Ziolkowski (ed.) 2002, p. 10.

69 It can also be found in the *Speculum theologiae* that contains the *Lignum Vitae*. Beinecke MS 41. See n. 33 above. Carruthers & Ziolkowski 2002, pp. 83-102. This six-winged seraph was seen by St. Francis in the vision where he received his stigmata, as depicted in Gaddi's fresco. The vision and the stigmatisation are treated in all the *lives* of St. Francis: Thomas of Celano's *First life of St.*

Francis, II, 3; St. Bonaventure's *Major Life*, XIII & *Minor Life*, VI. See Habig 1973.

70   *ST* II-II, Q. 49.

71   Recent studies in cognitive science seem to confirm this understanding. A study carried out at Lund University in Sweden shows that the person's eye movements reflect the positions of objects while they were listening to a spoken description, retelling it or describing a previously seen picture. The effect was equally strong when retelling from memory, irrespective of whether the original elicitation was spoken or optically seen. See Johansson et al. 2006.

72   Cicero *De oratore*, II, 87, 357. Cicero 1979, p. 469.

73   Cicero *De oratore*, II, 87, 357. Cicero 1979, p. 469.

74   Carruthers 1996B, p. 45.

75   Carruthers 1999, p. 4.

76   Carruthers 1999, p. 9.

77   Mitchell 1994, p. 107.

78   Mitchell 2005, p. 257.

79   *De memoria*. Lectio II, 311. Thomas Aquinas 1949, p. 91. Carruthers & Ziolkowski 2002, p. 160.

80   Carruthers 1996, p. 54.

81   *De memoria*. Lectio II, 326. Thomas Aquinas 1949, p. 94. Carruthers & Ziolkowski 2002, p. 165.

82   *ST* I, Q. 78, art. 4.

83   See Carruthers 1996, pp. 51-54.

84   As formulated in his working notes dated June 1960. See Merleau-Ponty 1968, p. 259. Merleau-Ponty's discussions on this are interesting and clearly inspired by medieval (and catholic) thinking, as pointed out by Biernoff 2005.

85   Miles 1983, p. 126.

86   See references in n. 1 above.

87   St. Augustine: *Confessions*, X, 9; see Augustine 2002B, pp. 180-181.

88   The relation between the sign and what it signifies is purely conventional according to St. Augustine. Meaning has meaning only in communities. This highlights the communal aspects, or familiarity (oikonomia), of memory. On St. Augustine's understanding of signs: see Markus 1996, particularly chapters 3-4, pp. 71-124.

89   On the synaesthetic understanding of the medieval sensoria, see the very interesting reflections in Baert 2013.

90   See Miles 1983, p. 129. St. Augustine: *Confessions*, VII, 17 & IX, 10.

91   Hale 1995, p. 3.

92   Hale 1995, p. 11.

93   Laugerud 2007.

94   Leclercq 2003, p. 16.

95   There were two main theories: The *extramission* theory and the *intromission* theory. The first theory states that the eye *sends out* 'rays' or 'sense particles' towards an object and these 'rays' or 'particles' are then reflected back to the eye. The intromission theory states in contrast, that the eye *receives* 'rays' or 'sense particles' which the object of the gaze *emits* towards the eye. The standard

reference on medieval optics is Lindberg 1976, particularly pp. 104-121. See also Mitchell 2005, p. 263.

96 Biernoff 2005, p. 42. See also Bennett 2001.

97 Biernoff 2005, p. 43. See Habig 1973, pp. 729-736.

98 Bennett 2001, p. 6.

99 Woolgar 2006, p. 2.

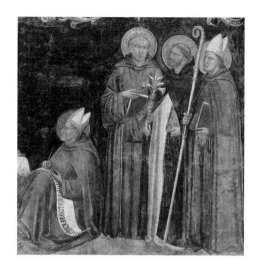

Aavitsland, Kristin B.: "Materialiet og teofani, Om bruken av kostbare materialer i romansk alterut-smykning", *Kunst og kultur*, 2, 2007, pp. 78-91.

Aavitsland, Kristin B.: "Visual orders in the golden altar from Lisbjerg", *Ornament and Order, Essays on Viking and Northern Medieval Art*, ed. Margrethe Stang & Kristin B. Aavitsland, Trondheim: Tapir Academic Press, 2008, pp. 73-95.

Aavitsland, Kristin B.: "Visual Splendour and Verbal Argument in Romanesque Golden Altars", *Inscriptions in Liturgical Spaces, Acta ad archaeologiam et artium historiam pertinentia*, 24, 10, ed. Kristin B. Aavitsland & Turid Karlsen Seim, Rome: Scienze e lettere, 2011, pp. 205-226.

Aavitsland, Kristin B.: *Imagining the Human Condition in Medieval Rome*, Aldershot: Ashgate, 2012.

Ælfric's Letter to the Monks of Eynsham, ed. & trans. Christopher A. Jones, Cambridge: Cambridge University Press, 1998.

Alain of Lille: "Rhytmus alter, quo graphice natura hominis fluxa et caduca depingitur", *Patrologia Latina, Cursus Completus*, vol. CCX, ed. Jacques-Paul Migne, Turnhout: Brepols, 1844-65.

Amalarius of Metz, "Liber Officialis," *Amalarii Episcopi opera liturgica Omnia*, vol. II, ed. Iohanne Michaele Hanssens, Città del Vaticano: Biblioteca Apostolica Vaticana, 1948.

Ambrose: *Ambroise de Milan, Des Sacrements, Des Mystères, Explication du symbole – Introduction, texte, traduction, notes et index*, ed. Bernard Botte, Sources Chrétiennes 25, Paris: Cerf, 1950, 1980, 2007.

Andersen, Flemming G.: *Popular Drama in Northern Europe in the Later Middle Ages, A Symposium*, ed. Julia McGrew, Tom Pettitt & Reinhold Schröder, Odense: Odense University Press, 1988.

Andersen, Kasper H. & Pajung, Stefan (ed.): *Drikkekultur i middelalderen*, Aarhus: Aarhus University Press, 2014.

Andersson, Carolina & Hållans, Ann-Mari: "No Trespassing, Physical and Mental Boundaries in Agrarian Settlement", *Visions of the Past, Trends and Traditions in Swedish Medieval Archaeology*, ed. Hans Andersson, Peter Carelli & Lars Ersgård, Stockholm: Central Board of National Antiquities, 1997, pp. 583-596.

Andrén, Anders: "Landscape and settlement as utopian space", *Settlement and Landscape*, ed. Charlotte Fabech & Jytte Ringved, Aarhus: Jysk Arkæologisk Selskab, 1999, pp. 383-393.

Andrén, Anders: *"Ad sanctos* – de dödas plats under medeltiden", *Hikuin*, 27, 2000, pp. 6-26.

Appel, Hans Henrik: *Tinget, magten og æren – Studier i sociale processer og magtrelationer i et jysk bondesamfund i 1600-tallet*, Odense: Odense University Press, 1999.

Armstrong, Robert P.: *The Affecting Presence, An Essay in Humanistic Anthropology*, Urbana & Chicago: University of Illinois Press, 1971.

Arnulf, Arwed (ed.): *Kunstliteratur in Antike und Mittelalter, Eine kommentierte Anthologie*, Darmstadt: Wissenschaftliche Buchgesellschaft, 2008.

Arvidson, Jens; Askander, Mikael; Bruhn, Jørgen & Führer, Heidrun (ed.): *Changing Borders, Contemporary Positions in Intermediality*, Lund: Intermedia Studies Press, 2007.

Assunto, Rosario: *Die Theorie des Schönen im Mittelalter*, Cologne: DuMont, 1963, 1982.

Attwater, Donald: *The Penguin Dictionary of Saints*, Harmondsworth: Penguin, 1980.

Auerbach, Erich: *Mimesis*, Princeton: Princeton University Press, 1946, 2003.

Augustine: *De Doctrina Christiana*, ed. & trans. R.P.H. Green, Oxford: Clarendon Press, 1995.

Augustine: *On Genesis, The Works of Saint Augustine*, vol. I/XIII, New York: New City Press, 2002A.

Augustine: *The Confessions of St. Augustine*, New York: Dover Publications, 1955, 2002B.

Augustine: *Confessions*, Cambridge, Mass.: Harvard University Press, 1912, 2006.

Augustine: *On the Trinity, A Select Library of the Nicene and Post-Nicene Fathers of the Christian Church*, vol. III, ed. Philip Schaff, Edinburgh: T&T Clark & Michigan: Eerdmans Publishing Company, 1998.

Augustine: *The Trinity*, vol. I/V, ed. John E. Rotelle & trans. Edmund Hill, New York: New City Press, 1991, 2012.

Babb, Warren (trans.) & Palisca, Claude V. (ed.): *Hucbald, Guido, and John on Music, Three Medieval Treatises*, New Haven: Yale University Press, 1978.

Backman, E. Louis: *Religious Dances in the Christian Church and in Popular Medicine*, trans. E. Classen, London: George Allen & Unwin, 1952.

Baert, Barbara: *Interspaces between Word, Gaze and Touch – The Bible and the Visual Medium in the Middle Ages, Collected essays on 'Noli me tangere', the Woman with the Haemorrhage, the Head of John the Baptist*, Leuven: Peeters, 2011.

Baert, Barbara: "An Odour, A Taste, A Touch, Impossible to Describe, *Noli me tangere* and the Senses", *Religion and the Senses in Early Modern Europe*, ed. Christine Göttler, Leiden: Wietse de Boer, 2013, pp. 111-151.

Bagnoli, Martina: "The Stuff of Heaven, Materials and Craftsmanship in Medieval Reliquaries", *Treasures of Heaven – Saints, Relics and Devotion in Medieval Europe*, New Haven & London: Yale University Press, 2010, pp. 137-148.

Baldini, Umberto: *Santa Croce – Kirche, Kapellen, Kloster, Museum*, Stuttgart: Urachhaus, 1985.

Banning, Knud (ed.): *A Catalogue of Wall-Paintings in the Churches of Medieval Denmark 1100-1600, Scania, Halland, Blekinge*, vol. I-IV, Copenhagen: Akademisk Forlag, 1976-1982.

Barsalou, Lawrence; Barbey, Aron K.; Simmon, Kyle W. & Santos, Ava: "Embodiment in Religious Knowledge", *Journal of Cognition and Culture*, 5, 2005, pp. 14-57.

Bartels, Michiel: *Steden in scherven, Vondsten uit beerputten in Deventer, Dordrecht, Nijmegen en Tiel (1250-1900)*, Zwolle: Stechting Promotie Archeologie, 1999.

Bartz, Gabriele: *Guido di Piero, known as fra Angelio, ca. 1395-1455*, Potsdam: H.F. Ullmann Verlag, 2007.

Bell, Catherine: *Ritual – Perspectives and Dimensions*, Oxford: Oxford University Press, 1997.

Belting, Hans: *Likeness and Presence, A History of the Image before the Era of Art*, Chicago: University of Chicago Press, 1997.

Benedict of Nursia: *Benedikts Regel*, trans. Brian Møller Jensen, Copenhagen: Museum Tusculanum Press, 1998.

Benjamin, Walter: "The Work of Art in the Age of Mechanical Reproduction", *Illuminations*, New York: Harcourt, Brace & World, 1968.

Bennett, Jill: "Stigmata and Sense Memory, St. Francis and the Affective Image", *Art History*, 24, 1, 2001, pp. 1-16.

Bernard of Clairvaux: *Sermones in Cantica, On the Song of Songs*, vol. I, trans. Kilian Walsh, Kalamazoo: Cistercian Publications, 1977.

Bertelsen, Thomas: "Desorienterede kirketårne – praktiske løsninger og arkitektoniske idealer i senmiddelalderens kirkebyggeri", *Hikuin*, 33, 2006, pp. 11-28.

Biblia Sacra, Iuxta Vulgatam Versionem, Stuttgart: Deutsche Bibelgesellschaft, 1994.

Biernoff, Suzannah: "Carnal Relations, Embodied Sight in Merleau-Ponty, Roger Bacon and St. Francis", *Journal of Visual Culture*, 4, 1, 2005, pp. 39-52.

Bille, Mikkel & Sørensen, Tim F.: "An Anthropology of Luminosity, The Agency of Light", *Journal of Material Culture*, 12, 3, 2007, pp. 263-284.

Bille, Mikkel; Hastrup, Frida & Sørensen, Tim F.: "Introduction, An Anthropology of Absence", *An Anthropology of Absence, Materializations of Transcendence and Loss*, ed. Mikkel Bille, Frida Hastrup & Tim F. Sørensen, New York: Springer, 2010, pp. 3-22.

Bille, Mikkel & Sørensen, Tim F.: "In Visible Presence, The Role of Light in Shaping Religious Atmospheres", *The Oxford Handbook of Light in Archaeology*, ed. Konstantinos Papadopoulos & Greame Earl, Oxford: Oxford University Press (in press).

Bille, Mikkel; Bjerregaard, Peter & Sørensen, Tim F.: "Staging atmospheres – Materiality, culture, and the texture of the in-between", *Emotion, Space and Society*, 13, 2015 (in press).

Bisgaard, Lars: "Det religiøse liv i senmiddelalderen, En tabt dimension i dansk historieskrivning", *Danmark i Senmiddelalderen*, ed. Per Ingesman & Jens Villiam Jensen, Aarhus: Aarhus University Press, 1994, pp. 342-362.

Bisgaard, Lars: "Det religiøse liv", *Middelalderens Danmark, Kultur og samfund fra trosskifte til reformation*, ed. Per Ingesman, Ulla Kjær, Per Kristian Madsen & Jens Vellev, Copenhagen: Gad, 1999, pp. 118-135.

Bisgaard, Lars: "Religion, gilder og identitet i den senmiddelalderlige by", *Middelalderbyen*, ed. Søren Bitsch Christensen, Aarhus: Aarhus University Press, 2004, pp. 249-269.

Blick, Sarah & Tekippe, Rita (ed.): *Art and Architecture of Late Medieval Pilgrimage in Northern Europe and the British Isles*, vol. I-II, Leiden: Brill, 2005.

Boertjes, Katja: "Pilgrim Ampullae from Vendôme, Souvenirs from a Pilgrimage to the Holy Tear of Christ", *Art and Architecture of Late Medieval Pilgrimage in Northern Europe and the British Isles*, ed. Sarah Blick & Rita Tekippe, Leiden: Brill, 2005, vol. I, pp. 443-472.

Boitani, Piero & Torti, Anna (ed.): *The Body and the Soul in Medieval Literature*, Cambridge: D.S. Brewer, 1998.

277

Bolter, Jay D. & Grusin, Richard: *Remediation, Understanding New Media*, Cambridge, Mass. & London: MIT Press, 1999.

Bolvig, Axel: *Danmarks kalkmalerier*, Copenhagen: Gyldendal, 2002.

Bonaventure: *Opera Omnia Sancti Bonaventuræ*, vol. XII, ed. Adolphe C. Peltier, Paris: Ludovico Vives, 1864.

Bonaventure: *St. Bonaventurae Opera omnia*, vol. VIII, Quaracchi: Collegium S. Bonaventurae, 1898.

Bonaventure: *The Works of Bonaventure*, vol. I, *Mystical Opuscula*, trans. José de Vinck, Paterson, N. J.: St. Anthony Guild Press, 1960.

Bonaventure: "Itinerarium mentis in Deum", *Bonaventure, The Soul's Journey into God, The Tree of Life, The Life of St Francis*, trans. Ewert Cousins, Mahwah: Paulist Press, 1978.

Boncompagno da Signa: *Rhetorica Novissima, Bibliotheca Iuridica Medii Aevi*, vol. II, ed. Augusto Gaudentio, Bologna, 1892.

Bonne, Jean-Claude: "Entre l'image et la matière, La choséité du sacré en Occident", *Bulletin de l'Institut historique Belge de Rome*, 69, 1999, pp. 77-112.

Bourcier, Paul: *Histoire de la dance en Occident*, Paris: Éditions du Seuil, 1978.

Bourdieu, Pierre: *Outline of a Theory of Practice*, Cambridge: Cambridge University Press, 2003.

Boyle, Leonard E.: *A Short Guide to St. Clement's in Rome*, Rome: Collegio San Clemente, 1972.

Boynton, Susan: *Shaping a Monastic Identity – Liturgy and History at the Imperial Abbey of Farfa, 1000-1225*, Ithaca: Cornell University Press, 2006.

Braun, Joseph: *Der christliche Altar in seiner geschichtlichen Entwicklung*, vol. I-II, Munich: Koch, 1924.

Brendalsmo, A. Jan: "De dødes landskap, Måtte man begraves ved sognekirken i middelalderen?", *Hikuin*, 27, 2000, pp. 27-42.

Broadbridge, David: *Treading the Dance, Danish Medieval Ballads*, Gylling: Hovedland, 2011.

Browe, Peter: *Die Verehrung der Eucharistie im Mittelalter*, Rome: Herder, 1933, 1967.

Brown, Peter: "The Rise and Function of the Holy Man in Late Antiquity", *The Journal of Roman Studies*, 61, 1971, pp. 80-101.

Brown, Peter: *The Cult of the Saints, Its Rise and Function in Latin Christianity*, London: SCM Press & Chicago: University of Chicago Press, 1981, 1982.

Bruhn, Jørgen: "Tristan Transformed, Bodies and Media in the Historical Transformation of the Tristan and Iseut-Myth", *Changing Borders, Contemporary Positions in Intermediality*, ed. Jens Arvidson, Mikael Askander, Jørgen Bruhn & Heidrun Führer, Lund: Intermedia Studies Press, 2007, pp. 339-360.

Bruhn, Jørgen: *Lovely Violence, Chrétien de Troyes' Critical Romances*, Newcastle on Tyne: Cambridge Scholars Publishing, 2010.

Bryer, Anthony & Herrin, Judith (ed.): *Iconoclasm, Papers given at the ninth Spring Symposium of Byzantine Studies, University of Birmingham, March 1975*, Birmingham: Centre for Byzantine Studies, 1977.

Buc, Philippe: *The Dangers of Ritual, Between Early Medieval Texts and Social Scientific Theory*, Princeton: Princeton University Press, 2001.

Buchan, David: *The Ballad and the Folk*, London & Boston: Routledge & Kegan Paul, 1972.

Buchli, Victor: "Presencing the Im-Material", *An Anthropology of Absence, Materializations of*

Transcendence and Loss, ed. Mikkel Bille, Frida Hastrup & Tim F. Sørensen, New York: Springer, 2010, pp. 185-203.

Burke, Peter: *Popular Culture in Early Modern Europe*, London: Temple Smith, 1979, 2009.

Bynum, Caroline Walker: "Introduction, The Complexity of Symbols", *Gender and Religion, On the Complexity of Symbols*, ed. Caroline Walker Bynum, Steven Harall & Paula Richman, Boston: Beacon Press, 1986, pp. 1-20.

Bynum, Caroline Walker: *Holy Feast and Holy Fast, The Religious Significance of Food to Medieval Women*, Berkeley: University of California Press, 1987.

Bynum, Caroline Walker: "The Female Body and Religious Practice in the Later Middle Ages", *Fragments for a History of the Human Body, Part One*, ed. Michel Feher et al., New York: Zone Books, 1989, pp. 160-219.

Bynum, Caroline Walker: *Fragmentation and Redemption, Essays on Gender and the Human Body in Medieval Religion*, New York: Zone Books, 1992.

Bynum, Caroline Walker: *The Resurrection of the Body in Western Christianity, 200-1336*, New York: Columbia University Press, 1995.

Bynum, Caroline Walker: *Wonderful Blood, Theology and Practice in Late Medieval Northern Germany and Beyond*, Philadelphia: University of Pennsylvania Press, 2007.

Bynum, Caroline Walker: *Christian Materiality, An Essay on Religion in Late Medieval Europe*, New York: Zone Books, 2011.

Caldwell, John: "Do We Still Need 'Liturgy'?", *Cantus Planus, Papers Read at the 9th Meeting, Esztergom & Visegrád 1998*, ed. L. Dobszay, Budapest: Hungarian Academy of Sciences, 2001, pp. 585-592.

Camille, Michael: "The Image and the Self, Unwriting Late Medieval Bodies", *Framing Medieval Bodies*, ed. Miri Rubin & Sarah Kay, Manchester: Manchester University Press, 1994, pp. 62-99.

Camille, Michael: *Gothic Art, Glorious Visions*, London: Prentice Hall, 1996.

Camille, Michael: *The Medieval Art of Love, Objects and Subjects of Desire*, London: Laurence King, 1998.

Camille, Michael: "Mimetic Identification and Passion Devotion in the Later Middle Ages, A Double-sided Panel by Meister Francke", *The Broken Body, Passion Devotion in Late-Medieval Culture*, ed. Alasdair A. MacDonald, H.N. Bernhard Ridderbos & Rita M. Schlusemann, Groningen: Egbert Forsten, 1998, pp. 183-210.

Camille, Michael: "Adam's House at Angers – Sculpture, Signs and Contrasts on the Medieval Street", *Kontraste im Alltag des Mittelalters*, ed. Gerhard Jaritz, Wien: Verlag der Österreichischen Akademie der Wissenschaften, 2000, pp. 143-178.

Carey, James W.: *Communication as Culture, Essays on Media and Society*, New York: Routledge, 1989, 2009.

Carruthers, Mary: *The Book of Memory, A Study of Memory in Medieval Culture*, Cambridge: Cambridge University Press, 1996A.

Carruthers, Mary: "Boncompagno at the Cutting-edge of Rhetoric, Rhetorical *Memoria* and the Craft of Memory", *The Journal of Medieval Latin*, 61, 1996B, pp. 44-69.

279

Carruthers, Mary: *The Craft of Thought – Meditation, Rhetoric, and the Making of Images, 400-1200*, Cambridge: Cambridge University Press, 1999.

Carruthers, Mary: "The concept of *ductus*, or journeying through a work of art", *Rhetoric beyond Words, Delight and Persuasion in the Arts of the Middle Ages*, ed. Mary Carruthers, Cambridge: Cambridge University Press, 2010, pp. 190-213.

Carruthers, Mary & Ziolkowski, Jan M. (ed.): *The Medieval Craft of Memory*, Philadelphia: University of Pennsylvania Press, 2002.

Caviness, Madeline H.: "Images of Divine Order and the Third Mode of Seeing", *Gesta*, 22, 2, 1983, pp. 99-120.

Cawley, Martinus (trans.): *Bernard of Clairvaux, Early Biographies*, Lafayette: Guadalupe Translations, 2000.

Chambers, Raymond Wilson: *A Fifteenth Century Courtesy Book*, London: Early English Text Society, 1914.

Chenu, Marie-Dominique: *Nature, man and society in the twelfth century, Essays on new theological perspectives in the Latin West*, Toronto: University of Toronto Press & Medieval Academy of America, 1997.

Chrétien de Troyes: *Arthurian Romances*, trans. William W. Kibler, London: Penguin Books, 1991.

Chrétien de Troyes: *Oeuvres completes*, ed. Daniel Poirion, Paris: Nouvelle Revue Francaise & Gallimard, 1994.

Chrétien, Jean-Louis: *The Call and the Response*, New York: Fordham University Press, 1992, 2004.

Christie, Neil: *From Constantine to Charlemagne, An Archaeology of Italy, AD 300-800*, Aldershot: Ashgate, 2006.

Ciardi, Anna Minara: *Lundakanikernas levnadsregler, Aachenregeln och Consuetudines canonicae*, Lund: Lunds universitets kyrkohistoriska arkiv, 2003.

Cicero: *De oratore*, vol. I, trans. Edward W. Sutton & Harris Rackham, London: Heinemann, 1942, 1979.

Clark, Elizabeth A.: *History, Theory, Text – Historians and the Linguistic Turn*, Cambridge, Mass.: Harvard University Press, 2004.

Classen, Constance: *Worlds of Sense, Exploring the Senses in History and Across Cultures*, London: Routledge, 1993.

Classen, Constance: "Foundations for an anthropology of the senses", *International Social Science Journal*, 49, 153, 1997, pp. 401-412.

Classen, Constance: *The Deepest Sense, A Cultural History of Touch*, Urbana, Chicago & Springfield: University of Illinois Press, 2012.

Cline, Ruth H.: "Heart and Eyes", *Romance Philology*, 25, 2, 1971, pp. 263-297.

Cohen, Meredith: "An Indulgence for the Visitor, The Public at the Sainte-Chapelle of Paris", *Speculum*, 83, 4, 2008, pp. 840-883.

Colbert, David W.: *The Birth of the Ballad, The Scandinavian Medieval Genre*, Stockholm: Svenskt visarkiv, 1989.

Colby, Alice M.: *The Portrait in Twelfth-Century French Literature, An Example of the Stylistic Originality of Chrétien de Troyes*, Genève: Droz, 1965.

Colgrave, Bertram & Mynors, R.A.B. (ed.): *Bede's Ecclesiastical History of the English People*, Oxford: Clarendon Press, 1969, 1992.

Colpe, Carsten: "Sacred and the Profane", *Encyclopedia of Religion*, vol. XII, ed. Lindsay Jones, Detroit: Macmillan Reference USA, 2005, pp. 7964-7978.

Congar, Yves: *The Meaning of Tradition*, San Francisco: Ignatius, 1964, 2004.

Consuetudines lundenses, Statutter for kannikesamfundet i Lund c. 1123, ed. Erik Buus, Copenhagen: C.A. Reitzels Boghandel, 1978.

Coolman, Boyd Taylor: *The Theology of Hugh of St. Victor*, Cambridge: Cambridge University Press, 2010.

Cooper, Helen: *The Canterbury Tales*, Oxford: Oxford University Press, 1989, 1996.

Crook, John: *English Medieval Shrines*, Woodbridge, Suffolk: Boydell Press, 2011.

Cumberpatch, Chris: "Face to face with medieval pottery, Some observations on medieval anthropomorphic pottery in north-east England", *Assemblage, The Sheffield Graduate Journal of Archaeology*, 9, 2006, accessed: 14/11/2014, http://www.assemblage.group.shef.ac.uk/issue9/cumberpatch.html

Curtius, Ernst Robert: *European Literature and the Latin Middle Ages*, Princeton: Princeton University Press, 1953, 1973.

Cyril of Jerusalem: *On the Mysteries*, ed. Philip Schaff, *A Select Library of the Nicene and Post-Nicene Fathers of the Christian Church*, ser. II, vol. VII, Edinburgh: T&T Clark & Michigan: Eerdmans Publishing Company, 1893.

Dahl, Ellert: "Kirkeutsmykningen i middelalderen, Bernard av Clairvaux og Suger av St. Denis som representanter for to motsatte åndsidealer", *Lumen*, 14, 1971, pp. 100-109.

Dahlerup, Pil: *Dansk litteratur, Middelalder*, vol. I, *Religiøs litteratur*, Copenhagen: Gyldendal, 1998.

Dahlerup, Pil: *Sanselig Senmiddelalder, Litterære perspektiver på danske tekster 1482-1523*, Aarhus: Aarhus University Press, 2010.

Damasio, Antonio: *Descartes' Error – Emotion, Reason, and the Human Brain,* New York: Putnam, 1994.

Damasio, Antonio: *The Feeling of What Happens, Body and Emotion in the Making of Consciousness,* New York: Harcourt, 1999.

Damasio, Antonio: *Self Comes to Mind, Constructing the Conscious Brain,* New York: Pantheon Books, 2010.

Daniel, Walter: *Vita Ailredi, The Life of Ailred of Rievaulx*, trans. Maurice Powicke, Oxford: Clarendon Press, 1978.

Danske Magazin, 4. R. II, 1873.

Danske Samlinger, 2. Række, 6, 1877-79.

Dante Alighieri: *The Divine Comedy*, trans. Henry Wadsworth Longfellow, Boston: James R. Osgood & Company, 1871.

Dante, Alighieri: *De vulgari eloquentia, Über das Dichten in der Muttersprache*, trans. Franz Dornseif & Josef Balloch, Darmstadt: Wissenschaftliche Buchgesellschaft, 1966.

Davies, Glyn: *Medieval and Renaissance Art – People and Possessions*, London: V&A, 2009.

de Bruyne, Edgar: *Études d'Esthétique Médiévale*, vol. I-III, Brugge: Rijksuniversiteit te Gent, 1946.

de Bruyne, Edgar: *The Esthetics of the Middle Ages*, trans. Eileen B. Hennessy, New York: Frederick Ungar, 1969.

Dinshaw, Carolyn: *Getting Medieval – Sexualities and Communities, Pre- and Postmodern*, Durham: Duke University Press, 1999.

Dinzelbacher, Peter: *Angst im Mittelalter – Teufels-, Todes- und Gotteserfahrung, Mentalitätsgeschichte und Ikonographie*, Paderborn: Ferdinand Schöningh, 1996.

Dinzelbacher, Peter: *Himmel, Hölle, Heilige – Visionen und Kunst im Mittelalter*, Darmstadt: Primus-Verlag, 2002.

Duby, Georges: "À propos de l'amour dit courtois", *Féodalité*, Paris: Gallimard, 1996.

Duby, Georges: "Les trois ordres ou l'imaginaire du féodalisme", *Féodalité*, Paris: Gallimard, 1996, pp. 451-825.

Duby, Georges: "Que sait-on de l'amour en France au XIIeme siècle?", *Féodalité*, Paris: Gallimard, 1996, pp. 1413-1420.

Duerr, Hans Peter: *Nacktheit und Scham, Der Mythos vom Zivilisationsprozess*, Frankfurt am Main: Suhrkamp, 1988.

Duerr, Hans Peter: *Nakenhed och Skam*, Stockholm: Brutus Östlings Bokförlag Symposion, 1994.

Duffy, Eamon: *The Stripping of the Altars, Traditional Religion in England c. 1400-1580*, New Haven & London: Yale University Press, 1992, 2005.

Dufrenne, Mikel: *In the Presence of the Sensuous, Essays in Aesthetics*, Atlantic Highlands, N.J.: Humanities Press International, 1987.

Dumoutet, Édouard: *Le Désir de voir l'Hostie et les Origines de la Dévotion au Saint-Sacrement*, Paris: Gabriel Beauchesne, 1926.

Durandus, Guillaume: *Durandus' Rationale in spätmittelhochdeutscher Übersetzung, das vierte Buch nach der Hs*, ed. G.H. Buijssen, Assen: van Gorcum, 1966.

Dyer, Christopher: *Standards of Living in the Later Middle Ages, Social Change in England c. 1200-1520*, Cambridge: Cambridge University Press, 1998.

Dyggve, Ejnar: "The origin of the urban churchyard", *Classica et mediaevalia, Revue danoise de philologie et d'histoire*, 13, 1952, pp. 147-158.

Eco, Umberto: *Art and Beauty in the Middle Ages*, trans. Hugh Bredin, New Haven: Yale University Press, 1959, 1986.

Eden, Kathy: *Hermeneutics and the Rhetorical Tradition, Chapters in the Ancient Legacy and Its Humanist Reception*, New Haven & London: Yale University Press, 1997.

Eliade, Mircea: *Das Heilige und das Profane, Vom Wesen des Religiösen*, Hamburg: Rowohlt, 1957.

Elias, Norbert: *The Civilizing Process, The History of Manners and State Formation and Civilization*, Oxford: Blackwell, 1939, 1994.

Elleström, Lars (ed.): *Media Borders, Multimodality and Intermediality*, Houndmills: Palgrave Macmillan, 2010.

Elleström, Lars: "The Modalities of Media, A Model for Understanding Intermedial Relations", *Media Borders, Multimodality and Intermediality*, ed. Lars Elleström, Houndmills: Palgrave Macmillan, 2010, pp. 11-48.

Elleström, Lars (ed:): *Intermediala perspektiv på medeltida ballader*, Stockholm: Gidlunds, 2011.

Elleström, Lars & Kværndrup, Sigurd: "Den intermediala balladen", *Intermediala perspektiv på medeltida ballader*, ed. Lars Elleström, Stockholm: Gidlunds, 2011, pp. 13-39.

Engberg, Nils & Kieffer-Olsen, Jacob: "Kirkegårdens grøft, Om den ældste indhegning af Danmarks kirkegårde", *Nationalmuseets Arbejdsmark*, Copenhagen: The National Museum, 1992, pp. 168-177.

Engberg, Nils: "De kristne begravelsers religiøse og sociale manifestation", *Religion från stenålder till medeltid*, ed. Kerstin Engdahl & Anders Kaliff, Linköping: Riksantikvarämbedet, pp. 149-158.

Engelke, Matthew: *A Problem with Presence, Beyond Scripture in an African Church*, Berkeley: University of California Press, 2007.

Engelke, Matthew: "Material religion", *Cambridge Companion to Religious Studies*, ed. Robert A. Orsi, Cambridge: Cambridge University Press, 2012, pp. 209-229.

Engelke, Matthew & Tomlinson, Matt (ed.): *The Limits of Meaning, Case Studies in the Anthropology of Christianity*, Oxford: Berghahn Books, 2007.

Erickson, Carolly: *The Medieval Vision, Essays in History and Perception*, New York: Oxford University Press, 1978.

Exordium magnum cisterciense, ed. Bruno Griesser, Rome: Editiones Cistercienses, 1961.

Fassler, Margot: *Gothic Song, Victorine Sequences and Augustinian Reform in Twelfth-Century Paris*, Notre Dame: University of Notre Dame Press, 1993, 2011.

Faulstich, Werner: *Medien und Öffentlichkeiten im Mittelalter 800-1400*, Göttingen: Vandenhoeck & Ruprecht, 1996.

Faupel-Drevs, Kristin: *Vom rechten Gebrauch der Bilder im liturgischem Raum, Mittelalterliche Funktionsbestimmungen bildener Kunst im* Rationale Divinorum Officiorum *des Durandus von Mende (1230/1-1296)*, Leiden, Boston & Cologne: Brill, 2000.

Favreau, Robert: *Epigraphie médiévale*, Turnhout: Brepols, 1997.

Ferrari, Michele C.: "Die Wende zum Körper, Dialektik und Eukaristie im 11. Jahrhundert", *Canossa 1077, Erschütterung der Welt – Geschichte, Kunst und Kultur am Aufgang der Romanik*, vol. I, ed. Christoph Stiegemann & Matthias Wemhof, Munich: Hirmer Verlag, 2006, pp. 266-276.

Finucane, Ronald C.: *Miracles and Pilgrims, Popular Beliefs in Medieval England*, London: J.M. Dent & Sons, 1977.

Fischer, Genevieve & DiPaolo Loren, Diana: "Embodying Identity in Archaeology", *Cambridge Archaeologica Journal*, 13, 2, 2003, pp. 225-230.

Fischer-Lichte, Erika: *Ästhetische Erfahrung, Das Semiotische und das Performative*, Tübingen: A. Francke Verlag, 2001.

Flanigan, C. Clifford, "The Fleury *Playbook*, the Traditions of Medieval Latin Drama, and Modern Scholarship," *The Fleury Playbook:* Essays and Studies, ed. Thomas P. Campbell and Clifford Davidson, Kalamazoo: Medieval Institute Publications, 1985, pp. 1-25.

Flanigan, C. Clifford, "Medieval Latin Music-Drama," *The Theatre of Medieval Europe: New Research in Early Drama*, ed. Eckehard Simon, Cambridge: Cambridge University Press, 1991, pp. 21-41.

283

Flanigan, C. Clifford: "Medieval Liturgy and the Arts, Visitatio Sepulchri as Paradigm", *Liturgy and the Arts in the Middle Ages, Studies in Honour of C.Clifford Flanigan*, ed. Eva Louise Lillie & Nils Holger Petersen, Copenhagen: Museum Tusculanum Press, 1996, pp. 9-35.

Flanigan, C. Clifford; Ashley, Kathleen M. & Sheingorn, Pamela: "Liturgy as Social Performance, Expanding the Definitions", *The Liturgy of the Medieval Church*, ed. Thomas J. Heffernan & E. Ann Matter, Kalamazoo: Medieval Institute Publications, 2001, pp. 695-714.

Foley, John Miles: *The Singer of Tales in Performance*, Bloomington & Indianapolis: Indiana University Press, 1995.

Forgeais, Arthur: *Collection de Plombs Historiés trouvés dans la Seine*, vol. IV, *Imagerie Religieuse*, Paris: Aubry, 1865.

Fourrier, Anthime: *Le courant réaliste dans le roman courtois en France au Moyen-Âge*, vol. I, *Les débuts (XIIe siècle)*, Paris: A.G. Nizet, 1960.

France, James: *Medieval Images of Saint Bernard of Clairvaux*, Kalamazoo: Cistercian Publications, 2007.

France, Marie de: *Les lais de Marie de France*, ed. Jean Rychner, Paris: Les classiques français du moyen âge, 1966.

Freedberg, David: *The Power of Images, Studies in the History and Theory of Response*, Chicago: University of Chicago Press, 1989.

Fritzbøger, Bo: *A Windfall for the Magnates, The Development of Woodland Ownership in Denmark c. 1150-1830*, Odense: University Press of Southern Denmark, 2004.

Gaimster, David R.M.: *German Stoneware 1200-1900, Archaeology and Cultural History*, London: British Museum Press, 1997.

Gaimster, David R.M.: "The Baltic Ceramic Market 1200-1600, Measuring Hanseatic Cultural Transfer and Resistance", *Cultural Exchange in Early Modern Europe, Forging European Identities 1400-1700*, ed. Herman Roodenburg, Cambridge: Cambridge University Press, 2007, vol. IV, pp. 30-58.

Gaimster, David R.M. & Stamper, Paul: *The Age of Transition, The Archaeology of English Culture 1400-1600*, Oxford: Oxbow, 1997.

Ganshorn, Jørgen: "Hus og Bolig", *Middelalderens Danmark, Kultur og samfund fra trosskifte til reformation*, ed. Per Ingesman, Ulla Kjær, Per Kristian Madsen & Jens Vellev, Copenhagen: Gad, 1999, pp. 188-207.

Ganz, Davis & Lentes, Thomas (ed.): *Ästhetik des Unsichtbaren, Bildteorie und Bildgebrauch der Vormoderne*, Berlin: Dietrich Reimer Verlag, 2004.

Gaunt, Simon: "Between Two (or More) Deaths – Tristan, Lancelot, Cligès", *Love and Death in Medieval French and Occitan Courtly Literature*, Oxford & New York: Oxford University Press, 2006, pp. 104-137.

Geertz, Clifford: "Religion as a Cultural System", *Anthropological Approaches to the Study of Religion*, ed. Michael Banton, London: Tavistock Publications, 1966, pp. 1-46.

Gell, Alfred: "The Language of the Forest, Landscape and Phonological Iconism in Umeda", *The Anthropology of Landscape, Perspectives on Place and Space*, ed. Eric Hirsch & Michael E.

O'Hanlon, Oxford: Clarendon Press, 1995, pp. 232-254.

Gell, Alfred: *Art and Agency, An Anthropological Theory*, Oxford: Oxford University Press, 1998.

Gerson, Jean: *Jean Gerson, Early Works*, ed. Brian Patrick McGuire, Mahwah: Paulist Press, 1998, pp. 75-127.

Gilson, Etienne: *The Philosophy of St. Thomas Aquinas*, New York: Dorset Press, 1929.

Gregory of Tours: *Glory of the Martyrs*, trans. Raymond van Dam, Liverpool: Liverpool University Press, 1988.

Grimbert, Joan Tasker: "Cligès and the Chansons, A Slave to Love", *A Companion to Chrétien de Troyes*, ed. Norris J. Lacy & Joan Tasker Grimbert, Rochester: D.S. Brewer, 2005, pp. 120-136.

Grundtvig, Svend et al. (ed.): *Danmarks gamle Folkeviser*, vol. I-XII, Copenhagen: Universitets-Jubilæets danske Samfund, 1853-1976.

Gumbrecht, Hans Ulrich: "Modern, Modernität, Moderne", *Geschichtliche Grundbegriffe, Historisches Lexikon zur politisch-sozialen Sprache in Deutschland*, vol. IV, ed. Reinhart Koselleck, Werner Conze & Otto Brunner, Stuttgart: Klett-Cotta, 1978, 2004, pp. 93-131.

Gumbrecht, Hans Ulrich: *The Production of Presence, What Meaning Cannot Convey*, Stanford: Stanford University Press, 2004.

Gumbrecht, Hans Ulrich: "Presence Achieved in Language (With Special Attention Given to the Presence of the Past)", *History and Theory*, 45, 2006, pp. 317-327.

Gummere, Francis B.: *The Popular Ballad*, Boston: Houghton, Mifflin, 1907.

Gurevich, Aron: *Medieval Popular Culture, Problems of Belief and Perception*, Cambridge: Cambridge University Press, 1981, 1990.

Haastrup, Niels: "Esrom – et kloster nær ødemarken?", *Danske Studier*, 1985, pp. 99-102.

Haastrup, Ulla: "The wall paintings in the parish church of Bellinge (dated 1496) explained by parallels in contemporary European theatre", *Medieval Iconography and Narrative, A Symposium*, ed. Flemming G. Andersen, Odense: Odense University Press, 1980, pp. 135-156.

Haastrup, Ulla (ed.): *Danske kalkmalerier, Tidlig gotik 1275-1375*, Copenhagen: The National Museum & Christian Ejlers Forlag, 1989.

Haastrup, Ulla (ed.): *Danske kalkmalerier, Sengotik 1500-1536*, Copenhagen: The National Museum & Christian Ejlers Forlag, 1992.

Habig, Marion A.: *St. Francis of Assisi, Writings and Early Biographies, English Omnibus of the Sources for the Life of St. Francis*, Chicago: Franciscan Herald Press, 1973.

Haidu, Peter: *Aesthetic Distance in Chrétien de Troyes, Irony and Comedy in Cliges and Perceval*, Genève: Minard, 1968.

Hale, Rosemary D.: *"Taste and See for God is Sweet*, Sensory Perception and Memory in Medieval Christian Mystical Experience", *Vox Mystica, Essays on Medieval Mysticism*, ed. Anne C. Bartlett, Cambridge: Brewer, 1995.

Hall, Stuart: "The Work of Representation", *Representation, Cultural Representations and Signifying Practices*, London: Sage Publications, 1997, pp. 13-74.

Hamburger, Jeffrey F.: *The Visual and the Visionary, Art and Female Spirituality in Late Medieval Germany*, New York: Zone Books, 1998.

Hamburger, Jeffrey F.: "'The Various Writings of Humanity', Johannes Tauler on Hildegaard of Bingen's *Liber Scivias*", *Visual Culture and the German Middle Ages*, ed. Kathryn Starkey & Horst Wenzel, New York & Hampshire: Palgrave Macmillan, 2005, pp. 161-205.

Hamburger, Jeffrey F. & Bouche, Anne-Marie (ed.): *The Mind's Eye, Art and Theological Argument in the Middle Ages*, Princeton: Princeton University Press, 2006.

Hamm, Berndt: "'Gott berühren', Mystische Erfahrung im ausgehenden Mittelalter, Zugleich ein Beitrag zur Kläring der Mystikbegriffs", *Gottes Nähe unmittelbar erfahren, Mystik im Mittelalter und bei Martin Luther*, ed. Berndt Hamm & Volker Leppin, Tübingen: Mohr Siebeck, 2007, pp. 111-137.

Hammer, Karen E.: *Sakrale Wandmalerei in Dänemark und Norddeutschland im ausgehenden Mittelalter, Eine Studie zu den Malereien der Elmelundegruppe in Sakralräumen Süddänemarks unter besonderer Berücksichtigung der Kirche zu Fanefjord sowie der norddeutschen Wandmalerei*, Ammersbek bei Hamburg: Verlag an der Lottbek, 1990.

Hansen, Birgit A.: "Arkæologiske spor efter døbefontens placering i kirkerummet gennem middelalderen", *Hikuin*, 22, 1995, pp. 27-40.

Harris, Oliver J.T. & Sørensen, Tim F.: "Re-thinking emotion and material culture", *Archaeological Dialogues*, 17, 2, 2010, pp. 145-163.

Harvey, Susan Ashbrook: *Scenting Salvation, Ancient Christianity and the Olfactory Imagination*, Berkeley: University of California Press, 2006.

Hasse, Dag Nikolaus & Bertolacci, Amos (ed.): *The Arabic, Hebrew and Latin Reception of Avicenna's Metaphysics*, Berlin & Boston: De Gruyter, 2012.

Hatfield, Rab: "The Tree of Life and the Holy Cross", *Christianity and the Renaissance, Image and Religious Imagination in the Quattrocento*, ed. Timothy Verdon & John Henderson, Syracuse: Syracuse University Library, 1990, pp. 132-160.

Haupt, Barbara: "Die Kemenate der hochmittelalterlichen Burg im Spiegel der zeitgenössigen (volkssprachlichen) Literatur", *Burg und Schloss als Lebensorte in Mittelalter und Renaissance*, ed. Wilhelm G. Busse, Düsseldorf: Droste, 1995, pp. 129-145.

Heffernan, Thomas J. & Matter, E. Ann (ed.): *The Liturgy of the Medieval Church*, Kalamazoo: Medieval Institute Publications, 2001.

Heidegger, Martin: *Being and Time*, New York: Harper & Row, 1927, 1962.

Heller-Roazen, Daniel: *The Inner Touch, Archaeology of a Sensation*, New York: Zone Books, 2007.

Heller-Roazen, Daniel: "Common Sense – Greek, Arabic, Latin", *Rethinking the Medieval Senses – Heritage, Fascinations, Frames*, ed. Stephen Nichols, Andreas Kablitz & Alison Calhoun, Baltimore: The Johns Hopkins University Press, 2008, pp. 30-50.

Hermansen, Victor & Nørlund, Poul (ed.): *Danmarks Kirker, Sorø Amt*, Copenhagen: The National Museum & Gads Forlag, 1938.

Hesbert, René-Jean: *Corpus antiphonalium officii*, vol. I-VI, Rome: Herder, 1963-79.

Hibbs, Thomas S.: *Thomas Aquinas On Human Nature*, Indianapolis & Cambridge: Hackett Publishing Company, 1999.

Historisches Wörterbuch der Philosophie, vol. I-XIII, ed. Joachim Ritter & Karlfried Gründer, Basel: Schwabe, 1971-2007.

Hjort, Øystein: *Ecclesia Christi, Ecclesia Virens – Mosaikkerne i San Clemente i Rom*, Copenhagen: University of Copenhagen, 1990 (unpublished dissertation).

Holmberg, Rikard: *Kyrkobyggnad, kult och samhälle – Landskyrkan i Lunds forna ärkestift genom tiderna*, Stockholm: Almqvist & Wiksell International, 1990.

Honorius Augustodunensis: "Gemma animae", *Patrologia Latina, Cursus Completus*, vol. CLXXII, ed. Jacques-Paul Migne, Turnhout: Brepols, 1844-65.

Howes, David: "Nose-wise, Olfactory Metaphors in Mind", *Olfaction, Taste and Cognition*, ed. Catherine Rouby, Benoist Schaal & A. Holley, Cambridge: Cambridge University Press, 2002, pp. 67-81.

Howes, David: "Architecture of the Senses", *Sense of the City, An Alternate Approach to Urbanism*, ed. Mirko Zardini, Montréal: Canadian Centre for Architecture & Lars Müller Publishers, 2005, pp. 322-331.

Howes, David (ed.): *Empire of the Senses, The Sensual Culture Reader*, Oxford & New York: Berg, 2006.

Howes, David: "Anthropology and Multimodality, The Conjugation of the Senses", *The Routledge Handbook of Multimodal Analysis*, ed. Carey Jewitt, New York: Routledge, 2009A, pp. 225-235.

Howes, David: "Introduction, The Revolving Sensorium", *The Sixth Sense Reader*, ed. David Howes, Oxford: Berg, 2009B, pp. 1-52.

Hugh of St. Victor: *On the Sacraments of the Christian Faith (De sacramentis)*, Cambridge, Mass.: The Mediaeval Academy of America, 1951.

Hugh of St. Victor: "De sacramentis Christiane fidei", *Patrologia Latina*, vol. CLXXV, ed. Jacques-Paul Migne, Patrologia Latina Database, Oxford: ProQuest-CSA LLC, 1996-2014.

Husserl, Edmund: *The Crisis of European Sciences and Transcendental Phenomenology, An Introduction to Phenomenological Philosophy*, Evanston: Northwestern University Press, 1936, 1970.

Illich, Ivan: *In the Vineyard of the Text, A Commentary to Hugh's 'Didascalicon'*, Chicago & London: University of Chicago Press, 1996.

Isaksson, Sven: *Food and Rank in Early Medieval Time*, Stockholm: Theses and Papers in Scientific Archaeology, 2000.

Jacobus de Voragine: *The Golden Legend*, trans. Granger Ryan & Helmut Ripperger, New York: Arno Press, 1969.

Jacobus de Voragine: *The Golden Legend, Readings on the Saints*, vol. I-II, trans. William Granger Ryan, New Jersey: Princeton University Press, 1993.

James, Liz: "Senses and Sensibility in Byzantium", *Art History*, 27, 4, 2004, pp. 522-537.

Jansson, Sven-Bertil: "Vad hörde Albertus? Om målaren och folkdikten", *Albertus Pictor, Målare av sin tid*, vol. I, ed. Pia Melin, Stockholm: Kungl. vitterhets historie och antikvitets akademien, 2009, pp. 81-91.

Jaritz, Gerhard: "Der Alltag der Kontraste, Muster von Argumentationen und Perzeptionen im Spätmittelalter", *Kontraste im Alltag des Mittelalters*, ed. Gerhard Jaritz, Wien: Verlag der österreichischen Akademie der Wissenschaften, 2000, pp. 9-24.

Jessen, Mads D.: "The Hall and the Church During Christianization", *Excavating the Mind – Cross-sections through Culture, Cognition and Materiality*, ed. Niels Johannsen, Mads Jessen & Helle Juel Jensen, Aarhus: Aarhus University Press, 2012A, pp. 133-160.

Jessen, Mads D.: "Material Culture, Embodiment and the Construction of Religious Knowledge", *Embodied Knowledge, Historical Perspectives on Technology and Belief, Part I, Beliefs*, ed. Marie Louise Stig Sørensen & Katharina Rebay-Salisbury, Oxford: Oxbow Books, 2012B, pp. 40-51.

Jessen, Mads D.: "Religion and the Extra-somatics of Conceptual Thought", *Origins of Religion, Cognition and Culture*, ed. Amin W. Geertz, Durham: Acumen, 2013, pp. 319-340.

Jewitt, Carey (ed.): *The Routledge Handbook of Multimodal Analysis*, New York: Routledge, 2009.

Johannsen, Hugo & Smidt, Claus M.: *Danmarks Arkitektur, Kirkens huse*, Copenhagen: Gyldendal, 1985.

Johansson, Jan: *Kyrkogårdens hägn i det medeltida Sverige, Om bogård, balk och stiglucka*, Antikvariskt Arkiv, 76, Stockholm: Almqvist & Wiksell, 1993.

Johansson, Roger; Holsanova, Jana & Holmqvist, Kenneth: "Pictures and Spoken Descriptions Elicit Similar Eye Movements During Mental Imagery, Both in Light and in Complete Darkness", *Cognitive Science, A Multidisciplinary Journal*, 30, 6, 2006, pp. 1053-1079.

John of Salisbury: *The Metalogicon of John of Salisbury, A Twelfth-Century Defence of the Verbal and Logical Arts of the Trivium*, trans. & ed. Daniel D. McGarry, Gloucester, Mass.: Peter Smith, 1971.

Johnson, Matthew: *Behind the Castle Gate, From Medieval to Renaissance*, New York: Routledge, 2002.

Johnson, Maxwell E.: *The Rites of Christian Initiation, Their Evolution and Interpretation*, Collegeville, Minn.: Liturgical Press, 1999, 2007.

Jones, Caroline A.: "The Mediated Sensorium", *Sensorium – Embodied Experience, Technology, and Contemporary Art*, ed. Caroline A. Jones, Cambridge, Mass.: MIT Press, 2006, pp. 5-49.

Jones, John N.: "Sculpting God, The Logic of Dionysian Negative Theology", *The Harvard Theological Review*, 89, 4, 1996, pp. 355-371.

Jonsson, Bengt R.; Solheim, Svale & Danielson, Eva: *The Types of the Scandinavian Medieval Ballad, A Descriptive Catalogue*, Stockholm: Svenskt visarkiv & Oslo: Universitetsforlaget, 1978.

Jørgensen, Hans Henrik Lohfert: "*Velatio* and *Revelatio*, Hagioscopic Vision in Early Medieval Architecture on the Iberian Peninsula", *The Enduring Instant, Time and the Spectator in the Visual Arts & Der bleibende Augenblick, Betrachterzeit in den Bildkünsten*, ed. Antoinette Roesler-Friedenthal & Johannes Nathan, Berlin: Gebr. Mann Verlag, 2003, pp. 177-191.

Jørgensen, Hans Henrik Lohfert: "Cultic Vision – Seeing as Ritual, Visual and Liturgical Experience in the Early Christian and Medieval Church", *The Appearances of Medieval Rituals, The Play of Construction and Modification*, ed. Jeremy Llewellyn et al., Turnhout: Brepols, 2004A, pp. 173-197.

Jørgensen, Hans Henrik Lohfert: "Middelalderlige metabilleder, Billedskepsis og skærpet billed-bevidsthed i tidlig vestlig middelalder", *Transfiguration, Nordisk tidsskrift for kunst og kristendom*, 1, 2004B, pp. 7-38.

Jørgensen, Hans Henrik Lohfert: "Middelalderens rum og sansning, Om sanselige strukturer i middelalderens kristne og islamiske rumdannelser", *Middelalderens Verden – Verdensbilledet*, *tænkningen, rummet og religionen,* ed. Ole Høiris & Per Ingesman, Aarhus: Aarhus University Press, 2010, pp. 169-193.

Jørgensen, Hans Henrik Lohfert: "The Image as *Contact Medium* – Mediation, Multimodality, and Haptics in Medieval Imagery", *Medieval Iconography, Means and Methods for the Interpretation of Medieval Images,* ed. Lena Liepe, Oslo (forthcoming).

Jütte, Robert: *A History of the Senses, From Antiquity to Cyberspace,* Cambridge: Polity Press, 2005.

Kaiser, Gert: *Der tanzende Tod,* Frankfurt am Main: Insel Verlag, 1983.

Kamerick, Kathleen: *Popular Piety and Art in the Late Middle Ages, Image Worship and Idolatry in England 1350-1500,* New York: Palgrave, 2002.

Kapstein, Matthew T. (ed.): *The Presence of Light, Divine Radiance and Religious Experience,* Chicago: University of Chicago Press, 2004.

Karg, Sabine: *Medieval Food Traditions in Northern Europe,* Copenhagen: The National Museum of Denmark, 1998.

Kaspersen, Søren: "Kalkmaleri og samfund 1241-1340/50", *Kulturblomstring og samfundskrise i 1300-tallet,* ed. Brian Patrick McGuire, Copenhagen: C.A. Reitzel, 1979, pp. 108-165.

Kaspersen, Søren: "Bildende Kunst, Theater und Volkstümlichkeit im mittelalterlichen Dänemark, Zur Wechselwirkung von Wandmalerei und Spielkultur", *Popular Drama in Northern Europe in the Later Middle Ages, A Symposium,* ed. F.G. Andersen et al., Odense: Odense University Press, 1988, pp. 201-250.

Kaspersen, Søren: "Narrative 'Modes' in the Danish Golden Frontals", *Decorating the Lord's Table, On the Dynamics between Image and Altar in the Middle Ages,* ed. Søren Kaspersen & Erik Thunø, Copenhagen: Museum Tusculanum Press, 2006, pp. 79-128.

Kaspersen, Søren: "'Birgittine' Wall-Paintings? – A Reconsideration of a Disputed Phenomenon", *The Birgittine Experience, Papers from a Birgitta Conference in Stockholm 2011,* ed. Mia Åkestam & Roger Andersson, Stockholm: Kungl. vitterhets historie och antikvitets akademien, 2013, pp. 209-226.

Kaspersen, Søren; Kværndrup, Sigurd; Lönnroth, Lars & Olsen, Thorkil Damsgaard (ed.): *Dansk litteraturhistorie,* vol. I, *Fra runer til ridderdigtning o. 800-1480,* Copenhagen: Gyldendal, 1984, 2000.

Keane, Webb: "Signs Are Not the Garb of Meaning, On the Social Analysis of Material Things", *Materiality,* ed. Daniel Miller, London: Duke University Press, 2005.

Kensinger, Kenneth M.: *How Real People Ought to Live, The Cashinahua of Eastern Peru,* Prospect Heights: Waveland Press, 1995.

Kessler, Herbert L.: *Seeing Medieval Art,* Peterborough: Broadview Press, 2004.

Kieffer-Olsen, Jakob: *Grav og gravskik i det middelalderlige Danmark, Otte kirkegårdsudgravninger,* Højbjerg: Middelalderarkæologisk Nyhedsbrev, 1993.

Kornerup, Jens: "Om Middelalderens Begravelsesmaade i Danmark", *Aarbøger for Nordisk Old-kyndighed og Historie,* 1873, pp. 251-276.

Köster, Egon P.: "The Specific Characteristics of the Sense of Smell", *Olfaction, Taste and Cognition,* ed. Catherine Rouby, Benoist Schaal & A. Holley, Cambridge: Cambridge University Press, 2002, pp. 27-43.

Kragh, Birgitte: *Til jord skal du blive... Dødens og begravelsens kulturhistorie i Danmark 1780-1990*, Sønderborg: Aabenraa Museum, 2003.

Krautheimer, Richard: "Introduction to an 'Iconography of Medieval Architecture'", *Studies in Early Christian, Medieval, and Renaissance Art*, ed. Richard Krautheimer, London: University of London Press, 1969, pp. 115-150.

Kretzmann, Norman: "Philosophy of mind", *The Cambridge Companion to Aquinas*, ed. Norman Kretzmann & Eleonore Stump, Cambridge: Cambridge University Press, 1994.

Krogh, Knud J. & Voss, Olfert: "Fra hedenskab til kristendom i Hørning, En vikingetids kammergrav og en trækirke fra 1000-tallet under Hørning kirke", *Nationalmuseets Arbejdsmark*, Copenhagen: The National Museum, 1961, pp. 5-34.

Krueger, Roberta L.: "Marie de France", *The Cambridge Companion to Medieval Women's Writing*, ed. Carolin Dinshaw & David Wallace, Cambridge: Cambridge University Press, 2003, pp. 172-183.

Kurth, Betty: *Die deutschen Bildteppiche des Mittelalters*, vol. I-III, Wien: Anton Schroll & Co., 1926.

Kus, Susan: "Towards an Archaeology of Body and Soul", *Representations in Archaeology*, ed. Jean-Claude Gardin & Christopher S. Peebles, Bloomington: Indiana University Press, 1992, pp. 168-177.

Kværndrup, Sigurd: *Den østnordiske ballade, Oral teori og tekstanalyse, Studier i Danmarks gamle Folkeviser*, Copenhagen: Museum Tusculanum Press, 2006.

Kværndrup, Sigurd: "'Media' before 'Media' were invented, The Medieval Ballad and the Romanesque Church", *Media Borders, Multimodality and Intermediality*, ed. Lars Elleström, Houndmills: Palgrave Macmillan, 2010, pp. 99-110.

Kværndrup, Sigurd: "Karen Brahes Folio, Textualisering och medialisering av orale ballader", *Intermediala perspektiv på medeltida ballader*, ed. Lars Elleström, Stockholm: Gidlunds, 2011, pp. 102-145.

Kværndrup, Sigurd & Olofsson, Tommy: *Medeltiden i ord och bild, Folkligt och groteskt i nordiska kyrkmålningar och ballader*, Stockholm: Atlantis Förlag, 2013.

Ladis, Andrew: *Taddeo Gaddi, Critical Reappraisal and Catalogue Raisonné*, Columbia & London: University of Missouri Press, 1982.

Ladner, Gerhardt B.: "Medieval and Modern Understanding of Symbolism, A Comparison", *Speculum*, 54, 2, 1979, pp. 223-256.

Larson, Laurence Marcellus (trans.): *The King's Mirror*, New York: The American-Scandinavian Foundation, 1917.

Laugerud, Henning: "Some remarks on the Sacredness or the Sanctity of Images according to the Council of Trent and St. Thomas Aquinas", *Categories of Sacredness in Europe 1500-1800, Conference at the Norwegian Institute in Rome 11-14 October 2001*, ed. Arne Bugge Amundsen & Henning Laugerud, Oslo, 2003, pp. 111-130.

Laugerud, Henning: *Det hagioskopiske blikk – Bilder, syn og erkjendelse i høy- og senmiddelalder*, Bergen: University of Bergen, 2005 (unpublished dissertation).

Laugerud, Henning: "Polysemi og den dynamiske tradisjon", *Passepartout, Skrifter for kunsthistorie*, 25, 2005, pp. 94-103.

Laugerud, Henning: "Visuality and Devotions in the Middle Ages", *Instruments of Devotion, The Practices and Objects of Religious Piety from the Late Middle Ages to the 20th Century*, ed. Henning Laugerud & Laura K. Skinnebach, Aarhus: Aarhus University Press, 2007, pp. 173-188.

Laugerud, Henning: "Memory Stored and Reactivated, Some Introductory Reflections", *ARV, Nordic Yearbook of Folklore Studies*, 66, Uppsala: Swedish Science Press, 2010A, pp. 7-20.

Laugerud, Henning: "To See with the Eyes of the Soul, Memory and Visual Culture in Medieval Europe", *ARV, Nordic Yearbook of Folklore Studies*, 66, Uppsala: Swedish Science Press, 2010B, pp. 43-68.

Le Goff, Jacques: *La civilisation de l'occident medieval*, Paris: Flammarion, 1982.

Le Roy Ladurie, Emmanuel: *Montaillou, Village occitan de 1294 à 1324*, Paris: Gallimard, 1975.

Leclercq, Henri: "Mandatum", *Dictionnaire d'archéologie chrétienne et de liturgie*, vol. X, Paris: Librarie Letouzey et Ané, 1931, col. 1387-88.

Leclercq, Jean: *The Love of Learning and the Desire for God, A Study of Monastic Culture*, New York: Fordham University Press, 1957, 2003.

Leder, Drew: *The Absent Body*, Chicago: Chicago University Press, 1990.

Legendre, Olivier (ed.): *Collectaneum exemplorum et visionum Clarevallense*, Corpus Christianorum, Continuatio Mediaevalis, Turnhout: Brepols, 2005.

Les Ecclesiastica Officia, Cisterciens du XIIème siècle, ed. Danièle Choisselet & Placide Vernet, Reiningue: Les Éditions de la Documentation Cistercienne, 1989.

Levi-Strauss, Claude: *Introduction to Marcel Mauss*, London: Routledge, 1987.

Liebgott, Niels-Knud: *Middelalderen – Kirke og Konge*, Copenhagen: Sesam, 1994.

Liepe, Lena: *Den medeltida kroppen, Kroppens och könets ikonografi i nordisk medeltid*, Lund: Nordic Academic Press, 2003.

Liepe, Lena: "Body and Space in the Ølst Frontal", *Decorating the Lord's Table, On the Dynamics between Image and Altar in the Middle Ages*, ed. Søren Kaspersen & Erik Thunø, Copenhagen: Museum Tusculanum Press, 2006, pp. 129-146.

Liepe, Lena: "The Multimateriality of Bernt Notke's St. George and the Dragon", *Art, Cult and Patronage, Die visuelle Kultur im Ostseeraum zur Zeit Bernt Notkes*, ed. Uwe Albrecht & Anu Mänd, Kiel: Verlag Ludwig, 2013, pp. 199-207.

Linaa, Jette: *Kar i hvermands eje, Køkken- og bordtøjets brug og betydning i senmiddelalder og renæssance*, Aarhus: University of Aarhus, 2000 (unpublished dissertation).

Linaa, Jette: *Keramik, kultur og kontakter – Køkken- og bordtøjets brug og betydning 1350-1650*, Højbjerg: Jysk Arkæologisk Selskab, 2006.

Linaa, Jette: *Coast, Culture, Contacts & Consumption – The Coastal Culture, Its Provisions and Alterations around the Sound-Region ca. 1150-1700*, Højbjerg: Jysk Arkæologisk Selskab (in press).

Linaa, Jette & Skov, Hans: "Boligmiljø på byernes parceller – især i Aarhus", *Bolig og Familie i Danmarks Middelalder*, ed. Else Roesdahl, Højbjerg: Jysk Arkæologisk Selskab, 2004, pp. 119-128.

Lindberg, David C.: *Theories of Vision from al-Kindi to Kepler*, Chicago: University of Chicago Press, 1976.

Liturgiczne aciskie dramatyzacje Wielkiego Tygodnia XI-XVI, ed. Julian Lewaski, Lublin: Towarzystwo Naukowe, 1999.

Löffler, Anette: "Die Liturgie des Deutschen Ordens in Preussen, Ritus und Heiligenverehrung am Beispiel des Festes Visitatio Mariae anhand der Königsberger Fragmentüberlieferung", *Zeitschrift für Ostmitteleuropa-Forschung*, 47, 3, 1998, pp. 371-382.

Löffler, Anette: "The Manuscripts in Danzig's St. Mary's Church and their Importance for the Liturgy of the Teutonic Order", *Pfarrkirchen in Städten des Hanseraumes, Archäologie und Geschichte im Ostseeraum & Archeology and History of the Baltic*, vol. I, ed. Felix Biermann, Manfred Schneider & Thomas Terberger, Rahden: Verlag Marie Leidorf, 2006, pp. 227-237.

Lukàcs, Georg: *Theorie des Romans, Ein geschichtsphilosophischer Versuch über die Formen der grossen Epik*, Berlin: Verlag Paul Cassirer, 1920.

MacDonald, Scott: "Theory of knowledge", *The Cambridge Companion to Aquinas*, ed. Norman Kretzmann & Eleonore Stump, Cambridge: Cambridge University Press, 1994.

Mackeprang, Mouritz: *Danmarks middelalderlige døbefonte*, Højbjerg: Hikuin, 1941, 2003.

Madsen, Per K.: "Han ligger under en blå sten, Om middelalderens gravskik på skrift og i praksis", *Hikuin*, 17, 1990, pp. 113-134.

Madsen, Per K.: "Gravens vellugt", *Skalk*, 5, 1981, pp. 27-30.

Malden, A.R. (ed.): *The Canonization of Saint Osmund from the Manuscript Records in the Muniment Room of Salisbury Cathedral*, Wiltshire: Wiltshire Record Society, 1901.

Map, Walter: *De nugis curialium, Courtiers' Trifles*, ed. M.R. James, Oxford: Clarendon Press, 1983.

Marks, Richard: *Image and Devotion in Late Medieval England*, Stroud: Sutton Publishing, 2005.

Markus, Robert A.: *Signs and Meanings, World and Text in Ancient Christianity*, Liverpool: Liverpool University Press, 1996.

McBrien, Richard P.: *Catholicism*, San Francisco: Harper Collins, 1980, 1994.

McGinn, Bernard: *The Presence of God, A History of Western Christian Mysticism*, vol. I-II, London: SCM Press, 1992-1995.

McGinn, Bernard: *The Harvest of Mysticism in Medieval Germany*, New York: The Crossroad Publishing Company, 2005.

McGuire, Brian Patrick: *The Difficult Saint, Bernard of Clairvaux and his Tradition*, Kalamazoo: Cistercian Publications, 1991.

McGuire, Brian Patrick: *Da himmelen kom nærmere, Fortællinger om Danmarks kristning 700-1300*, Frederiksberg: Alfa, 2008.

McGuire, Brian Patrick: *Den første europæer, Bernhard af Clairvaux*, Frederiksberg: Alfa, 2009.

McGuire, Brian Patrick: *Friendship and Community, The Monastic Experience 350-1250*, Ithaca: Cornell University Press, 2010.

McGuire, Brian Patrick (ed.): *The Brill Companion to Bernard of Clairvaux*, Leiden: Brill, 2010.

McGuire, Brian Patrick: *Hjælp mig Herre, Bøn i 1000 År*, Frederiksberg: Alfa, 2011.

McLuhan, Marshall: *Understanding Media, The Extensions of Man*, New York: McGraw-Hill & London: Routledge, 1964, 1965, 1997.

Melin, Pia: *Fåfängans förgänglighet, Allegorin som livs- och lärospegel hos Albertus Pictor*, Stockholm: Stockholmia förlag, 2006.

Melin, Pia (ed.): *Albertus Pictor, Målare av sin tid*, Stockholm: Kungl. vitterhets historie och antikvitets akademien, 2009.

Merleau-Ponty, Maurice: "Eye and Mind", *The Primacy of Perception and Other Essays on Phenomenological Psychology, the Philosophy of Art, History, and Politics*, Evanston: Northwestern University Press, 1964, pp. 159-192.

Merleau-Ponty, Maurice: *The Visible and the Invisible*, Evanston: Northwestern University Press, 1968.

Merleau-Ponty, Maurice: *Phenomenology of Perception*, London: Routledge, 1962, 2002.

Metcalf, Peter: "Wine of the Corpse – Endocannibalism and the Great Feast of the Dead in Borneo", *Representations*, 17, 1, 1987, pp. 96-109.

Miles, Margaret: "Vision – The Eye of the Body and the Eye of the Mind in Saint Augustine's *De trinitate* and *Confessions*", *The Journal of Religion*, 63, 2, 1983, pp. 125-142.

Miller, Daniel: *Material Culture and Mass Consumption*, Cambridge: Basil Blackwell, 1987, 2005.

Miller, Daniel: "Why Some Things Matter", *Material Cultures, Why Some Things Matter*, ed. Daniel Miller, Chicago: University of Chicago Press, 1998, pp. 3-20.

Mitchell, W.J.T.: *Iconology – Image, Text, Ideology*, Chicago: University of Chicago Press, 1987.

Mitchell, W.J.T.: *Picture Theory, Essays on Verbal and Visual Representation*, Chicago: University of Chicago Press, 1994.

Mitchell, W.J.T.: "There Are No Visual Media", *Journal of Visual Culture*, 4, 2, 2005, pp. 257-266.

Møller, Bente Ahlers & Buus, Erik: *Herre, vasker du mine fødder? Mandatumliturgien i Marbach og Lund*, Copenhagen: Museum Tusculanum Press, 1987.

Møller, Jens S.: *Fester og Højtider i gamle Dage, Skildringer fra Nordvestsjælland med Forsøg paa Tydninger, 2den Levering, Død og Begravelse*, Holbæk: P. Haase & Søn, 1929.

Moltke, Erik: *Bernt Notkes altertavle i Århus Domkirke og Tallinntavlen*, vol. I-II, Copenhagen: Gad, 1970.

Montagu, Ashley: *Touching, The Human Significance of the Skin*, New York: Harper & Row, 1971, 1986.

Morgan, David: *The Sacred Gaze, Religious Visual Culture in Theory and Practice*, Berkeley: University of California Press, 2005.

Morini, Luginia (ed.): *Bestiari medievali*, Turin: Giulio Einaudi editore, 1996.

Mortet, Victor: *Recueil de textes relatifs à l'histoire de l'architecture et à la condition des architectes en France au Moyen Age*, Paris: A. Pickard et fils, 1911.

Moser, Johann & Anderson, Robert (ed.): *Devoutly I adore Thee, The prayers and hymns of St Thomas Aquinas*, Manchester: Sophia Institute Press, 1993.

Mulryne, J.R. (ed.): *Europa Triumphans, Court and Civic Festivals in Early Modern Europe*, vol. II, Farnham: Ashgate, 2004.

Necrologium Lundense, Lunds Domkyrkas Nekrologium, ed. Lauritz Weibull, Lund: Berlingska Boktryckeriet, 1923.

293

Nichols, Stephen G.; Kablitz, Andreas & Calhoun, Alison (ed.): *Rethinking the Medieval Senses –
Heritage, Fascinations, Frames*, Baltimore: The Johns Hopkins University Press, 2008.

Nielsen, Karl Martin (ed.): *Middelalderens Danske Bønnebøger*, vol. I-IV, Copenhagen: Gyldendal,
1945-1982.

Nilsson, Bertil: "Död och begravning, Begravningsskicket i Norden", *Tanke och Tro, Aspekter på
medeltidens tankevärld och fromhetsliv*, ed. Inger Estham, Olle Ferm & Göran Tegnér, Stockholm:
Riksantikvarämbedet, 1987, pp. 133-150.

Nilsson, Bertil: *De Sepulturis, Gravrätten i Corpus Iuris Canonici och i medeltida nordisk lagstiftning*,
Kyrkovetenskapliga Studier, 44, Stockholm: Almqvist & Wiksell International, 1989.

Nørlund, Poul: "Les plus anciens retables danoises", *Acta archaeologica*, 1, 1930, pp. 147-163.

Nørlund, Poul: *Gyldne Altre, Jysk Metalkunst fra Valdemarstiden*, Aarhus: Wormianum, 1926, 1968.

Norn, Otto & Skovgaard Jensen, Søren: *The House of Wisdom & Visdommen i Vestjylland*,
Copenhagen: Christian Ejlers' Forlag, 1990.

Norton, Michael L.: *The Type II Visitatio Sepulchri, A Repertorial Study*, Ohio: Ohio State University,
1983 (unpublished dissertation).

Nykrog, Per: *Chrétien de Troyes, Romancier discutable*, Paris: Droz, 1996.

Nyrop, C. (ed.): *Danmarks Gilde- og Lavsskråer fra Middelalderen*, vol. I-II, Copenhagen: Selskabet for
Udgivelse af Kilder til dansk Historie, 1895-1904.

Öberg, Jan; Sandquist, Christina & Melin, Pia (ed.): *Albertus Pictor, Målare av sin tid, Samtliga
bevarade motiv och språkband med kommentarer och analyser*, vol. II, Stockholm: Kungl. vitterhets
historie och antikvitets akademien, 2009.

Odgaard, Bent V. & Nielsen, Anne Birgitte: "Udvikling i arealdækning i perioden 0-1850, Pollen
og landskabshistorie", *Danske Landbrugslandskaber gennem 2000 år, Fra digevoldinger til støtte-
ordninger*, ed. Bent V. Odgaard & Jørgen R. Rømer, Aarhus: Aarhus University Press, 2009,
pp. 41-58.

Olden-Jørgensen, Sebastian: "Hoffet til hverdag og fest", *Danmark og renæssancen 1500-1650*,
ed. Carsten Bach-Nielsen, Johan Møhlenfeldt Jensen, Jens Vellev & Peter Zeeberg, Copenhagen:
Gad, 2000, pp. 62-77.

Ong, Walter J.: *The Presence of the Word, Some Prolegomena for Cultural and Religious History*,
New Haven: Yale University Press, 1967.

Ong, Walter J.: *Orality and Literacy, The Technologizing of the Word*, New York: Routledge, 1982.

Ousterhout, Robert: "The Holy Space – Architecture and the Liturgy", *Heaven on Earth, Art and the
Church in Byzantium*, ed. Linda Safran, University Park: Pennsylvania State University Press,
1998, pp. 81-120.

Oxtoby, Willard G.: "Holy, Idea of the", *Encyclopedia of Religion*, vol. VI, ed. Lindsay Jones, Detroit:
Macmillan Reference USA, 2005, pp. 4095-4101.

Palazzo, Éric: *Histoire des Livres Liturgique, Le Moyen Âge, Des origines au XIIIe siècle*, Paris: Beachesne,
1993.

Palazzo, Éric: *Liturgie et société au Moyen Âge*, Paris: Aubier, 2000.

294

Palazzo, Éric: "Les cinq sens au Moyen Âge, état de la question et perspectives de recherche", *Cahiers de civilisation médiévale, Xe-XIIe siècles*, 55, 2012, pp. 339-366.

Palazzo, Éric: *L'invention chrétienne des cinq sens dans la liturgie et l'art au Moyen Âge*, Paris: Éditions du Cerf, 2014.

Pallasmaa, Juhani: *The Eyes of the Skin, Architecture and the Senses*, Chichester: John Wiley & Sons, 2005.

Pálsson, Gisli: *The Textual Life of Savants – Ethnography, Iceland and the Linguistic Turn*, London: Routledge, 1995.

Panofsky, Erwin: *Gothic Architecture and Scholasticism*, Latrobe: Archabbey Publications, 1967, 2005.

Parshall, Peter & Schoch, Rainer (ed.): *Origins of European Printmaking, Fifteenth-Century Woodcuts and their Public*, Washington, Nuremberg & New Haven: National Gallery of Art, Germanisches Nationalmuseum & Yale University Press, 2005.

Patrologia Latina, Cursus Completus, ed. Jacques-Paul Migne, Turnhout: Brepols, 1844-1865.

Pentcheva, Bissera V.: "The Performative Icon", *Art Bulletin*, 88, 4, 2006, pp. 631-655.

Pentcheva, Bissera V.: *The Sensual Icon – Space, Ritual, and the Senses in Byzantium*, University Park: Pennsylvania State University Press, 2010.

Pentcheva, Bissera V.: "Hagia Sophia and Multisensory Aesthetics", *Gesta*, 50, 2, 2011, pp. 93-111.

Peter Damian: "Sermones", *Corpus Christianorum, Continuatio Medievalis*, vol. LVII, ed. G. Lucchesi, Turnhout: Brepols, 1983.

Petersen, Nils Holger: "Carolingian Music, Ritual, and Theology", *The Appearances of Medieval Rituals, The Play of Construction and Modification*, ed. Nils Holger Petersen et al., Turnhout: Brepols, 2004, pp. 13-31.

Petersen, Nils Holger: "Representation in European Devotional Rituals, The Question of the Origin of Medieval Drama in Medieval Liturgy", *The Origins of Theater in Ancient Greece and Beyond, From Ritual to Drama*, ed. Eric Csapo & Margaret C. Miller, Cambridge: Cambridge University Press, 2007A, pp. 329-360.

Petersen, Nils Holger: "Ritual and Creation, Medieval Liturgy as Foreground and Background for Creation", *Creations – Medieval Rituals, the Arts, and the Concept of Creation*, ed. Sven Rune Havsteen et al., Turnhout: Brepols, 2007B, pp. 89-120.

Petersen, Nils Holger: "Biblical Reception, Representational Ritual, and the Question of 'Liturgical Drama'", *Sapientia et Eloquentia, Meaning and Function in Liturgical Poetry, Music, Drama, and Biblical Commentary in the Middle Ages*, ed. Gunilla Iversen & Nicolas Bell, Turnhout: Brepols, 2009, pp. 163-201.

Petersen, Nils Holger: "Il Doge and Easter Processions at San Marco in Early Modern Venice", *Ritual Dynamics and the Science of Ritual*, vol. V, *Transfer and Spaces*, ed. Gita Dharampal-Frick, Robert Langer & Nils Holger Petersen, Wiesbaden: Harrassowitz Verlag, 2010, pp. 301-311.

Petersen, Nils Holger: "The *Quarant' Ore*, Early Modern Ritual and Performativity", *Performativity and Performance in Baroque Rome*, ed. Mårten Snickare & Peter Gillgren, Farnham: Ashgate, 2012A, pp. 115-133.

Petersen, Nils Holger: "Liturgical Drama", *Oxford Bibliographies Online, Medieval Studies*, ed. Paul E. Szarmach, Oxford: Oxford University Press, 2012B.

Porsmose, Erland: "Middelalder, o. 1000-1536", *Det danske landbrugs historie*, vol. I, ed. C. Bjørn, Odense: Landbo Historisk Selskab, 1988, pp. 207-417.

Poulsen, Bjørn: "Daglivets fællesskaber", *Middelalderens Danmark, Kultur og samfund fra trosskifte til reformation*, ed. Per Ingesman, Ulla Kjær, Per Kristian Madsen & Jens Vellev, Copenhagen: Gad, 1999, pp. 188-207.

Poulsen, Bjørn: "Krydderier og klæde, Statusforbrug i senmiddelalderens Danmark", *Danmark og Europa i senmiddelalderen*, ed. Per Ingesman & Bjørn Poulsen, Aarhus: Aarhus University Press, 2000A, pp. 64-94.

Poulsen, Bjørn: "Samfundet set af en 1500-tals borger, Om typer og social mobilitet i Hans Christensen Sthens 'Kort Vending'", *Mark og menneske, Studier i Danmarks historie 1500-1800*, ed. Bjørn Poulsen, Claus Bjørn & Benedicte Fonnesbech-Wulf, Ebeltoft: Skippershoved, 2000B, pp. 123-139.

Poulsen, Bjørn: "Middelalderens fødsel – tiden 1000-1400 – avl og købstæder", *Det Sønderjyske Landbrugs Historie – Jernalder, Vikingetid og Middelalder*, ed. Per Ethelberg, Nis Hardt, Bjørn Poulsen & Anne Birgitte Sørensen, Haderslev: Haderslev Museum, 2003, pp. 458-537.

Poulsen, Bjørn: "Privatliv i middelalderens huse", *Bolig og Familie i Danmarks Middelalder*, ed. Else Roesdahl, Højbjerg: Jysk Arkæologisk Selskab, 2003, pp. 31-54.

Poulsen, Bjørn: "Trade and Consumption among Late Medieval and Early Modern Danish Peasants", *Scandinavian Economic History Review*, 52, 2004, pp. 52-68.

Poulsen, Bjørn: "Meeting the King in Late Medieval Denmark", *Power and Persuasion, Essays on the Art of Statebuilding in Honour of W.P. Blockmans*, ed. Peter Hoppenbrouwers, Antheun Janse & Robert Stein, Turnhout: Brepols, 2010, pp. 141-156.

Poulsen, Bjørn: "Bauern als Händler, Ökonomische Diversifizierung und soziale Differenzierung bäuerlicher Agrarproduzenten (15.-19. Jahrhundert)", *Quellen und Forschungen zur Agrargeschichte*, 52, 2011, pp. 57-76.

Poulsen, Bjørn & Hybel, Niels: *The Danish Resources c. 1000-1550, Growth and Recession*, Leiden: Brill, 2007.

Poulsen, Niels J.: "De græsklædte grave, Landsbykirkegården fra grønning til haveanlæg", *Nationalmuseets Arbejdsmark*, Copenhagen: The National Museum, 2003, pp. 49-65.

Pound, Louise: *Poetic Origins and the Ballad*, New York: Macmillan, 1921.

Prendergast, Christopher: *The Triangle of Representation*, New York: Columbia University Press, 2000.

Raff, Thomas: "Materia superat opus, Materialen als Bedeutungsträger bei mittelalterlichen Kunstwerken", *Studien zur Geschichte der Europäischen Skulptur im 12. und 13. Jahrhundert*, vol. I, ed. Herbert Beck & Kerstin Hengevoss-Dürkop, Frankfurt: Liebieghaus, 1994, pp. 17-28.

Regularis Concordia, The Monastic Agreement, ed. & trans. Thomas Symons, London: Thomas Nelson & Sons, 1953.

Reineking-von Bock, Gisela: *Steinzeug, Kataloge des Kunstgewerbemuseums Köln*, vol. IV, Cologne: Kunstgewerbemuseum der Stadt Köln, 1975.

Reno, Stephen J.: *The Sacred Tree as an Early Christian Literary Symbol*, Saarbrücken: Homo et Religio, 1978.

Roer, Hanne: "Dantes rumrejse år 1300", *Undervejs mod Gud, Rummet og rejsen i middelalderlig religiøsitet*, ed. Mette Birkedal Bruun & Britt Istoft, Copenhagen: Museum Tusculanum Press, 2004, pp. 115-137.

Rosenfeld, Hellmut: *Der mittelalterliche Totentanz – Entstehung, Entwicklung, Bedeutung*, Münster: Böhlau Verlag, 1956.

Rubin, Miri: *Corpus Christi, The Eucharist in Late Medieval Culture*, Cambridge: Cambridge University Press, 1991.

Runia, Eelco: "Presence", *History and Theory*, 45, 2006, pp. 1-29.

Rupert von Deutz: *Liber de divinis officiis*, trans. Helmut & Ilse Deutz, Freiburg: Herder, 2001.

Ryan, Salvador: "The Most Traversed Bridge, A Reconsideration of Elite and Popular Religion in Late Medieval Ireland", *Elite and Popular Religion*, ed. Kate Cooper & Jeremy Gregory, Suffolk & New York: Ecclesiastical History Society, 2006, pp. 120-129.

Sandler, Lucy Freeman: *The Psalter of Robert de Lisle*, London: Harvey Miller, 1983, 1999.

Schleif, Corine: "Medieval Memorials – Sights and Sounds Embodied; Feelings, Fragrances and Flavors Re-membered", *Senses & Society*, 5, 1, 2010, pp. 73-92.

Schlink, Wilhelm: *Saint-Benigne in Dijon, Untersuchungen zur Abteikirche Wilhelms von Volpiano (962-1031)*, Berlin: Gebr. Mann, 1978.

Schmitt, Jean-Claude: *Le corps des images, Essais sur la culture visuelle du Moyen Âge*, Paris: Gallimard, 2004.

Schnitzler, Norbert: "Illusion, Taüschung und Schöner Schein", *Frömmigkeit im Spätmittelalter*, ed. Klaus Schreiner, Munich: Fink Verlag, 2002, pp. 221-242.

Scholliers, Peter: "Meals, Food Narratives and Sentiments of Belonging in Past and Present", *Food, Drink and Identity – Cooking, Eating and Drinking in Europe since the Middle Ages*, ed. Peter Scholliers, Oxford: Berg, 2001, pp. 3-23.

Scholz, Bernhard F.: "A Whale That Can't Be Cotched? On Conceptualizing Ekphrasis", *Changing Borders, Contemporary Positions in Intermediality*, ed. Jens Arvidson, Mikael Askander, Jørgen Bruhn & Heidrun Führer, Lund: Intermedia Studies Press, 2007, pp. 283-320.

Schreiner, Klaus (ed.): *Gepeinigt, begehrt, vergessen – Symbolik und Sozialbezug des Körpers im späten Mittelalter und in der frühen Neuzeit*, Munich: Wilhelm Fink, 1992.

Searle, John R.: *Speech Acts, An Essay in the Philosophy of Language*, Cambridge & London: Cambridge University Press, 1974.

Sears, Elizabeth: "Sensory perception and its metaphors in the time of Richard of Fournival", *Medicine and the Five Senses*, ed. W.F. Bynum & Roy Porter, Cambridge: Cambridge University Press, 1993, pp. 17-39.

Shailor, Barbara et al. (ed.): *Catalogue of Medieval and Renaissance Manuscripts in the Beinecke Rare Book and Manuscript Library*, Yale University, accessed: 6/12/2014, http://brbl-net.library.yale.edu/pre1600ms/

Siegwart, Josef (ed.): *Die Consuetudines des Augustiner-Chorherrenstiftes Marbach im Elsass (12. Jahrhundert)*, Spicilegium Friburgense, 10, Freiburg: Universitätsverlag Freiburg, 1965.

Simon-Muscheid, Katharina: "Der Umgang mit Alkohol, Männliche Soziabilität und Weibliche

Tugend", *Kontraste im Alltag des Mittelalters*, ed. Gerhard Jaritz, Wien: Verlag der österreichischen Akademie der Wissenschaften, 2000, pp. 35-60.

Skaarup, Bi: *Renæssancemad, Opskrifter og køkkenhistorie fra Christian 4.'s tid*, Copenhagen: Gyldendal, 2006.

Skemer, Don C.: *Binding Words, Textual Amulets in the Middle Ages*, University Park: Pennsylvania State University Press, 2006.

Skinnebach, Laura Katrine: "Forestillingen om 'periodens enhed' og begrebet 'habitus' i den kunsthistoriske praksis", *Talende Bilder, Tekster om kunst og visuell kultur*, ed. Sigrid Lien & Caroline Serck-Hanssen, Oslo: Spartacus, 2010, pp. 55-68.

Skinnebach, Laura Katrine: *Practices of Perception – Devotion and the Senses in Late Medieval Northern Europe*, Bergen: University of Bergen, 2013 (unpublished dissertation).

Smith, Mark M.: *Sensing the Past – Seeing, Hearing, Smelling, Tasting, and Touching in History*, Berkeley: University of California Press, 2008.

Snyder, Jane McIntosh: "The Web of Song, Weaving Imagery in Homer and the Lyric Poets", *The Classic Journal*, 76, 3, 1981, pp. 193-196.

Sommer, Anne-Louise: *De dødes haver, Den moderne storbykirkegård*, Odense: University Press of Southern Denmark, 2003.

Sonne de Torrens, Helene: "The Stadil Altar Frontal – a Johannine Interpretation of the Nativity of Christ and the Advent of Ecclesia", *Decorating the Lord's Table, On the Dynamics between Image and Altar in the Middle Ages*, ed. Søren Kaspersen & Erik Thunø, Copenhagen: Museum Tusculanum Press, 2006, pp. 147-170.

Sørensen, Tim F.: "The Presence of the Dead – Cemeteries, Cremation and the Staging of Non-place", *Journal of Social Archaeology*, 9, 1, 2009, pp. 110-135.

Sørensen, Tim F.: *An Archaeology of Movement – Materiality, Affects and Cemeteries in Prehistoric and Contemporary Odsherred, Denmark*, Aarhus: University of Aarhus, 2010 (unpublished dissertation).

Spearing, A.C.: *The Medieval Poet as Voyeur*, Cambridge & New York: Cambridge University Press, 1993.

Spiegel, Gabrielle M.: "Paradoxes of the Senses", *Rethinking the Medieval Senses*, ed. Stephen Nichols, Andreas Kablitz & Alison Calhoun, Baltimore: The Johns Hopkins University Press, 2008, pp. 186-193.

Spinks, Bryan D.: *Early and Medieval Rituals and Theologies of Baptism, From the New Testament to the Council of Trent*, Aldershot: Ashgate, 2006.

Steele, Robert: *Three Prose Versions of the Secreta Secretorum*, London: Early English Text Society, 1898.

Steiner, Wendy: *The Colors of Rhetoric, Problems in the Relation between Modern Literature and Painting*, Chicago: Chicago University Press, 1982.

Stephan, Hans-Georg: "Spätmittelalterliche Gesichtsgefässe aus Mitteleuropa", *Everyday and Exotic Pottery from Europe c. 650-1900, Studies in honour of John G. Hurst*, ed. David R.M. Gaimster & Mark Redknap, Oxford: Oxbow Books, 1988, pp. 127-156.

Stephan, Hans-Georg: "Deutsche Keramik im Handelsraum der Hanse, Überlegungen zur mittelalterlichen Exportkeramik, zur Nachwirkung von Wirtschaftsverbindungen in der Neuzeit und zur kultureller Prägung", *Nahrung und Tischkultur im Hanseraum*, ed. Günter Wiegelmann & Ruth-Elisabeth Mohrmann, Münster: Waxmann Verlag, 1996, pp. 95-124.

Steward, Dana: *The Arrow of Love – Optics, Gender, and Subjectivity in Medieval Love Poetry*, Lewisburg: Bucknell University Press, 2003.

Stiesdahl, Hans: "Grøngaard, Hertug Hans den Ældres Jagtslot", *Nationalmuseets Arbejdsmark*, Copenhagen: The National Museum, 1956, pp. 115-127.

Stump, Eleonore: *Aquinas*, London & New York: Routledge, 2003.

Suger, Abbot: "De rebus in administratione sua gestis", *On the Abbey Church of St.-Denis and Its Art Treasures*, ed. Erwin Panofsky, Princeton: Princeton University Press, 1946, 1979.

Sulpicius, Severus: *Life of Martin of Tours*, ed. Carolinne White, *Early Christian Lives*, London: Penguin, 1998.

Syndergaard, Larry E.: *English Translations of the Scandinavian Medieval Ballads, An Analytical Guide and Bibliography*, Turku: The Nordic Institute of Folklore, 1995.

Tatarkiewicz, Władysław: *History of Aesthetics*, vol. II, *Medieval Aesthetics*, Warszawa: Polish Scientific Publishers, 1970.

Tatton-Brown, Tim & Crook, John: *Salisbury Cathedral, The Making of a Medieval Masterpiece*, London: Scala, 2009.

Tellkamp, Jörg Alejandro: *Sinne, Gegenstände und Sensibilia, Zur Wahrnehmungslehre des Thomas von Aquin*, Leiden: Brill, 1999.

Thaastrup-Leth, Anne K.: "Trækirker i det middelalderlige Danmark indtil ca. 1100, Hvornår blev de bygget?", *Kristendommen i Danmark før 1050, Et symposium i Roskilde den 5.-7. februar 2003*, ed. Niels Lund, Roskilde: Roskilde Museum, 2004, pp. 207-214.

Thacker, Alan: "Loca Sanctorum, The Significance of Place in the Study of the Saints", *Local Saints and Local Churches in the Early Medieval West*, ed. Alan Thacker & Richard Sharpe, Oxford: Oxford University Press, 2002, pp. 1-43.

The Cloud of Unknowing, ed. James Walsh, Mahwah: Paulist Press, 1981.

The Lais of Marie de France, trans. Judith P. Shoaf, 1991-1996, accessed: 12/07/2014, http://www.clas.ufl. edu/users/jshoaf/Marie/

The Manuscript 541 of the Bibliothèque Mazarine Paris, The Processional of Châlons-en-Champagne, ed. Orsolva Csomó, Budapest: Institute of Musicology of the Hungarian Academy of Sciences, 2010.

Thomas a Kempis: *The Inner Life*, London: Penguin Books, 2005.

Thomas Aquinas: *Summa Theologica*, ed. & trans. Fathers of the English Dominican Province, London: Burns, Oates & Washbourne, 1920.

Thomas Aquinas: *Summa Theologica*, vol. I-IV, Allen, Texas: Christian Classics, 1911, 1981.

Thomas Aquinas: *S. Thomae Aquinatis in Aristotelis libros De sensu et sensato, De memoria et reminiscentia commentarium*, ed. Raymundi M. Spiazzi, Turin & Rome: Marietti, 1949.

Thomas Aquinas: *A Commentary on Aristotle's De Anima*, trans. Kenelm Foster & Silvester Humphries, New Haven: Yale University Press, 1951.

Thomas Aquinas: *Commentary on Aristotle's De Anima*, trans. Kenelm Foster & Silvester Humphries, Notre Dame, Indiana: Dumb Ox Books, 1951, 1994.

Thomas Aquinas: *A Commentary on Aristotle's De Anima*, trans. Robert Pasnau, New Haven & London: Yale Library of Medieval Philosophy, 1999.

Thomas Aquinas: *Truth* (*Quaestiones disputatae de veritate*), vol. I-III, Indianapolis & Cambridge: Hackett, 1954, 1994.

Thunø, Erik: "The Golden Altar of Sant'Ambrogio in Milan – Image and Materiality", *Decorating the Lord's Table, On the Dynamics between Image and Altar in the Middle Ages*, ed. Søren Kaspersen & Erik Thunø, Copenhagen: Museum Tusculanum Press, 2006, pp. 63-78.

Tilander, Gunnar (ed.): "Les livres du roy Modus et de la royne Ratio", *Société des anciens textes français*, vol. I, Paris, 1932.

Toynbee, Jocelyn & Ward Perkins, John: *The Shrine of St. Peter and the Vatican Excavations*, London, New York & Toronto: Longmans, Green & Co., 1956.

Tugwell, Simon: *The Nine Ways of Prayer of St. Dominic*, Rome: Missionary Society of St. Paul the Apostle in the State of New York, 1982.

Unger, Richard W.: *Beer in the Middle Ages and the Renaissance*, Philadelphia: University of Pennsylvania Press, 2004.

Vacandard, Elphège: *Vie de Saint Bernard, abbé de Clairvaux*, vol. II, Paris: Librairie Victor Lecoffre, 1902.

van Dijk, Ann: "'Domus Sanctae Dei Genetricis Mariae' – Art and Liturgy in the Oratory of Pope John VII", *Decorating the Lord's Table, On the Dynamics between Image and Altar in the Middle Ages*, ed. Søren Kaspersen & Erik Thunø, Copenhagen: Museum Tusculanum Press, 2006, pp. 13-42.

van Engen, John H.: *Rupert of Deutz*, Berkeley: University of California Press, 1983.

van Os, Henk: *Sienese Altarpieces 1215-1460*, vol. I-II, Groningen: Egbert Forsten, 1988-1990.

Vance, Eugene: "Seeing God – Augustine, Sensation, and the Mind's Eye", *Rethinking the Medieval Senses – Heritage, Fascinations, Frames*, ed. Stephen G. Nichols, Andreas Kablitz & Alison Calhoun, Baltimore: The Johns Hopkins University Press, 2008, pp. 13-29.

Vauchez, André: *Sainthood in the Later Middle Ages*, Cambridge: Cambridge University Press, 1997.

Vinzent, Markus: "Rome", *The Cambridge History of Christianity, Origins to Constantine*, ed. Margaret M. Mitchell & Frances M. Young, Cambridge: Cambridge University Press, 2006, pp. 397-412.

Vogel, Cyrille & Elze, Reinhard (ed.): *Le pontifical romano-germanique du dixième siècle*, vol. I-III, Citta del Vaticano: Biblioteca Apostolica Vaticana, 1963-72.

von Achen, Henrik: "Piety, Practice and Process", *Instruments of Devotion, The Practices and Objects of Religious Piety from the Late Middle Ages to the 20th Century*, ed. Henning Laugerud & Laura Katrine Skinnebach, Aarhus: Aarhus University Press, 2007, pp. 23-44.

Waddell, Helen (trans.): *The Desert Fathers, Translations from the Latin*, Ann Arbor: University of Michigan Press, 1966.

Wade, Mara R.: *Triumphus Nuptialis Danicus – German Court Culture and Denmark, The Great Wedding of 1634*, Wiesbaden: Otto Harrassowitz, 1996.

Wainwright, Geoffrey: *Doxology, A Systematic Theology*, London: Epworth Press, 1980.

Wall, J. Charles: *Shrines of British Saints*, London: Methuen & Co., 1905.

Wandhoff, Haiko: *Ekphrasis, Kunstbeschreibungen und virtuelle Räume in der Litteratur des Mittelalters*, Berlin: De Gruyter, 2003.

Ward, Benedicta: "The Desert Myth, Reflections on the Desert Ideal in Early Cistercian Monasticism", *One Yet Two, Monastic Tradition East and West*, ed. Basil Pennington, Kalamazoo: Cistercian Publications, 1976, pp. 183-199.

Ward, Benedicta & Savage, Paul: *The Great Beginning of Cîteaux, A Narrative of the Beginning of the Cistercian Order, The* Exordium Magnum *of Conrad of Eberbach*, ed. E. Rozanne Elder, Collegeville, Minn.: Liturgical Press, 2012.

Wartofsky, Marx W.: "Picturing and Representing", *Perception and Pictorial Representation*, ed. Calvin F. Nodine & Dennis F. Fisher, New York: Praeger, 1979, pp. 272-283.

Watts, Alan W.: *Myth and Ritual in Christianity*, London: Thames & Hudson, 1954, 1983.

Webb, Heather: "Cardiosensory Impulses in Late Medieval Spirituality", *Rethinking the Medieval Senses – Heritage, Fascinations, Frames*, ed. Stephen G. Nichols, Andreas Kablitz & Alison Calhoun, Baltimore: The Johns Hopkins University Press, 2008, pp. 265-285.

Webb, Heather: *The Medieval Heart*, New Haven: Yale University Press, 2010.

Webster, Leslie: "Visual Literacy in a Protoliterate Age", *Literacy in Medieval and Early Modern Scandinavian Culture*, ed. Pernille Hermann, Odense: University Press of Southern Denmark, 2005, pp. 21-46.

Webster's New World Dictionary, New York: Prentice Hall, 1994.

Westermann-Angerhausen, Hiltrud: "Incense in the Space between Heaven and Earth, The Inscriptions and Images on the Gozbert-Censer in the Cathedral Treasury of Trier", *Inscriptions in Liturgical Spaces, Acta ad archaeologiam et artium historiam pertinentia*, 24, 10, ed. Kristin B. Aavitsland & Turid Karlsen Seim, Rome: Scienze e lettere, 2011, pp. 227-242.

Whitaker, E.C.: *Documents of the Baptismal Liturgy*, ed. Maxwell E. Johnson, London: SPCK, 2003.

Whitehouse, Harvey: "Modes of Religiosity, Towards a Cognitive Explanation of the Sociopolitical Dynamics of Religion", *Method & Theory in the Study of Religion*, 14, 2002, pp. 293-315.

William of Saint Thierry: "Vita Prima Bernardi", *Patrologia Latina, Cursus Completus*, vol. CLXXXV, ed. Jacques-Paul Migne, Turnhout: Brepols, 1844-1865.

Wirth, Jean: *L'image à l'époque romane*, Paris: Cerf, 1999.

Wittgenstein, Ludwig: *Philosophical Investigations*, Malden, Oxford & Carlton, Victoria: Blackwell Publishing, 1953, 2007.

Wolfson, Harry A.: "The Internal Senses in Latin, Arabic, and Hebrew Philosophic Texts", *Harvard Theological Review*, 28, 2, 1935, pp. 69-133.

Woolgar, Chris M.: "Fast and Feast, Conspicuous Consumption and the Diet of the Nobility in the Fifteenth Century", *Revolution and Consumption in Late Medieval England*, ed. Michael Hicks, Woodbridge & Rochester: Boydell Press, 2001, pp. 7-25.

Woolgar, Chris M.: *The Senses in Late Medieval England*, New Haven: Yale University Press, 2006.

Woolgar, Chris M.: "Food and the Middle Ages", *Journal of Medieval History*, 36, 1, 2010, pp. 1-19.

Wright, Thomas: *A History of Domestic Manners and Sentiments in England during the Middle Ages*, London: Chapman & Hall, 1862.

Yates, Frances: *The Art of Memory*, London: Pimlico, 1966, 1994.

Young, Karl: *The Drama of the Medieval Church*, vol. I-II, London: Clarendon Press, 1933, 1967.

302

INDEX

drama 10, 12, 35, 58, 60, 137, 146

Duccio di Buoninsegna (c. 1255-c.1318) 201

ear 12, 13, 15, 30, 40, 162-164, 166, 172, 251

effluvium 41, 45

ekphrasis 124, 125

elevation, Elevation of the Host 52, 76, 156, 227, 232

eloquent, *eloquentia* 136, 153

Elsinore 234, 238

embody 29, 49, 77, 228, 240

emotion 11, 13, 14, 47, 96, 209, 116, 222, 230, 235, 252, 270

environment, church environment 11, 130, 206-211, 213, 215, 216, 218-223

Erec et Enide (Chrétien de Troyes) 125

eschatology 28, 31, 75, 87

Esrum, North of Zealand, Denmark 97, 103, 106

Etymologies (Isidore of Seville) 41

Eucharist 30, 42, 49, 50, 52, 68, 69, 72, 77-79, 81, 84, 85, 87, 88, 182, 194, 200, 202, 205, 216, 217, 221, 227, 230, 231, 237, 241, 243, 254, 258, 260, 261

Eugenius III (d. 1153) 108

euphony 14, 15

exempla 107

exemplary 17, 34, 65, 183, 190

exposition, *Expositio* 45, 50, 51, 54, 74, 81

Exordium magnum cisterciense (Conrad of Eberbach) 103

external senses 11, 19, 26, 38, 175

extramission 121, 124, 271, see also intromission

extrasensory 11, 29, 36, 38, 50, 51

faeces 140

Fall of Man 75, 116, 148, 231, 232, 243, 256, 269

Henri de Férrières (d. 1093-1100), 74

figure, *figura* 15, 20, 45, 54, 62, 78, 81, 103, 107, 161, 179, 239, 241, 247-249, 250, 261

figuration, *figuratur* 15, 54, 81, 133, 170, 223, 248

flesh 72, 254

Floda church 138

Florence 246, 248, 252, 254

foramina 54, 56, 58, 60, 61, 62, 69, 70

formation 165, 206

Francis of Assisi (1181/82-1226) 254, 258, 261, 262, 266, 267, 270

Friis, Johan 233

ritual, rite 10, 11, 19, 21, 29, 30, 32, 34, 45, 50, 52, 57, 85, 180-184 188, 190-193, 195-202, 209, 211, 212, 214-217, 219-221, 223, 226, 227, 230, 234, 236, 237, 241, 242, 260, ritualised 57, 60, 181, 196, 226, 227, 232, 234, 242

Robert Grosseteste (1170-1253) 13

Roman German Pontifical 184

Rome 33, 211

Rosborg castle, Denmark 239

Roskilde 140

Rule of Saint Benedict (Benedict of Nursia) 97

Rupert of Deutz (c. 1075-c. 1130) 200-202

sacrament, *sacramentum* 11, 20, 21, 29, 30, 42, 50, 78, 86, 114, 180, 182, 193-202 , 217, 230, 231, 254, 261 sacramental 19, 28, 29, 30, 43, 49-52, 72, 77, 180, 194, 195, 197, 199, 200, 216, 260, 269 sacramentality 19, 23, 28

sacred 10, 17, 20, 21, 24-26, 28-38, 41-45, 47, 50-52, 54, 57, 58, 60-66, 73, 74, 76, 77, 85, 86, 93, 104, 168, 193, 194, 197, 209, 212, 216, 217, 220, 221, 251, 258, 259 , sacred impact 35, sacred transformation 35

Saint Ruf 190

Sainte-Chapelle 54, 69

Sainte Larme 64

Salisbury 56, 57, 60, 70

sanctification 31, 63, 66

sanctity 11, 16, 20, 21, 25, 27, 29-36, 38, 41, 43-45, 47, 52, 54, 58, 61, 62-65, 92-94, 190

sanctuaria 63

sanctus 52, 93, 110, 179

Santa Croce, Florence 246, 248, 252, 254, 258

saturation 10-14, 16-18, 21, 25, 26, 35, 39, 44, 63, 77, 169, 172, 175, 222

savour 13, 30, 41, 68, savoury 29, 40

scent 17, 29, 41, 45, 218, 257, 264, 269

Scete 96

Schaubild 16

see 14, 16, 18, 28, 30-32, 38, 42, 44, 47, 50-52, 74, 75, 77, 78, 84-86, 94, 96, 121, 126, 162, 163, 168, 172, 182, 209, 229, 248, 259-262, 266, behold, beholding 51, 57, 85, 86, 162, 164, 166, 169, see also *visum*

sense, *sensus* 9-21, 24-45, 47, 49-52, 54, 56-58, 60-65, 72-78, 81, 82, 85, 87, 88, 92-96, 100-104, 108, 112-116, 118-120, 122, 124-127, 132, 134, 137, 141, 148, 152, 154, 155, 161-170, 172, 174, 175, 179-182, 191, 192, 196-200, 202, 206-209, 212, 216-222, 223, 226-230, 232, 235-237, 241-243, 246-249, 251, 252, 257-267, sensory transformation 35, sensory model 27, sensory paradigm il nsory paradigm (jf. kplicit 27, 81, 88 *see also perception*

sensibles, *sensibilia* 37-39, 41, 162, 164-166, 170, 172, 175, see also common sensibles

317

AUTHORS

Kristin Bliksrud Aavitsland, Dr. Art., is Professor in Medieval Culture and Church History at the MF Norwegian School of Theology, Oslo (Norway). Her research interests include image use and religious practices in medieval and early modern cultures, as well as cultural memory and uses of the medieval past in modernity and postmodernity. Relevant publications include *Imagining the Human Condition in Medieval Rome*, Aldershot: Ashgate Publishing, 2012; "Nationalism, Age Values and Cultural Capital: Harry Fett and Heritage Preservation in 20th Century Norway", *Future Anterior* 6 (2), New York: Columbia University, 2011; "Visual Orders in the Golden Altar from Lisbjerg", in: M. Stang & K. Aavitsland (eds), *Ornament and Order: Essays on Viking and Northern Medieval Art*, Trondheim: Tapir Academic Press, 2008.

Jørgen Bruhn, PhD, is a Professor in the Department of Film and Literature at Linnæus University, Växjö (Sweden). His research interests include medieval literature, media studies, and intermediality. Relevant publications include *Changing Borders, Contemporary Positions in Intermediality*, co-edited with J. Arvidson, M. Askander & H. Führer, Lund: Intermedia Studies Press, 2007; "Heteromediality", in: L. Elleström (ed.), *Media Borders, Multimodality and Intermediality*, Houndmills: Palgrave Macmillan, 2010; *Lovely Violence, Chrétien de Troyes' Critical Romances*, Newcastle on Tyne: Cambridge Scholars Publishing, 2010; *Adaptation Studies – New Perspectives, New Approaches*, co-edited with Eirik Frisvold Hanssen & Anne Gjelsvik, London: Bloomsbury Academic, 2013. He is currently finishing a book on intermedial literary analysis.

Mads Dengsø Jessen, PhD, is a Project Researcher in Ancient Cultures of Denmark and the Mediterranean at The National Museum of Denmark. His research focuses on the ideological transitions taking place in the first millennium AD, in particular the Christianization of Southern Scandinavia during the Viking Age and later, including ritual buildings, the material culture of ritual, and cultural history in combination with cognitive studies. He is co-editor of the *Danish Journal of Archaeology* (Taylor & Francis). Relevant publications include "Religion and the Extra-somatics of Conceptual Thought", in: A. Geertz (ed.), *Origins of Religion, Cognition and Culture*, Oxford: Routledge, 2013; "Material Culture, Embodiment and the Construction of Religious Knowledge", *Embodied Knowledge: Technology and Beliefs*, Oxford: Oxbow, 2013.

Hans Henrik Lohfert Jørgensen, PhD, is Associate Professor of Art History and Visual Culture in the Department of Aesthetics and Communication at Aarhus University (Denmark). His current research focuses on intermedia, multimodal imagery, and the cultural history of the senses and the body, as well as cultic media, architecture, and visuality in the Middle Ages. Relevant publications include *AMAMM – All Media Are Mixed Media, Intersensorisk og intermedial analyse i kunsten*, with Astrid B. Steffensen & Camilla S. Paldam, Aarhus: Aarhus University, 2012; "Anti-Ritual", *Creations – Medieval Rituals, the Arts, and the Concept of Creation*, Turnhout: Brepols, 2007; "Middelalderlige metabilleder", *Transfiguration*, 6 (1), 2006; "Cultic Vision – Seeing as Ritual", *The Appearances of Medieval Rituals*, Turnhout: Brepols, 2004; "Prostheses of Pious Perception, On the Instrumentalization and Mediation of the Medieval Sensorium", *The Materiality of Devotion in Late Medieval Northern Europe*, Dublin: Four Courts Press (forthcoming).

Sigurd Kværndrup, PhD and DPhil, was formerly an Assistant Professor in the Institute for Nordic Philology at the University of Copenhagen (Denmark), and also at Linnæus University (Sweden). His research interests include medievalism, the literary and media history of Scandinavia, and medieval popular ballads. He is co-editor of *Dansk Litteraturhistorie* (The History of Danish Literature), vols 1–9, Copenhagen: Gyldendal, 1984–1986. Relevant publications include various articles about intermediality and medieval popular ballads, published in Sweden; *Den østnordiske ballade, Oral teori og tekstanalyse*, Copenhagen: Museum Tusculanum Press, 2006 (with English summary); *Medeltiden i ord och bild, Folkligt och groteskt i nordiska kyrkmålningar och ballader*, with Tommy Olofsson, Stockholm: Atlantis Förlag, 2013; *Den nordiske Løveridder*, Copenhagen: Museum Tusculanum Press, 2014.

Henning Laugerud, Dr. Art., is an Associate Professor in the Department of Linguistics, Literary and Aesthetic Studies at the University of Bergen (Norway). His research interests include the medieval and early modern period, cultural history, visual studies, rhetoric, mnemology, and theories of interpretation. Relevant publications include *The Materiality of Devotion in Late Medieval Northern Europe: Images, Objects and Practices*, co-edited with Salvador Ryan & Laura Skinnebach, Dublin: Four Courts Press (forthcoming); *Devotional Cultures of European Christianity, c. 1789–c. 1960*, co-edited with Salvador Ryan, Dublin: Four Courts Press, 2012; *Instruments of Devotion, The Practices and Objects of Religious Piety from the Late Middle Ages to the 20th Century*, co-edited with Laura Skinnebach, Aarhus: Aarhus University Press, 2007.

Jette Linaa, PhD, is a Senior Researcher in the Department of Archaeology, Moesgaard Museum (Denmark). Her research interests include the medieval and early modern period, cultural history, consumption studies, studies of medieval and early modern communities, and the agency of materiality. She is leader of the research projects "Urban Diaspora: Diaspora Communities and Materiality in Early Modern Denmark" and "Urban Consumption 1000–1800". Relevant publications include "In Memory of Merchants: The Consumption and Cultural Meetings of a Wealthy Dutch Immigrant in Early Modern Elsinore", *Across The North Sea: Later Historical Archaeology in Britain and Denmark, c. 1500–2000 AD*, Odense: University Press of Southern Denmark, 2012; *Keramik, kultur og kontakter: Køkken- og bordtøjets brug og betydning 1350–1650*, Højbjerg: Jysk Arkæologisk Selskab, 2006; *Coast, Culture, Contacts & Consumption: The Coastal Culture, Its Provisions and Alterations around the Sound ca. 1150–1700*, Højbjerg: Jysk Arkæologisk Selskab (forthcoming).

Brian Patrick McGuire, DPhil Oxon., was an Associate Professor in the Institute for Greek and Latin at the University of Copenhagen (Denmark) between 1975 and 1996, and Professor of Medieval History at Roskilde University (Denmark) between 1996 and 2012. Relevant publications include *Conflict and Continuity at Øm Abbey*, Copenhagen: Museum Tusculanum Press, 1976; *The Cistercians in Denmark*, Kalamazoo, MI: Cistercian Publications, 1982; *Friendship and Community: The Monastic Experience 350–1250*, Cistercian Publications, 1988, Ithaca, NY: Cornell University Press, 2010; *The Difficult Saint: Bernard of Clairvaux and his Tradition*, Cistercian Publications, 1991; *Jean Gerson and the Last Medieval Reformation*, Philadelphia, PA: Penn State University Press, 2005; *Den første europæer: Bernard af Clairvaux*, Frederiksberg: Alfa, 2009; *Det kristne Europas fødsel: Sankt Bonifacius*, Alfa, 2014.

Nils Holger Petersen, PhD, is Associate Professor of Church History in the Faculty of Theology at the University of Copenhagen (Denmark). He has been leader of the Centre for the Study of the Cultural Heritage of Medieval Rituals (established as a centre of excellence by the Danish National Research Foundation, 2002–2010) and project leader for an international interdisciplinary project on medieval saints' cults and their later receptions in the arts under the European Science Foundation, 2010–2014. He is editor for the musical reception of the Bible (*Encyclopedia of the Bible and its Reception*, Berlin: De Gruyter, 2009–) and main editor for the book series *Ritus et Artes: Traditions and Transformations*, Turnhout: Brepols. Relevant publications include *Medieval Ritual and Early Modern Music*, co-authored with Eyolf Østrem, Turnhout: Brepols, 2008, as well as numerous articles and co-edited volumes on medieval liturgy and its reception into the arts.

Laura Katrine Skinnebach, PhD, currently holds a postdoctoral position in the Department of Aesthetics and Communication at Aarhus University (Denmark), financed by the Danish Council for Independent Research. Her research interests include the medieval and early modern periods, devotional practice, prayer books, practices of perception, materiality, and theories of interpretation. Relevant publications include *Instruments of Devotion, The Practices and Objects of Religious Piety from the Late Middle Ages to the 20th Century*, co-edited with Henning Laugerud, Aarhus: Aarhus University Press, 2007; *The Materiality of Devotion in Late Medieval Northern Europe: Images, Objects and Practices*, co-edited with Henning Laugerud & Salvador Ryan, Dublin: Four Courts Press (forthcoming).

Tim Flohr Sørensen, PhD, is an Assistant Professor in the Saxo Institute at the University of Copenhagen (Denmark). He was an Assistant Professor at Aarhus University (Denmark) between 2012 and 2014, and Marie Curie Fellow in the McDonald Institute for Archaeological Research at the University of Cambridge between 2010 and 2012. As an archaeologist, he is interested in materiality, affect, space, and movement with reference to architecture and mortuary practice in the past and the present. Relevant publications include *An Anthropology of Absence: Materializations of Transcendence and Loss*, co-edited with Mikkel Bille & Frida Hastrup, New York: Springer, 2010; "In Visible Presence: The Role of Light in Shaping Religious Atmospheres", *The Oxford Handbook of Light in Archaeology* (forthcoming); *Staging Atmospheres*, a special issue of *Emotion, Space and Society* (forthcoming); "Delusion and Disclosure: Human Disposal and the Aesthetics of Vagueness", *Embodied Knowledge: Technology and Beliefs*, Oxford: Oxbow, 2013.